SURFACTANTS IN PERSONAL CARE PRODUCTS AND DECORATIVE COSMETICS

THIRD EDITION

SURFACTANT SCIENCE SERIES

SURFACTANTS IN PERSONAL CARE PRODUCTS AND DECORATIVE COSMETICS

THIRD EDITION

Linda D. Rhein
Fairleigh Dickinson University
Teaneck, New Jersey, U.S.A.

Mitchell Schlossman
Kobo Products, Inc.
South Plainfield, New Jersey, U.S.A.

Anthony O'Lenick
Siltech LLC
Dacula, Georgia, U.S.A.

P. Somasundaran
Columbia University
New York, New York, U.S.A.

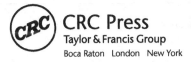

CRC Press
Taylor & Francis Group
Boca Raton London New York

CRC Press is an imprint of the
Taylor & Francis Group, an informa business

CRC Press
Taylor & Francis Group
6000 Broken Sound Parkway NW, Suite 300
Boca Raton, FL 33487-2742

First issued in paperback 2020

© 2007 by Taylor & Francis Group, LLC
CRC Press is an imprint of Taylor & Francis Group, an Informa business

No claim to original U.S. Government works

ISBN-13: 978-0-367-57778-0 (pbk)
ISBN-13: 978-1-57444-531-2 (hbk)

Library of Congress Cataloging-in-Publication Data

Surfactants in personal care products and decorative cosmetics. -- 3rd ed. / [edited by] Linda D. Rhein ... [et al.].
   p. cm.
   Rev. ed. of: Surfactants in cosmetics. 2nd ed., rev. and expanded / edited by Martin M. Rieger, Linda D. Rhein. c1997.
   Includes bibliographical references and index.
   ISBN 1-57444-531-6 (acid-free paper)
   1. Surface active agents. 2. Cosmetics. I. Rhein, Linda D. II. Surfactants in cosmetics. III. Title.

TP994.S8763 2006
668'.55--dc22   2006049168

Visit the Taylor & Francis Web site at
http://www.taylorandfrancis.com

and the CRC Press Web site at
http://www.crcpress.com

Preface

This is the third edition of *Surfactants in Cosmetics*. The first edition focused on such topics as the types of surfactants used in cosmetics, why they are needed, what functions the different structures serve, and the problems associated with their use in personal care products. The second edition covered fundamental physical chemical principles of surfactants in cosmetic emulsions, introducing multiple emulsions, phase inversion emulsions, microemulsions, vesicles, liposomes, solubilization in emulsions, and emulsion stability. The chemistry of interaction of surfactants with the substrates — skin and hair — and strategies to provide milder formulations or optimal cleansing were also provided in the second edition.

This edition now focuses, for the first time, on the use of surfactants in decorative cosmetics. The first few chapters cover fundamental aspects of the use of surfactants in personal care products and decorative cosmetics, discussing surfactant solution properties, surfactant emulsions, nanotechnology, cleanser/conditioner systems, and pigment dispersions. A review of fundamental skin science, including the rapidly advancing area of skin lipids, is included. Additionally, the measurement of skin color and the use of state-of-the-art non-invasive instrumental technology to measure efficacy of skin care cosmetic products are reviewed. Also provided is a chapter detailing strategies to assess consumer acceptability of cosmetic formulations.

The second part of this edition covers the role of surfactants in pigmented products such as nail enamel, lipsticks, makeup/foundations, sunscreens, self-tanners, and hair care products. The final section covers the use of specific surfactants with application to the formulation of decorative cosmetics and personal care products.

The editors thank the authors for their contributions and apologize for the significant delay in obtaining all the submissions. We also thank Taylor & Francis for inviting us to edit this new edition. We hope the readers find the edition valuable in their quest for providing more consumer-acceptable technologies for decorative cosmetics in the marketplace.

Editors

Linda D. Rhein, Ph.D., received her M.S. and Ph.D. in biochemistry and neurobiology from the University of Maryland and completed postdoctoral training at the University of Pennsylvania. She has worked in the cosmetic and OTC pharmaceutical industries for many companies for 25 years. She has been serving as editor of *Surfactants in Cosmetics*, part of the Surfactant Science Series. She has served as editor of the *Journal of Cosmetic Science* and as monograph editor for the society for several years. Currently, she is president-elect of the Society of Cosmetic Chemists and has served on their Committee on Scientific Affairs for numerous years. She was the recipient of the Women in Industry Award in 1987, as well as several awards from the Society of Cosmetic Chemists: the merit award in 2004, two best paper awards in 1985 and 1999, and the literature award in 1999. She is a member of the New York Academy of Sciences, American Association for the Advancement of Science, and the Scientific Society of Sigma Xi. Currently, she is an adjunct professor for the master's degree in cosmetic science program at Fairleigh Dickinson University, teaching biochemistry of skin, hair, and nails. She is best known for her innovative research contributions in skin lipid biophysical structure and its relevance to barrier function, and also mechanisms of surfactant damage to skin, prevention, and repair. Her research has resulted in more than 50 publications in scientific journals, and she has given over 25 invited lectures in her field.

Mitchell L. Schlossman received his B.A. from New York University and his M.A. from Kean University. Mitch was cofounder of Kobo Products, Inc. He has been part owner of Presperse, Inc., Tevco, Inc., Emery Industries, Inc., Pfizer, Inc., and Revlon, Inc. He is a member of the Society of Cosmetic Chemists (fellow) and past chairman of the New York Chapter of SCC (fellow). He has served as past director–east merit awardee and is also a member of the American Chemical Society, AIC (fellow), Chemist's Club, CIBS, and AAAS. He has served as editor of *Chemistry and Manufacture of Cosmetics*, third edition, has coauthored several books in the field of cosmetic chemistry, including publishing articles in numerous professional journals and trade magazines, and is the patentee of various U.S. and foreign patents.

P. Somasundaran, Ph.D., received his M.S. and Ph.D. from the University of California at Berkeley. Initially employed by the International Minerals and Chemical Corporation and Reynolds Industries, he was then appointed in 1983 as the first La von Duddleson Krumb Professor in the Columbia University School of Engineering and Applied Science. In 1987, he became the first director of the Langmuir Center for Colloids and Interfaces, and in 1998, the founding director of the National Science Foundation Industry/University Cooperative Center for Advanced Studies in Novel Surfactants. He was also elected chairman of the Henry Krumb School at Columbia University in 1988 and 1991, and chair of the chemical engineering, material science, and mineral engineering department in 1992 and 1995. He was inducted in 1985 into the National Academy of Engineering, the highest professional distinction that can be conferred to an engineer at that time, in 1998 to the Chinese National Academy of Engineering, in 1999 to the Indian National Academy of Engineering and in 2000 to the Russian Academy of Natural Sciences. He is the recipient of the Antoine M. Gaudin Award (1982), the Mill Man of Distinction Award (1983), the Publication Board Award (1980), the Robert H. Richards Award (1987), the Arthur F. Taggart Award for best paper (1987), and Henry Krumb Lecturer of the Year (1989) and is a distinguished member (1983) of AIME. He is the recipient of the "Most Distinguished Achievement in Engineering" Award from AINA (1980). In addition, he was awarded the "Ellis Island Medal of Honor" in 1990 and the Engineering Foundation's 1992 Frank F. Aplan Award. This year he won the AIME Education Award (2006). He is the author/editor of 15 books and over 500 scientific publications and patents. He is the honorary editor-in-chief of the international journal *Colloids and Surfaces*. He has served on many international, national, and professional committees and National Research Council panels. He served on the Congress's 28th Environmental Advisory Committee, several NSF research panels, and Engineering Research Center review panels. He was the chairman of the board of the Engineering Foundation (1993 to 1995). He was member of the Committee on Scientific Affairs (COSA) of the Society of Cosmetic Chemists from 2003 to 2005. He has served on the board of the SME/AIME (1982 to 1985). His research interests are in surface and colloid chemistry, nanogel particles, liposomes, polymer/surfactant/protein systems, environmental engineering, molecular interactions at surfaces using advanced spectroscopy, flocculation, and nanotechnology.

Anthony J. O'Lenick, Jr., received his B.S. and M.S. in chemistry at Rutgers University. Tony O'Lenick is president of Siltech LLC, a silicone and surfactant specialty company he founded in 1989. Prior to that, Tony held technical and executive positions at Alkaril Chemicals, Inc., Henkel Corporation, and Mona Industries. He has been involved in the personal care market for over 30 years. Tony is the author of *Surfactants Chemistry and Properties*, published in 1999, and *Silicones for Personal Care*, published in 2003. He teaches continuing education courses in silicones and patent law for the SCC. He has also published over 45 technical articles in trade journals, contributed chapters to 5 books, and is the inventor on over 250 patents. He has received a number of awards for his work in chemistry, including the 1996 Samuel Rosen Award given by the American Oil Chemists' Society, the 1997, Innovative Use of Fatty Acids Award given by the Soap and Detergents Association, and the Partnership to the Personal Care Award given by the Advanced Technology Group. Tony was a member of the Committee on Scientific Affairs of the Society of Cosmetic Chemists.

Contributors

Steven W. Amato
Coty, Inc.
Morris Plains, New Jersey

K.P. Ananthapadmanabhan
Unilever Research & Development
Trumbull, Connecticut

Svetlana Babajanyan
Fairleigh Dickinson University
Teaneck, New Jersey

Donna C. Barson
Barson Marketing, Inc.
Manalapan, New Jersey

Gina Butuc
Penreco
The Woodlands, Texas

Soma Chakraborty
NSF Industry/University Cooperative
  Research Center for Advanced
  Studies in Novel Surfactants
Langmuir Center for Colloids and
  Interface
Columbia University
New York, New York

Ratan K. Chaudhuri
EMD Chemicals, Inc.
Hawthorne, New York

Namita Deo
NSF Industry/University Cooperative
  Research Center for Advanced
  Studies in Novel Surfactants
Langmuir Center for Colloids and
  Interface
Columbia University
New York, New York

Puspendu Deo
NSF Industry/University Cooperative
  Research Center for Advanced
  Studies in Novel Surfactants
Langmuir Center for Colloids and
  Interface
Columbia University
New York, New York

Raymond Farinato
Cytec Industries, Inc.
Stamford, Connecticut

Nissim Garti
Casali Institute of Applied Chemistry
Hebrew University of Jerusalem
Givat Ram Campus
Jerusalem, Israel

E.D. Goddard
Cambridge, Maryland

Steven Harripersad
Beauty Avenues
New York, New York
and
Fairleigh Dickinson University
Teaneck, New Jersey

Jane Hollenberg
JCH Consulting
Red Hook, New York

X.Y. Hua
Unilever Research & Development
Trumbull, Connecticut

John A. Imperante
Phoenix Chemical, Inc.
Somerville, New Jersey

Carter LaVay
Zenitech LLC
Old Greenwich, Connecticut

A. Lips
Unilever Research & Development
Trumbull, Connecticut

Somil C. Mehta
Columbia University
New York, New York

David J. Moore
International Specialty Products
Wayne, New Jersey

Nicholas Morante
Nick Morante Consultants
Laboratory and Technical Center
Holbrook, New York

David S. Morrison
Penreco
The Woodlands, Texas

Stéphane Nicolas
Cosmetics Division
SunChemical Colors Group
Parsippany, New Jersey

Anthony J. O'Lenick, Jr.
Siltech LLC
Dacula, Georgia

Mark E. Rerek
Reheis, Inc.
Berkeley Heights, New Jersey

Linda D. Rhein
Fairleigh Dickinson University
Teaneck, New Jersey

Robert W. Sandewicz
Revlon Research Center
Edison, New Jersey

Mitchell L. Schlossman
Kobo Products
New York, New York

P. Somasundaran
NSF Industry/University Cooperative
    Research Center for Advanced
    Studies in Novel Surfactants
Langmuir Center for Colloids and
    Interface
Columbia University
New York, New York

Tamara Somasundaran
NSF Industry/University Cooperative
    Research Center for Advanced
    Studies in Novel Surfactants
Langmuir Center for Colloids and
    Interface
Columbia University
New York, New York

M. Vethamuthu
Unilever Research & Development
Trumbull, Connecticut

C. Vincent
Unilever Research & Development
Trumbull, Connecticut

Rick Vrckovnik
Siltech Corporation
Toronto, Canada

Randall Wickett
Department of Pharmacy
University of Cincinnati
Cincinnati, Ohio

Thomas H. Wines
Pall Corporation
Port Washington, New York

Alan Wohlman
The Fanning Corporation
Chicago, Illinois

L. Yang, Ph.D.
Unilever Research & Development
Trumbull, Connecticut

Contents

Part I

ASSESSMENT OF PERSONAL CARE AND DECORATIVE COSMETICS

1 Review of Skin Structure and Function with Special Focus on Stratum Corneum Lipid

Linda D. Rhein, Ph.D. and Svetlana Babajanyan, M.D.
Fairleigh Dickinson University

CONTENTS

1.1 INTRODUCTION

This chapter provides a review of the structure and function of skin. It will begin with a detailed discussion of the general structure of the epidermis and dermis, followed by the stratum corneum as a specialized part of the epidermis. Keratinization and epidermal renewel as an outcome of differentiation are detailed. After this, the primary focus is on lipids in the stratum corneum, namely, as a component of the protective membrane on the surface, i.e., the barrier that protects and retains moisture and interacts with topical products of interest to the cosmetic and pharmaceutical industry.

1.2 OVERVIEW OF THE STRUCTURE AND FUNCTION OF SKIN

Skin is a formidable physical barrier that protects us from the environment. It has become particularly adapted to withstand desiccation, allowing us to live in a nonaqueous environment, and is essential in thermal regulation of body temperature.

The skin is a continuous membrane or sheet covering the entire body surface. It is composed of two main layers:[1,2]

- Epidermis
- Dermis

The relative and total thickness of the two layers varies over different regions of the body.[1] The epidermis is thickest on the palms and soles of the feet. The dermis is thickest on the back and thinnest on the palms. The various layers of skin are shown in the histological cross section taken from a biopsy of skin in Figure 1.1.

The epidermis is the uppermost layer, and its purpose is to generate the stratum corneum, the so-called horny layer, which is the most superficial layer of dead cells and is the protective layer for the entire body — from dehydration and damage from foreign substances. The epidermis also interacts with stimuli from both the blood and the outside and is programmed to respond in various ways to the stimuli in an effort to preserve the protective function of the layer. It contains three main living cell types: keratinocytes, Langerhans cells, and melanocytes. Keratinocytes are the major cell type and eventually are converted by programmed cell death to corneocytes that make up the dead upper layer. The Langerhans cells are also called dendritic cells and provide the immune function in the epidermis, and the melanocytes provide the color of skin. These will be discussed later.

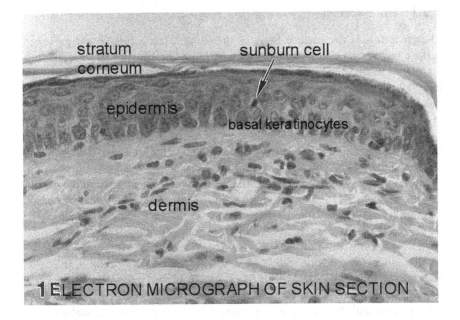

FIGURE 1.1 Cross section of the epidermis and dermis. The epidermis is a self-renewing stratified epithelium composed mostly of keratinocytes. It takes about 1 month from the time a basal cell leaves the bottom layer until it is desquamated or sloughed off from the surface. Differentiation is a genetically programmed event (apoptosis) that begins with a postmitotic keratinocyte and terminates with dead cells. The keratinocytes are organized into various layers that represent different stages of differentiation, as illustrated in the schematic. The events of cell differentiation include: appearance of new organelles, reorganization of existing organelles, and loss of organelles; synthesis and modification of structural proteins, especially keratins; change in cell size and shape; specialization of cellular metabolism; changes in the properties of cell membranes; dehydration; and formation of the barrier. (From Kligman, *J. Soc. Cosmet. Sci.* 47, 135, 1996. With Permission).

The dermis is the thick, fibrous layer beneath the epidermis, as shown in Figure 1.1. It provides structure to the membrane such that the membrane can cover the organs underneath and protect them from damage — mechanical or other. The dermis contains nerves and blood vessels and has one main living cell type: fibroblasts that generate the fibrous material. It contains several connective tissue proteins: collagens, elastin, and proteoglycans. Collagen is the rigid scaffold that covers the body. Elastin provides elasticity and strength, and proteoglycans are involved in damage repair.

The focus for the purposes of this chapter will be on the epidermis.

1.2.1 THE EPIDERMIS

The epidermis is the surface layer of the skin. It has a ridged and patterned surface — you can clearly see on your fingertips. The structure of the epidermis is complex. Cells in the epidermis form a multilayered system. These cells change morphologically as they migrate across the epidermis to fulfill their functions, i.e., form a barrier. The epidermis does not contain blood vessels, nerves, or sweat glands.

The epidermis is in a continual state of renewal as the keratinocytes, the major cell type within the epidermis, are formed, mature, and die.[1] It is estimated that the epidermis completely renews itself every 45 to 75 days.[1]

Keratinocytes are so called because they contain large amounts of the protein keratin.[1] Keratin is a tough, insoluble protein that provides physical protection and rigidity and strength to the cells. Keratin is the same substance that makes up the bulk of hair and nails, as well as animal claws and horns, hence the origin of the term *horny layer.*

Keratinocytes are formed by cell division from the stem cells in the basal layer of the epidermis, shown in Figure 1.1.[2] The newly formed keratinocytes move upward through the epidermis, continually maturing and changing structure via a process called differentiation (Figure 1.2).[1] This process is actually one of regulated cell death or apoptosis. This culminates in the formation of dead cells called corneocytes in the uppermost layer — the stratum corneum. The various differentiated states can be clearly seen when you look at a cross section schematic of the epidermis, such as that in Figure 1.2.[3]

The epidermis is composed of four distinct layers, as shown in Figure 1.1 and Figure 1.2:

- Stratum corneum — horny layer
- Stratum granulosum — granular layer
- Stratum spinosum — spiny layer
- Stratum basale — basal layer

Each layer represents a progressive stage in the life cycle of a keratinocyte. The histological cross section taken from skin can be seen in Figure 1.1, and the schematic in Figure 1.2 depicts the various cell types present in each layer.

As newly formed keratinocytes move upward, they flatten, lose their nucleus, and die. They also begin to produce increasing amounts of keratin, so that cells in the uppermost layer, the stratum corneum, are completely filled with keratins. This process of cell maturation and increased keratin production is known as *keratinization.*[2] The terminal differentiation of epidermal keratinocytes is characterized by development-specific gene expression. For example, the proliferating relatively undifferentiated basal keratinocytes (found in the stratum basale) express keratin proteins K5 (58 kD) and K14 (50 kD), whereas the keratin filaments specifically expressed in suprabasal keratinocytes — the upper, differentiated layers — are K1 (67 kD) and K10 (56.5 kD), along with K2 and K11,

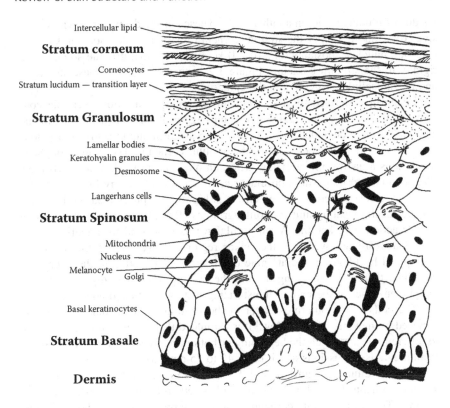

FIGURE 1.2 Fixed cross section of the outer layer of the skin, the epidermis, a stratified squamous epithelium, and the closely apposed sublayer, the dermis. It is from the malar eminence of a 20-year-old white woman. The majority of cells are keratinocytes, which are organized into layers. The layers are named for either their function or their structure. Cells interspersed among the keratinocytes may be lymphocytes (white blood cells), Langerhans cells (immune cells), melanocytes (pigment cells), or Merkel cells. The basal keratinocytes have cytoplasmic rootlets (serrations) that extend into the papillary dermis. In the malpighian layer, the keratinocytes gradually become flattened and are parallel to the surface. Keratohyalin granules develop in this layer. In the two to three layers of the stratum granulosum, the keratinocytes are stretched horizontally. The stratum lucidum is compact, and the stratum corneum appears lacy in its upper part. The stratum corneum has lipid in the intercellular space between proteinaceous corneocytes.

as well as retaining the basal keratinocyte-derived keratins K5 and K14.[4–6] The keratinocytes in the stratum granulosum are characterized by keratohyalin granules containing abundant quantities of profilaggrin and loricrin proteins.[5,6] As the terminally differentiated keratinocytes develop into corneocytes, their plasma membrane is transformed into the cornified envelope as a result of extensive cross-linking of involucrin and loricrin and other proline-rich structural proteins by the epidermal transglutaminases 1, 2, and 3 enzymes.[7] This calcium-dependent enzyme cross-links the ε-amino group of lysine on one chain to the γ-glytamyl residue of glutamic acid on another chain. These cornified envelopes with extensive cross-linking render the stratum corneum resistant to degradation. Corneocytes are anuclear, postapoptotic (dead) keratinocytes that provide strength and rigidity to the stratum corneum. Figure 1.2 further exemplifies these structures and the subcellular structures in the epidermis.

Filaggrin is derived from keratohyalin granules, as are other keratinaceous proteins, shown in Figure 1.2. Filaggrin helps aggregate or stack the keratin fibers[8] and is ultimately degraded in the upper layers to form amino acids, pyrrolidone carboxylic acid, and lactic acid in the stratum corneum. These are thought to function as a natural moisturizing factor, an old concept in skin moisturization. The precursor to filaggrin is profilaggrin, which contains many filaggrin chains joined by tyrosine-rich linker regions; it is highly phosphorylated on the serine residue. Each repeating unit of profilaggrin has 10 to 20 phosphates that prevent its interaction with keratin. When profilaggrin is processed to filaggrin, all the phosphates are removed and the linker regions cleaved. After the keratin is aggregated by filaggrin, the arginine of filaggrin is converted to the uncharged citrulline, thereby dissociating it from the keratin. Then it is digested by proteolytic enzymes to the natural moisturizing factors mentioned above.[9]

The cells in the outermost layer of the stratum corneum flake off and are replaced by new cells from below.[1] It is estimated that a new cell takes 28 days[1] to differentiate and reach the beginning or bottom of the stratum corneum (recall from previous discussions that it takes 45 to 75 days for a new cell to reach the top of the stratum corneum). It is also estimated that each day, one layer of the stratum corneum is shed and one is synthesized from the stratum granulosum below.[10] The entire stratum corneum is shed in approximately 14 days. The rate of addition of new keratinocytes to the stratum corneum is in balance with the rate of loss of dead keratinocytes from its surface. It is this balance in the rate of proliferation and differentiation that is thought to maintain a healthy skin barrier. When this balance is disturbed, such as in diseases like psoriasis, where cells proliferate much too fast,[11] the barrier becomes severely compromised and exhibits excessive scaling, itching, and ultimately inflammation.

This balance between proliferation and differentiation is thought to be regulated by nuclear hormone receptors such as the retinoid receptor, vitamin D receptor, peroxisome proliferator-activated receptor (PPAR), and others, along with the T-lymphocyte-derived cytokine balance. The details of this regulation are still not well understood.[12-14] Nuclear hormone receptors are transcription factors that regulate cellular functions, including differentiation and proliferation. Nuclear hormone receptors that heterodimerize with the retinoid receptor and the vitamin D receptor regulate expression of differentiation-specific genes coding for enzymes, proteins, and lipids that support differentiation and development of a healthy stratum corneum barrier. Some of these are transglutaminases, involucrin, loricrin, and the enzymes that form the barrier lipids. Agonists of these nuclear hormone receptors alter barrier formation.

Studies[12-14] have demonstrated that ligands that bind to PPAR receptors stimulate differentiation and inhibit proliferation in cultured human keratinocytes and accelerate epidermal development and permeability barrier formation in fetal rat skin explants. Topically applied PPARalpha ligands regulate keratinocyte differentiation in mouse epidermis *in vivo*. For example, topical treatment with PPARalpha activators resulted in decreased epidermal thickness. Furthermore, topically applied PPARalpha activators also decreased cell proliferation and accelerated recovery of barrier function following acute barrier abrogation. Expression of differentiation-specific structural proteins of the upper spinous/granular layers (involucrin, profilaggrin–filaggrin, loricrin) also increased. Studies with PPARalpha–/– knockout mice showed that these effects are specifically mediated via PPARalpha.[12] Additionally, in cultured human keratinocytes, this group has demonstrated that PPARalpha activators induce an increase in involucrin mRNA and an increase in gene expression that requires an intact AP-1 DNA response element. All studies support the role of PPARalpha in potentiating keratinocyte/epidermal differentiation and inhibiting proliferation.

Peroxisome proliferator-activated receptors (PPARs) are ligand-activated transcription factors that regulate the expression of target genes involved in many cellular functions, including cell proliferation, differentiation, and immune/inflammation response.[12–14] The PPAR subfamily consists of three isotypes: PPARalpha, PPARbeta/delta, and PPARgamma, which have all been identified in keratinocytes. PPARbeta/delta is the predominant subtype in human keratinocytes, whereas PPARalpha and PPARgamma are expressed at much lower levels and increase significantly upon keratinocyte differentiation. PPARbeta/delta is not linked to differentiation, but is significantly upregulated upon various conditions that result in keratinocyte proliferation, and during skin wound healing. *In vitro* and *in vivo* evidence suggest that PPARs appear to play an important role in skin barrier permeability, inhibiting epidermal cell growth, promoting epidermal terminal differentiation, and regulating skin inflammatory response by diverse mechanisms. These properties are pointing in the direction of PPARs being key regulators of skin conditions characterized by hyperproliferation, inflammatory infiltrates, and aberrant differentiation, such as psoriasis, but may also have clinical implications in inflammatory skin disease (e.g., atopic dermatitis), proliferative skin disease, wound healing, and acne.

It has been known for decades that the level of calcium *in situ* regulates growth vs. differentiation of epidermal keratinocytes. Mammalian epidermis normally displays a distinctive calcium gradient, with low levels in the basal/spinous layers and high levels in the stratum granulosum.[15] Changes in stratum granulosum calcium gradients regulate the lamellar body secretory response to permeability barrier alterations as well as the expression of differentiation-specific proteins *in vivo*. Elias et al.[15] has shown that acute barrier perturbations reduce calcium levels in stratum granulosum. Further studies showed that mouse epidermal differentiation can be regulated after loss of calcium due to acute barrier disruption by exposure of such acutely perturbed skin to either low ($0.03\ M$) or high ($1.8\ M$) calcium. For example, a few hours after acute barrier disruption, coincident with reduced calcium, there is ultrastructural evidence of accelerated lamellar body secretion and decreased mRNA levels for loricrin, profilaggrin, and involucrin in the outer epidermis. Moreover, exposure of disrupted skin to low-calcium solutions sustained the reduction in mRNA levels, whereas exposure to high-calcium solutions restored normal mRNA. Finally, with prolonged exposure to a low (<10%) relative humidity, calcium levels increased, but at high (>80%) relative humidity, calcium levels increased and then declined. Accordingly, mRNA and protein levels of the differentiation-specific markers increased at low and decreased at high relative humidities, respectively. These results provide direct evidence that acute and sustained fluctuations in epidermal calcium regulate expression of differentiation-specific proteins *in vivo*, and demonstrate that modulations in epidermal calcium coordinately regulate events late in epidermal differentiation that together form the barrier.

The roles of calcium and vitamin D are synergistic in the regulation of keratinocyte differentiation as reviewed by Bikle et al.[16] Both calcium and 1,25(OH) vitamin D promote the differentiation of keratinocytes *in vitro*. As discussed above, it is known that keratinocytes cultured in low calcium grow or proliferate, while keratinocytes grown in high calcium cease to grow and differentiate *in situ*. The production of 1,25(OH) vitamin D by keratinocytes, combined with the role of the epidermal calcium gradient in regulating keratinocyte differentiation *in vivo*, suggests the physiologic importance of this interaction. Calcium and 1,25(OH) vitamin D synergistically induce the differentiation-specific protein involucrin found in the cornified envelope. The involucrin promoter gene contains an AP-1 site essential for calcium and 1,25(OH)(2) vitamin D induction and an adjacent vitamin D receptor element essential for 1,25(OH)(2) vitamin D but not calcium induction. Calcium regulates coactivator complexes that bind to the vitamin D receptor. *In vivo* models support the importance of 1,25(OH) vitamin D–calcium interactions in epidermal differentiation. The epidermis of 1alphaOHase null mice fails to form a normal calcium gradient, has a reduced expression of proteins critical for barrier function, and shows little recovery of the permeability barrier when disrupted. Thus, *in vivo* and *in vitro*, calcium and 1,25(OH) vitamin D interact at multiple levels to regulate epidermal differentiation.

Retinoic acid receptors play a crucial role in tissue homeostasis, lipid metabolism, cellular differentiation, and proliferation.[17,18] These functions are in part controlled through the retinoid signaling pathway. Retinoids are compounds with pleiotropic functions and a relatively selective targeting of certain skin structures. They are vitamins, because retinol (vitamin A) is not synthesized in the body and must be derived from the diet, but also hormones with intracrine activity, because retinol is transformed into molecules that bind to nuclear receptors, exhibit their activity, and are subsequently inactivated. Retinoids are also therapeutically effective in the treatment of skin diseases (acne, psoriasis, and photoaging) and of some cancers.[17–22] Most of these effects are the consequences of retinoic acid activation of a series of nuclear hormone receptors, including RAR and RXR, which trigger transcriptional events leading to either transcriptional activation or suppression of retinoid-controlled genes. Synthetic ligands are able to mimic part of the biological effects of the natural retinoic acid receptors, all-trans retinoic acid. Therefore, retinoic acid receptors are valuable therapeutic targets, and limiting unwanted secondary effects due to retinoid treatment requires a molecular knowledge of retinoic acid receptors' biology.

For example, in the case of photodamage, ultraviolet (UV) irradiation of human skin sets in motion a complex sequence of events that causes damage to the dermal matrix.[19,20] When topical tretinoin is applied to human skin, any collagen deficiency existing in photoaged skin is remedied at least partially, and skin metabolic activity is primed to prevent further dermal matrix degradation induced by UV radiation. Production of procollagen is increased to augment the formation of types I and III collagen, and retinoids block expression of mediators of inflammation. Retinoids have therefore become essential in the treatment and prevention of photoaging.

Retinoids also play a vital role in the treatment of acne because they act on the primary preacne lesion, the microcomedo.[21,22] Several retinoid compounds are used for treating acne, in either topical or systemic form, for example, tretinoin (all-trans retinoic acid), isotretinoin (13-cis-retinoic acid), adapalene (derived from naphthoic acid), and tazarotene (acetylenic retinoid). They act mainly as comedolytics, but anti-inflammatory actions have also been recently discovered. The retinoids have great beneficial effects, but also some adverse effects, the main one being teratogenicity (causing birth defects). It is preferrable not to use them in topical form for pregnant women, although a pregnancy test is only compulsory for Accutane® and tazarotene. Only isotretinoin is used in systemic (oral tablet) form: Accutane. Isotretinoin acts on most of the factors causing acne (over active sebaceous glands, inflammation, and blocked pilosebaceous units) and offers long remissions, and sometimes complete cures. Precautions must be taken for women of childbearing age due to its teratogenicity. It is also important to be aware of its other adverse effects, explain them to the patient, and, if possible, deal with them in advance.

Although keratinocytes are the major cells within the epidermis, melanocytes (Figure 1.1 and Figure 1.2) also play an important role in skin barrier function and specifically confer skin color. There is approximately 1 melanocyte for every 36 keratinocytes in the human epidermis. Together these form an epidermal melanin unit.[23] Melanocytes synthesize melanin, a compound that absorbs UV light and is responsible for substantial protection against UV radiation.[23] Melanin is secreted by the melanocytes into the associated keratinocytes in the melanin unit. Melanocyte function is able to determine skin color. It is not dependent on melanocyte number (this is constant across racial groups), but upon the organization of the epidermal melanin unit.[23]

Of the four epidermal layers, the one of most importance in terms of topical treatment for skin disorders and enhancing appearance of skin is the stratum corneum.

1.2.2 THE STRATUM CORNEUM[10]

The stratum corneum is the outermost layer of the epidermis. It is made up of approximately 15 layers of flat, dead cells called corneocytes that are completely

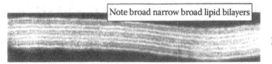

Expanded scale

Stratum corneum lipid bilayers

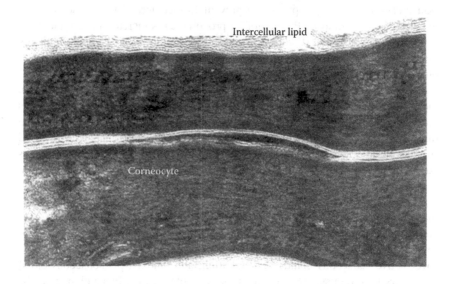

FIGURE 1.3 Transmission electron micrographs of stratum corneum of mammalian species depicting the intercellular lamellae. Note the multilayered repeat units (arrows). Postfixation is with ruthenium tetroxide to show lipid. (Modified from Rawlings, A.V., *J. Cosmet. Sci.* 47, 32, 1996. With permission.)

filled with keratin (Figure 1.3). For this reason, it is sometimes called the horny layer. The highly keratinized cells of the stratum corneum are packed tightly together and are surrounded by a multilayered lipid structure.[10] This tightly packed structure is often compared to bricks and mortar — providing structural strength through the keratin-filled bricks and waterproofing through the layer of lipid mortar (Figure 1.3).

The cells of the horny layer are constantly worn away and replaced by newly keratinized cells, in a continual cycle. The stratum corneum itself is replaced about every 14 days; that is, it takes about 14 days for a dead cell to move from the bottom of the stratum corneum to the surface of the membrane. This cycle of keratinization, cell loss, and replacement is important because a variety of skin problems, including ichthyosis, psoriasis, atopic eczema, and acne, involve disturbances of the normal sequence. The cycle may be disturbed by a variety of factors, including exposure to substances such as cosmetics, low relative humidity, cold weather, vitamin A, steroid hormones or drugs, as well as chemical messengers produced by the cells themselves or a disease, e.g., psoriasis, that is characterized by accelerated cell growth or proliferation.[11]

The stratum corneum is composed of lipids and proteins. Some of the proteins that originate from the differentiating keratinocyte and the keratohyalin granules visible in Figure 1.2 were discussed in the last section, but a detailed discussion of the lipids found in the stratum corneum is in order for the purposes of this chapter. Lipids constitute about ~10% of the wet weight or <30% of the dry weight of the stratum corneum. Lipids in the stratum corneum originate from the lamellar bodies shown in Figure 1.2. Lamellar bodies are secretory granules originating from the Golgi. The lamellar body attaches to the cell membrane of the differentiated keratinocytes, and their lipid contents are extruded into the intercellular spaces around the corneocytes (dead keratinocytes) in the upper part. They are then modified by enzymes present in the intercellular spaces to produce the intercellular lipids surrounding the corneocytes found in the upper layers of the stratum corneum.[24–26] Lipids in the upper layers contain predominantly cholesterol, ceramides, and free fatty acids in a ratio of approximately 25:50:15, as weight percent, with 10% other minor lipids.[24,25] They are unique because they do not contain phospholipids, which are typically found in other biological membranes. During the process of modification to produce the stratum corneum lipids, phospholipids present in the lamellar body secretions are completely abolished and converted to free fatty acids; glucosyl ceramides also present in the secretions are converted to ceramides, and cholesterol sulfate is converted to free cholesterol.[24,25]

Table 1.1 exemplifies this lipid modification process in the various layers of the epidermis.

Also, it is important to note that on the skin surface, the sebaceous lipids originating from the sebaceous glands will become an important entity, along with the interactions and mixing of sebaceous lipids with the epidermal lipids. Sebaceous lipids are enriched in triglycerides, wax esters, cholesterol, and free fatty acids; the latter can vary, depending on the enrichment of microorganisms on the skin surface that convert triglycerides to free fatty acids, primarily *Propionibacterium acnes*.[27–30]

TABLE 1.1
Lipid Composition in Different Epidermal Layers (as Weight Percent)

Lipid Class	Basal/Spinous Layers	Granular Layer	Stratum Corneum
Phosopholipid	63	25	0
Glucosyl ceramide	7	10	0
Ceramides	0	15	50
Cholesterol	10	21	25
Free fatty acids	7	17	15
Other	13	12	10

Source: Review by Abraham, W., in *Surfactants in Cosmetics*, Rieger, M. and Rhein, L., Eds., Marcel Dekker, New York, 1997, chap. 20.

The lipids are organized in a multilayered structure (see Figure 1.3). The lipid bilayers are attached hydrophobically to the corneocyte envelope on the surface of the corneocyte; this envelope contains covalently attached omega-hydroxy ceramide and fatty acids, lipids that serve as a template for the lipid bilayer attachment (see review by Abraham[24]). The carbon chain length of the acyl ceramides has been extensively studied by Wertz and Downing[26] and is on average 24 carbons, compared to the average chain length of 16 to 18 for phospholipids typically found in other biological membranes, again suggesting that stratum corneum lipids are unique. The need for increased hydrophobicity of this membrane is thus evident from the structure. Additionally, the fatty acids, both free and esterified to sphingolipids are highly enriched in saturated species (>70%), although linoleic acid is also a major fatty acid in ceramide (~14% and more). Details on their exact compositions can be found in additional references.[31,32] The enrichment of longer chains and saturation both attest to the hydrophobic nature of the barrier. More details on the lipids in skin can be found in a review by Wertz.[25]

In healthy skin, the stratum corneum is an effective barrier against UV light, heat or cold, bacteria, mechanical disruption, and many chemicals.[2] Some oils and alcohols, however, penetrate the stratum corneum layer quite well. This is why many skin preparations contain or are based on these components, to help carry the active ingredients into the deeper layers of cells. The stratum corneum is responsible for preventing both water loss from and environmental insult to the skin.[2]

A more definitive role of stratum corneum lipids in maintaining a healthy barrier is discussed in the next section.

1.3 ORIGIN AND FUNCTION OF STRATUM CORNEUM LIPIDS

Elias and Feingold[33] very effectively reviewed the origin of current concepts of stratum corneum and lipid structure. The old perception of mammalian stratum corneum, based on histological studies, was that of a loosely bound layer in various stages of disorganization and sloughing off. Table 1.2 displays the stages of understanding of the characteristics of this membrane.

This misleading image of a disorganized structure was refuted by physical-chemical, frozen-section, and freeze–fracture studies. The histological fixation

---

TABLE 1.2
Stages in the Understanding of Stratum Corneum Structure

Concepts	Approximate Date Observed
1. Disorganized, nonfunctional	Through 1950
2. Homogenous film	Up to the 1970s
3. Lipid–protein compartmentalization	1975–present
4. Metabolically active	1984–present

technique had resulted in destruction of the membrane. Thus, the ultrastructural preparations obscured further advances until the 1970s, therefore confusing recognition of the actual structure. Initially these studies showed a membrane film covering the stratum granulosum and led to the hypothesis that the stratum corneum was a homogeneous film. The freeze–fracture studies later refuted this and established that the layer was composed of tightly arrayed polyhedral structures in vertical interlocking columns. The initial awareness of lipid–protein segregation to specific tissue compartments came from freeze–fracture replication studies, which revealed the presence of multiple broad lamellations in the interstices of several types of mammalian keratinizing epithelia. X-ray diffraction studies previously demonstrated a highly ordered lipid structure in the stratum corneum that could account for the lamellations observed in freeze–fracture.

Definitive evidence for the compartmentalization of lipids came from the isolation of stratum corneum membrane "sandwiches" containing trapped intercellular lipids, reviewed by Elias and Feingold.[33] These structures that became visible with better staining techniques, i.e., ruthenium tetroxide postfixation, contained the same broad lamellae found in the interstices of the whole stratum structure (Figure 1.3). This came to be commonly referred to as the brick-and-mortar hypothesis for the stratum corneum structure, with the bricks being dead corneocytes and the mortar the intercellular lipid lamellae; this was discussed briefly earlier. Researchers from the Alza Corporation simultaneously reported the existence of lipophilic vs. hydrophilic pathways of percutaneous absorption,[34] which supported the idea of a protein pathway and an intercellular lipid pathway.

That the lipid part of the stratum corneum is metabolically active has also now been demonstrated by Elias and Feingold.[33] Co-localization of lipid catabolic enzymes within the intercellular lipid by both ultrastructural cytochemistry and enzyme biochemistry is further evidence for the structural heterogeneity of the stratum corneum. The fact that the phospholipids disappear in the stratum corneum and neutral lipids and sphingolipids (primarily ceramides) appear in abundance is now common knowledge (Table 1.1). The metabolic enzymes responsible for these changes are secreted along with the lipids into the intercellular spaces by the lamellar bodies (Figure 1.2 and Figure 1.4).[33,35] These enzymes are lipases, including acid lipase, phospholipase A, sphingomyelinase, steroid sulfatase, and acid phosphatase, and also proteases, like cathepsins and carboxypepidase. Figure 1.4 shows how the probarrier enzymes (phospholipase A, sphingomyelinase, and glucosidase) found both in the lamellar granules (except steroid sulfatase) and in the intercellular spaces work together to form the optimal intercellular lipids of the stratum corneum. Catabolic enzymes like acid phosphatase, proteases, other lipases, and glycosidases now work together to mediate normal desquamation of the stratum corneum.

Certain striking features of the modulation suggest that these alterations are necessary for optimal barrier function. Sphingolipids, in particular, have been cited as a critical molecule for barrier function because (1) they are the most abundant class of lipids, (2) they possess a long-chain hydrophobic base, (3) they have very long chain, highly saturated N-acylated fatty acids (such long chains

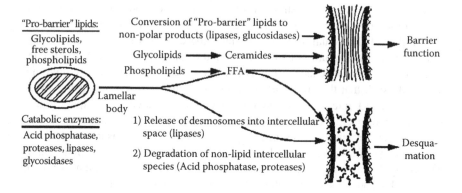

FIGURE 1.4 Scheme showing secretion of probarrier lipids and enzymes involved in lipid modulations and desquamation originating from lamellar body secretions.

have been postulated to span the bilayer), and (4) some species are the most abundant repository for an ester-linked linoleate residue (oleate substitution for linoleate is associated with a defective barrier in essential fatty acid deficiency).[24,36–38] The enrichment of longer chains and saturation both attest to the hydrophobic nature of the barrier. More details on the lipids in skin can be found in a review by Wertz.[25]

While these results allude to the importance of the sphingolipids in barrier function, they do not attest to the role of the neutral lipids, in particular free fatty acids and cholesterol. To establish a more definitive role of the lipids to barrier function, Elias took a more physiological approach. Elias studied hairless mice and damaged their skin barrier with either acetone or tape stripping. He tracked transepidermal water loss and the rate of its recovery along with the activity of enzymes involved in the synthesis of the three classes of stratum corneum lipids. After barrier abrogation, lipid synthesis increased rapidly, within 1 to 2 h. This paralleled the increase in activity of HMG-CoA reductase (rate-limiting enzyme in cholesterol biosynthesis), acetyl CoA carboxylase, and fatty acid synthase (the latter two are involved in fatty acid biosynthesis).[35,39] In contrast, the increase in sphingolipid synthesis and the activity of serine palmitoyl transferase (the first committed enzyme in sphingolipid biosynthesis) are delayed approximately 6 h after barrier disruption. Other studies have demonstrated that mRNA levels for HMG-CoA reductase, HMG-CoA synthase, farnesyl diphosphate synthase, squalene synthase, acetyl CoA carboxylate, and fatty acid synthase all increase soon after barrier abrogation. In contrast, sphingolipid synthesis and serine palmitoyl transferase, the first committed enzyme in sphingolipid biosynthesis, increase just a few hours later, suggesting regulation by a different mechanism.[35] As the mRNA levels for these proteins increase after either tape stripping or acetone treatment, these changes appear to be independent of the method of barrier perturbation. Moreover, the increase in mRNA levels for these enzymes is prevented by immediate occlusion with a plastic wrap, which provides an artificial permeability barrier. These data indicate that the increase in mRNA levels for these enzymes is regulated by barrier function rather than simply representing a response to injury.

The findings also suggest that actives can be identified that would alter the expression or activity of the barrier-forming enzymes to reconstruct a healthy barrier. Tanno et al.[40] studied the action of nicotinamide, one of the B vitamins, on the barrier. Their group studied the effects of nicotinamide on biosynthesis of sphingolipids, including ceramides and other stratum corneum lipids, in cultured normal human keratinocytes, and on the epidermal permeability barrier *in vivo*. The rate of sphingolipid biosynthesis was measured by the incorporation of [14C]-serine into sphingolipids. They found that the rate of ceramide biosynthesis was increased dose dependently by 4.1- to 5.5-fold on the sixth day compared with the control. Nicotinamide also increased the synthesis of glucosyl ceramide (sevenfold) and sphingomyelin (threefold) in the same concentration range effective for ceramide synthesis. Furthermore, the activity of serine palmitoyl transferase (SPT), the rate-limiting enzyme in sphingolipid synthesis, was increased in nicotinamide-treated cells. Nicotinamide increased the levels of human LCB1 and LCB2 mRNA, both of which encode subunits of SPT. This suggested that the increase in SPT activity was due to an increase in SPT mRNA. Nicotinamide increased not only ceramide synthesis, but also free fatty acid (2.3-fold) and cholesterol (1.5-fold) synthesis. Topical application of nicotinamide increased ceramide and free fatty acid levels in the stratum corneum and decreased transepidermal water loss in dry skin. Thus, nicotinamide improved the permeability barrier by stimulating *de novo* synthesis of ceramides, with upregulation of SPT and other intercellular lipids.

Below is summarized the evidence that barrier function regulates epidermal lipogenesis (Elias and Feingold[33]), and Table 1.3 summarizes support that epidermal lipids regulate barrier function.

- Dietary or solvent-induced barrier disruption stimulates epidermal lipogenesis
- Extent of lipid biosynthesis rates parallels severity of barrier defect
- Normalization of lipid biosynthesis rates parallels barrier recovery
- Occlusion with impermeable, but not vapor-permeable membrane after barrier disruption blocks acceleration of lipid biosynthesis
- Application of inhibitors of enzymes that synthesize all three classes of barrier lipids delays recovery of barrier after barrier disruption

Thus, Elias's research has demonstrated the importance of all three lipid classes to optimal barrier function, not just the sphingolipids. He has also shown that regulation of epidermal lipogenesis is controlled by conditions at the surface of the skin; i.e., the presence of plastic wrap on top can stop lipogenesis, and damage to the lipids by solvent extraction potentiates lipogenesis. Table 1.3 builds on this and summarizes evidence that it is the lipids that mediate epidermal barrier function.

TABLE 1.3
Evidence That Lipids Mediate Mammalian Epidermal Barrier Function

Solvent/Detergent Treatment

Removal of stratum corneum lipids by either organic solvents or detergents perturbs barrier function

The extent of the solvent-induced defect in barrier function correlates with both the amount and type of lipid removal

Recovery of barrier function correlates with return of lipid or artificial application of the natural lipid

Essential Fatty Acid Deficiency

The barrier defect in essential fatty acid-deficient epidermis is associated with loss of intercellular lipids

The barrier defect is corrected by topical application of natural and synthetic lipids that fix barrier function independent of eicosanoid generation

Topographic Differences in Barrier Function

The barrier to water transport across the stratum corneum of different body sites is inversely proportional to the lipid content of those sites

Dry vs. Moist Keratinizing Epithelia

Epidermal lipids are more polar, and constituent fatty acids are more unsaturated in marine mammals than in terrestrial mammals

The lipids of oral mucosa are more polar, and these compositional changes reflect permeability differences at these sites

Metabolic

Inhibitors of barrier lipid biosynthetic enzymes delay recovery of barrier function

Source: Modified from Elias, P.M. and Feingold, K., *Ann. N.Y. Acad. Sci.*, 548, 4–13, 1988.

That the stratum corneum is the main barrier to water transport was shown very elegantly by Smith et al.[41] Fragments of stratum corneum were reduced to single cells by grinding with a motor and pestle, followed by exhaustive extraction of the intercellular lipids with either ether or 2:1 chloroform:methanol and with the aid of a ground glass homogenizer. They found that >95% of the lipids were removed. When single cells were placed on water as a thin film in chloroform:methanol and the solvent left to evaporate, the cells showed no evidence of reaggregation into a sheet and provided no barrier to water transport. Upon addition of the extracted lipid, the single cells aggregated into a sheet and provided a barrier to water permeability as measured by its diffusional resistance. This was also dependent on the amount of lipid added. At the optimal lipid-to-cell ratio of greater than 4% lipid (wt/wt) the diffusional resistance was 1.0 mg/cm-h. This is close to the value for intact stratum corneum. The ability of cells to reaggregate was eliminated if the cells were trypsinized, suggesting certain proteins are involved in the aggregation, and we speculate that these are the desmosomes found in the intercellular spaces or the corneocyte envelopes that anchor the lipids' layers. Miriam Brysk et al. later found that triton X-100 also prevented reaggregation, and this may be caused by its binding to the covalently bound cell envelope lipid (omega-hydroxy ceramide) blocking the template upon which the bilayers are built.[42] Plantar cells were not as responsive to lipid reaggregation and offered a very poor barrier to water transport. Plantar skin is known for its excessive sweating, functionally supporting these findings and suggesting site differences.

Several authors also examined the water-holding capacity and skin condition before and after extraction of stratum corneum lipids from healthy adults (forearms) with organic solvents. Imokawa et al.[43] showed that removal of lipids increased with length of time of extraction with acetone ether and a dry scaly condition appeared that endured for more than 4 days. Shorter extraction times removed sebaceous lipids, and longer times removed stratum corneum lipids. The skin conductance went down, indicative of reduced water content. Application of extracted lipids from sebum (mostly wax esters and triglycerides) did not affect the conductance values, but application of the total stratum corneum epidermal lipid fraction or individual lipids (sterol ester, free fatty acid, cholesterol, ceramide, or glycolipids) significantly increased skin conductance, indicating an increase in water content of the membrane. Scaling also improved. Similar studies by Grubauer et al.[44] used hairless mice as the model and transepidermal water loss (TEWL) as the measure of barrier damage and came to similar conclusions regarding the importance of lipids to the water-holding capacity of the stratum corneum.

Using a structure activity study of 38 different ceramide derivatives, Imokawa et al.[45] showed that the presence of saturated straight alkyl chains with the absence of unsaturation or methyl branches in the ceramide species was optimal for water-retaining capacity after application to skin *in vivo*, as is characteristic of native stratum corneum ceramides. However, the preferred alkyl chains of C14 to C18 showed the greatest improvement in water-retaining capacity (measured by skin conductance); this differs from native ceramides, which tend to have very long chain lengths. Of course, one could argue that the barrier serves additional functions beyond water-holding capacity, i.e., normal desquamation, and it is possible that the longer chains are necessary for optimizing this function of the membrane.

1.4 SKIN LIPID MACROMOLECULAR STRUCTURE
AND PUTATIVE ORGANIZATION

Friberg and colleagues[46–49] have studied the macromolecular structure of the stratum corneum lipids. Friberg combined all of the lipids found in the surface layers of stratum corneum with 32% water and obtained a milky mixture of multiple phases. Upon adjusting the pH to be between 4.5 and 5.5, i.e., in the range of stratum corneum pH (done by neutralizing 41% of the fatty acid), a liquid crystalline phase emerged. This was verified by photomicroscopy and by small-angle x-ray diffraction. Diffraction patterns using small-angle measurements of the lipid model exhibited a broad reflection band with a maximum reflectance at 65 to 75 Å and were similar to that of intact isolated human stratum corneum. The microscopy patterns showed Maltese crosses and the typical light reflectance of a liquid crystal. Based on this effect, Friberg has proposed that the fatty acid/soap structure is the basis of the multilamellar structure. The layered structure formed even in the absence of all other lipids except the fatty acid/soap, but not with any of the other lipids alone, supporting the fatty acid/soap as the basis of the bilayer. However, this model does not contain the stratum corneum proteinaceous corneocytes with their covalently attached omega-hydroxy ceramide lipid template and the desmosomes and enzymes. Others have found a somewhat different pattern for murine stratum corneum; this will be discussed later.[36]

Friberg et al.[46-49] studied the effect of individually adding each of the lipids of stratum surface layers to the fatty acid/soap mixture on the initial interlayer spacing of the small-angle x-ray diffraction patterns generated by the fatty acid/soap. Changes in the interlayer spacing can provide information on the possible location of the specific lipids in the bilayer. They also varied the water content and tracked changes in the diffraction patterns upon dehydration of the lipid. Figure 1.5 shows the outcome of these experiments.

The lipids with polar head groups are postulated to be located between the chains, with the polar head group adjacent to the hydrophillic layer, e.g., fatty acid soaps and ceramides. Cholesterol also associates between the chains, and in fact, the data suggest that as more water is added to the bilayer, the cholesterol pushes some of the fatty acids out from between the chains to the hydrophobic methyl layer. This results in an increase in the interlayer spacing with added incremental water beyond what can be attributed only to the added water. Triglycerides and wax esters, surface lipids of mostly sebaceous origin, will exist in the hydrophobic layer along with squalene, and will therefore also increase the interlayer spacing upon their addition. The results shown in Figure 1.6 and Figure 1.7 for ceramides demonstrate its unique dependency on water content in

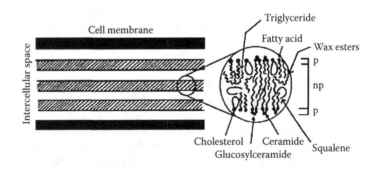

FIGURE 1.5 Schematic showing the putative location of stratum corneum lipids in the bilayer structure as predicted from x-ray diffraction studies.

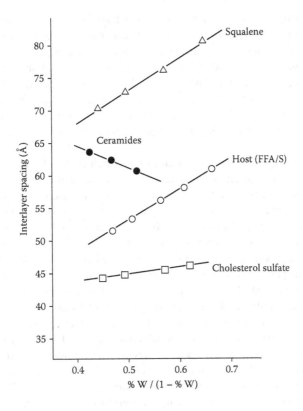

FIGURE 1.6 Addition of ceramide to the host fatty acid/soap lipid model; variations in interlayer spacing with increasing water content of the model lipid.

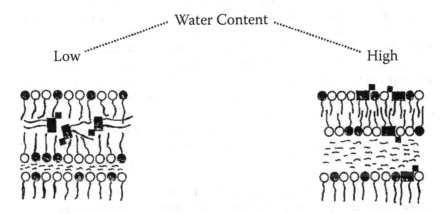

FIGURE 1.7 Illustration showing that the location of ceramides in the layered structure depends on moisture content. Note that at high moisture, ceramides move to the region between the chains. This will decrease the volume and concomitantly the interlayer spacing seen in Figure 1.6.

the layered structure. Figure 1.6 shows what happens to the interlayer spacing when ceramide is added to the fatty acid/soap model. The interlayer spacing decreases as the water content of the model lipid increases.

At low-moisture ceramide tended to reside in the hydrophobic methyl layer, giving an interlayer spacing of 65 Å, and at higher water content, it exists mostly between the chains of the palisade layer, resulting in a decrease in the interlayer spacing. Changes in moisture content can thus have a dramatic effect on the location of lipids in the ordered structure. This is illustrated schematically in Figure 1.7.

The other important learning from this research is that the lipids in at least part of the layered structure are dynamic, not static, and can move around in response to added compounds or environmental conditions, such as low relative humidity. The putative location of the lipids in the layered structure (Figure 1.5) is supported by the stratum corneum lipid extraction studies of Imokawa and Hattori discussed earlier.[51] They showed that with acetone extraction, triglycerides, waxes, and any hydrocarbons were removed in 30 sec, suggesting loose bonding by dispersion forces, while fatty acids, ceramides, and cholesterol continued to be removed after 15 min, suggesting they are more tightly bound by polar forces and hydrogen bonds and are partially ordered.

Accommodation of saturated fatty acids is problematic for the layered structure.[47] When saturated fatty acids were added to the model with only unsaturated fatty acid/soap, a phase change was observed. The unsaturated fatty acid/soap forms a liquid crystalline structure. Their combination with saturated fatty acids formed crystals suggestive of crystalline (orthorombic) character. The presence of sufficient crystals in the lipid structure perturbs the structure such that the barrier to water permeation is compromised. In fact, saturated fatty acids/soap alone offer no barrier to water permeation. Yet the stratum corneum barrier lipid is quite enriched in saturated fatty acids. Saturated fatty acids add rigidity and order to the layered structure. Extended studies show that once the other lipids are incorporated into the layered structure, the saturation becomes a nonissue. For example, addition of cholesterol to the unsaturated–saturated fatty acid/soap mixture returned the structure to the liquid crystalline form.[47] Similarly, ceramides, especially certain ceramides enriched in unsaturated fatty acids, will fluidize the structure. This is because cholesterol and unsaturated ceramides sufficiently disturb the order to fluidize the rigid structure. This research demonstrates the importance of the key lipids to the layered structure. It also shows the resulting delicate balance to help maintain the rigidity of the lipid macromolecular structure, yet ensures that it will be fluid enough to support mobility, permeability, and a water barrier function.

Friberg and colleagues also studied the effectiveness of various liquid crystalline structures at providing a barrier to water transport when reaggregated with delipidated corneocytes.[52] Table 1.4 shows the results for these various structures.

The data in Table 1.4 show that any of the liquid crystals establish a barrier to water transport through the reaggregated discs. Thus, it is the macromolecular structure that is essential for establishing a barrier to water transport, not the

TABLE 1.4
Permeability Constants (Kp)[a] of Reconstituted Stratum Corneum Samples Using Lyotropic Liquid Crystals, Model Lipid, Fatty Acid/Soap Model, and Natural Lipid

Aggregation Element (with Delipidated Corneocytes) (Structure Type)	$Kp \times 10^3$ cm-h^{-1}
% relative to corneocytes	
25% natural lipid	4.7 ± 0.2
25% lecithin:water	7.9 ± 0.07
(lamellar liquid crystal)	
25% SDS:$C_{12}(EO)_2$:water	7.6 ± 0.07
(lamellar liquid crystal)	
25% SDS:decanol:water	6.3 ± 0.21
(lamellar liquid crystal)	
25% Tween:water	6.2 ± 0.49
(hexagonal liquid crystal)	
20% model lipid	4.1 ± 0.6
(lamellar liquid crystal)	
20% unsaturated/saturated fatty acid mixture	3.9 ± 0.5
(lamellar liquid crystal)	
6% unsaturated/saturated fatty acid mixture	4.5 ± 0.6
(lamellar liquid crystal)	
Intact stratum corneum	0.7 ± 0.11

[a] Permeability constant determined at 93% RH and 31°C. Constants were determined for water vapor penetrating through five different reconstituted discs, and the values are means ± standard deviations.

Source: Taken and modified from Kayali, I. et al., *J. Pharm. Sci.*, 80, 428–431, 1991; Friberg, S.E. et al., *J. Invest. Dermatol.*, 94, 377–380, 1990.

composition or organization of the specific lipids. However, the natural lipid with the polar as well as the nonpolar components provided the better barrier to water transport compared to the surfactant:water liquid crystals, second only to intact stratum corneum. In the case of the unsaturated:saturated fatty acid mixture, which also provided an excellent barrier, the fatty acid is the nonpolar lipid and the soap is the polar species; this supports the role of fatty acid/soaps in creating the permeability barrier. However, the presence of unsaturated fatty acids like linoleic acid also fluidizes the barrier to get around the rigidity that may create a leaky barrier. The studies also show that one does not need a lamellar liquid crystal to provide a barrier to water transport in the reconstituted system; the hexagonal liquid crystal was also very effective.

Earlier studies showed that lipid crystals do not provide a barrier to water transport because a slurry of lipid crystal aggregates gave a barrier equal to an unprotected water surface, whereas liquid crystalline structures gave a barrier to water transport several orders of magnitude smaller.[54] Saturated fatty acids of 16 to 18 carbon chain lengths alone or partially saponified fatty acids in the soap form do not form liquid crystals.[47] However, in combination with the unsaturated species, like linoleic acid, they exist as a lamellar liquid crystal. That unsaturates provide this function is verified in essential fatty acid deficiency, where a scaly barrier persists and can be eliminated with topical treatment with linoleic acid, but not saturated fatty acids.

1.5 POLYMORPHISM IN THE STRATUM CORNEUM LIPID STRUCTURE

Other authors have examined the macromolecular structure of stratum corneum lipid further. Abraham and Downing[55] have used nuclear magnetic resonance (NMR) techniques and found polymorphism in the structure of the lipid. For example, thermal transitions were noted from lamellar to a hexagonal liquid crystal phase starting at 60 through 70°C. Schematic drawings of both lamellar and hexagonal phases are shown in Figure 1.8. The hexagonal phase of inverted micelles has a much more highly disordered hydrocarbon environment, but according to Friberg's research discussed above,[52] such phases do provide an effective barrier to water transport, and in some cases, it was as good as a lamellar phase. Downing also noticed that increasing ceramide and decreasing cholesterol lowers the energy barrier for the transition from lamellar to hexagonal phases to around 60°C, and also increases the disorder in the hexagonal phase; thus, the transition can be effected by changes in composition. Downing has suggested that the transitions to the hexagonal phase may have important implications in the reassembly of membrane discs extruded from the lamellar granules. During this stage there is a dramatic change in the composition of the lipids, predominantly catabolism of phospholipids and glucoceramides to free fatty acids and ceramides. There is also reduced water content and loss of polar head groups. These factors could regulate the structural preference of the lipids causing the transformation. Lipid molecules in membrane bilayers undergo momentary departure from bilayer organization at the point of contact and form intermediary structures such as inverted micelles during membrane fusion. Thus, the ability of stratum corneum lipids to form hexagonal phases establishes a plausible pathway for the reassembly of the membranous discs into extended lamellar sheets by membrane fusion processes involving transient nonlamellar intermediates, as mentioned by Abraham and Downing.[55]

1.5.1 ADDITIONAL SMALL-ANGLE X-RAY DIFFRACTION STUDIES SUGGESTING POLYMORPHISM

As discussed previously, Friberg studied the small-angle x-ray diffraction patterns of human stratum corneum and found a broad reflectance band that exhibited a maximum reflectance between 55 and 80 Å.[47] White et al.[50] reported studies of the x-ray diffraction patterns of isolated hairless mouse skin. He studied the

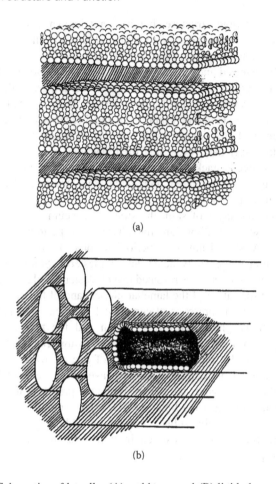

(a)

(b)

FIGURE 1.8 Schematics of lamellar (A) and hexagonal (B) lipid phases.

lamellar lipid domains and corneocyte envelopes. The diffraction pattern with the sample at 25°C showed a Bragg spacing of 131 Å for the repeat unit. The small-angle x-ray patterns of extracted lipids gave a repeat unit of 60 Å. Bouwstra et al.[56] also reported a low-angle diffraction spacing of 65 Å in human stratum corneum, but later reported that she was unsure if this was a first-order diffraction. She later reported a possible spacing of 130 Å in agreement with White above and concluded the huge background of the 65 Å peak may have obscured the first-order band. Upon heating, the pattern of intact stratum corneum became amorphous, but when cooled down, the repeat pattern returned, and thus the order returned. This suggests another component is present in the intercellular space that helps maintain the lamellar organization. It may in fact be attributed to the desmosomes that interconnect the corneocytes, and their degradation is key to desquamation or sloughing of the outer layers of corneocytes. It could also be some type of solid lipid structure, but it is not known. As discussed in the following sections, other authors are finding evidence for orthorhombic/gel lipid domains in the stratum corneum structure.

Hou et al.[57] reviewed and summarized the x-ray diffraction studies done and information that supports the findings. Cross-sectional images of the intercellular regions of mouse stratum corneum (in thin sections fixed with ruthenium tetroxide) are filled with lipid lamellae (Figure 1.3), and these images revealed a pattern with a periodicity of 128 Å, supporting White et al.'s findings[50] on murine stratum corneum. All the x-ray data reveal that the reflections occur in multiple orders of a given spacing due to stacking of repetitive lamellar units, supporting Friberg's original proposal of a multilayered intercellular lipid structure, also identified by the freeze–fracture studies.[33]

In the superficial layer of skin, the stratum corneum (SC), the lipids thus appear to form two crystalline lamellar phases with periodicities of 64 Å or 6.4 nm and 134 Å or 13.4 nm (long periodicity phase). The main lipid classes in SC are ceramides, free fatty acids, and cholesterol. Studies with mixtures prepared with isolated ceramides revealed that cholesterol and ceramides are very important for the formation of the lamellar phases, and of the nine ceramides in the stratum corneum, the presence of ceramide 1 is crucial for the formation of the long periodicity phase. This observation and the broad–narrow–broad sequence of lipid layers in the 13.4-nm phase led Bouwstra et al.[58] to propose a molecular model for this phase. This consists of one narrow central lipid layer with fluid domains on both sides of a broad layer with a crystalline structure. This is referred to as the sandwich model. While the presence of free fatty acids does not substantially affect the lipid lamellar organization, it is crucial for the formation of the orthorhombic sublattice, since the addition of free fatty acids to cholesterol/ceramide mixtures resulted in transition from a hexagonal to a crystalline lipid phase.

1.5.2 STUDIES WITH HIGH-ANGLE X-RAY DIFFRACTION AND OTHER TECHNIQUES SUPPORTING POLYMORPHISM

Hou et al.[57] reviewed that in biological membranes lateral packing of hydrocarbon chains of lipids also gives rise to high-angle reflections. Two spacings are commonly found: a sharp reflection at 4.0 to 4.2 Å indicative of crystalline packing and a broad diffuse reflection at 4.5 to 4.8 Å indicative of fluid-like packing. Longer-chain lipids in the solid state are known to give spacings of 4.2 and 3.8 Å. Stratum corneum lipid domains exhibit reflectance bands around 4.2 and 3.8 Å. In the liquid state, a reflectance band of 4.6 Å is also seen. The appearance or disappearance of these reflections is dependent on the transition temperatures. Table 1.5 and Table 1.6 (modified from their review paper) summarizes what is known about the reflection bands of stratum corneum in relation to temperature. The 4.2- and 3.8-Å bands disappear above 40°, indicating the crystalline structure has liquified. The 4.6-Å band persists as in Table 1.6; this is due to the liquid alkyl chains. Upon extraction of stratum corneum with solvent, the shorter bands

TABLE 1.5
Summary of Thermal Behavior of Lipid and Protein Domains in Stratum Corneum Using Wide-Angle X-Ray Diffraction: Assignment of Reflection Bands

Stratum Corneum Source	Assignment	Interlayer Spacing (Å) and Behavior as a Function of Temperature			
		25°C	40°C	69–70°C	80–90°C
Neonatal rat	Lipid	3.7	Absent		
		4.2	4.2	Absent	
	Protein	4.6	No change up to 77°C		
		9.8	No change up to 77°C		
Human	Lipid	3.7	Absent	Absent	Absent
		4.2	4.2	4.2	Absent
		4.6	4.6	4.6	Absent
	Protein	4.6	No change up to 77°C		
		9.8	No change up to 77°C		

Source: Assimilated from Hou, S.Y. et al., *Adv. Lipid Res.*, 24, 141–171, 1991.

TABLE 1.6
High-Angle Spacing (Å) Observed in Stratum Corneum as a Function of Temperature

Temperature			Interpretation
25°C	45°C	75°C	
9.4s	9.4s	9.4s	Both of the sharp lines, 9.4 and 4.6, originate from the
4.6s	4.6s	4.6s	protein in the corneocyte envelope
4.6b	4.6b	4.6b	Liquid alkyl chains
4.16s	Absent	Absent	Both 4.16 and 3.75 Å spacings are due to the crystalline alkyl chains organized as an orthorhombic perpendicular subcell; there may be a distribution of alkyl chains in the gel state because the 4.16 line is wide
Absent	4.12s	Absent	The 4.12-Å spacing is due to gel state alkyl chains organized as a hexagonal subcell — transition from crystalline state at 25°C (the 4.16- and 3.75-Å bands)
3.75s	Absent	Absent	Both 4.16- and 3.75-Å spacings are due to the crystalline alkyl chains organized as an orthorhombic perpendicular subcell

Note: s = sharp; b = broad, referring to the width of the reflection.

Source: Assimilated from Hou, S.Y. et al., *Adv. Lipid Res.*, 24, 141–171, 1991.

disappear; thus, they are attributed to the lipid part of the stratum corneum oriented perpendicular to the axis of the keratin fibers. Lipids in bilayers would have their hydorcarbon chains oriented perpendicular to the keratin. A halo present at 4.6 Å is attributed to protein along with the 9.8-Å band.

White et al.[50] obtained high-angle x-ray diffraction patterns (Table 1.6) of lipid extracts and intact stratum corneum at several temperatures and saw similar patterns in extracts and intact mouse stratum corneum; the patterns were consistent with both liquid and solidified alkyl chains present at 25 and 45°, while at 75° the chains are all in the liquid state. They report that at 25° the sharp lines appearing at 3.75 and 4.16 Å are crystalline alkyl chains characteristic of orthorhombic perpendicular subcells. By 45° these lines are replaced by a single line at 4.12 Å, which is expected of a gel state as alkyl chains ordered into hexagonal subcells. This band disappeared at 75° and was interpreted to be a gel-to-liquid crystalline transition. White's findings support coexistence of various macromolecular domains of the lipid.

Still, other authors[59–61] have used small-angle x-ray to study stratum corneum lipid domains and have reported the presence of two lamellar phases with periodicities of 13.4 and 6.4 nm, or same as 134 and 65 Å, as others found (above), and that may vary between species. The lateral lipid organization in stratum corneum has been studied by wide-angle x-ray diffraction as above by still others,[62–64] and spacings at 0.417 and 0.412/0.375 nm have been detected in humans by Garson[64] and Bouwstra et al.,[63] which they attributed to hexagonal (gel) and orthorhombic (crystalline) lipid lattices, respectively.

It seems that low- and high-angle x-ray diffraction can lead to somewhat different conclusions regarding the actual structure of the lamellar phases; the structures range from liquid crystal of the lamellar or hexagonal type to crystalline orthorhombic phases. It may depend on where in the stratum corneum structure one is looking. At lower levels in the stratum corneum, the structure may mirror the phospholipid-rich lamellar body secretions, while at the surface of the stratum corneum the sebum lipids may become intercalated into the membrane lipid and alter the structure. This is supported by recent studies investigating the role of ceramides in the phase behavior of stratum corneum. Deuterated NMR demonstrated that substitution of sphingomyelin for ceramide has dramatic effects on the physical properties of the model stratum corneum.[65,66] This result is of physiological significance, as ceramide in the stratum corneum is derived from the enzymatic cleavage of sphingomyelins at the lower levels and in lamellar granules. Further reports support this contention. Pilgram et al.[67] used the technique of cryoelectron diffraction to obtain local information about mixtures prepared from isolated pig ceramides, cholesterol, and long-chain fatty acids. It appeared that the addition of free fatty acids caused a transition from a hexagonal to an orthorhombic packing, and that electron diffraction can be applied to very nicely distinguish lattices. One comment is that no effort was make to study the fatty acid soap form of palmitic acid that would exist at a physiological pH of 4.5 of the stratum corneum. Of course, the pH will be closer to neutral at the lowest layers, near the living epidermis, and more acidic at the surface. Thus, as lipids are modified, such as by conversion of phospholipid to free fatty acids, as they approach the skin surface and prepare for desquamation, likely changes in the lipid domains may result. Bouwstra et al.[56] showed how incorporation of an azone completely altered the macromolecular structure of the lipid. So, the structure may be somewhat sensitive to the appearance of different lipid species during barrier development or artificially from exposure to substances on the outside. This technique can be used to track such regionally defined changes.

In fact, Pilgram et al.[68] have gone further and studied the relationship of lipid organization to depth in the stratum corneum using cryoelectron diffraction. Stratum corneum tape strips were prepared from native skin *in vivo* and *ex vivo*. They found that the lipid packing in samples prepared at room temperature is predominantly orthorhombic. In samples prepared at 32°C (the temperature of the outer layers of skin), the presence of a hexagonal packing is more pronounced in the outer layers of the stratum corneum. Gradually increasing the specimen temperature from 30 to 40°C (the inner temperature of skin is 37°C) induced a further transition from an orthorhombic to a hexagonal sublattice. At 90°C, all lipids were present in a fluid phase. These results are in good agreement with previously reported wide-angle x-ray diffraction and Fourier-transformed infrared spectroscopy studies. Thus, at the temperature of human skin, the hexagonal liquid crystal seems to predominate in the tape strip studies.

The research of Moore et al.[69,70] and Bouwstra et al.[71] examined artificial lipid combinations mirroring stratum corneum lipids. Both groups studied the role of certain ceramides in stratum corneum lipid organization. At least six to nine ceramides exist in the stratum corneum differing in either head group architecture or fatty acid chain length and degree of saturation. The fatty acid esterified to the sphingosine base can be either alpha-hydroxy or nonhydroxy acid. The chain length varies from C16 for ceramide 5 to C30 for ceramide 1. Furthermore, ceramide 1, assumed to be crucial for the characteristic organization of stratum corneum lipids, contains linoleic acid linked to the omega-hydroxy fatty acid. Linoleic acid is an essential fatty acid known to be crucial for normal barrier function, as shown in the condition of essential fatty deficiency discussed earlier. These structural lipids were reviewed previously (Wertz[25]).

To continue, Bouwstra et al.[71] studied the role of ceramide 1 and 2 further. They showed that to obtain the two lamellar phases reported for intact stratum corneum lipids at physiological amounts of cholesterol and ceramides, all of the ceramides together work much better. The complete ceramide mixture with lower amounts of cholesterol (ratio of 0.4 for cholesterol to ceramides) gave the two lamellar phases at x-ray periodicities of 5.6 and 12 nm. With cholesterol combinations with ceramide 1 and 2 alone, the ratio had to be greater than 1:1 cholesterol:ceramides 1 and 2. Solubility of the mixture of cholesterol with ceramides increased with ceramide 1 addition, suggesting its possible role. Incorporation of fatty acid (palmitic acid) in a physiological ratio of 1:1:1 cholesterol:ceramides 1 and 2:palmitic acid exhibited phase behavior less similar to that in intact stratum corneum than the cholesterol/ceramide 1 and 2 mixtures. An additional strong peak was found at 3.77 nm that was never seen before in stratum corneum and can be ascribed to the appearance of an additional phase. It is likely that the presence of only short-chain fatty acids like palmitic induces phase separation.

Moore et al.[70] used Fourier-transformed infrared (FTIR) spectroscopy to study the interactions of deuterated palmitic acid in the cholesterol/ceramide/palmitic acid model at pH 5.5 and hydrated. At physiologic temperatures, the CD2 scissoring mode of the palmitic acid and the rocking mode of the ceramide methylenes are each split into two components, suggesting that the components exist in separate conformationally ordered phases, probably orthorhombic perpendicular subcells. The magnitude of the splitting indicates that the domains are at least 100 chains in size. Overall, the FTIR observations suggest the following: Thermotropic studies at different temperatures show that from 10 to 40° a significant fraction of the palmitic acid in this model exists in a separate conformationally ordered orthorhombic phase of domain size greater than 100 chains, as stated above. This is consistent with the NMR studies of Kitson[65,66] showing, that 80% of the palmitic acid is in the solid phase at physiological temperatures. Between 40 and 50° the palmitic chains progressively disorder, but ceramide remains solid and there is significant phase separation; this is also consistent with the NMR studies above. Between 60 and 70° the ceramide disorders. The breadth of the phase transition suggests palmitic is mixing with cholesterol as it melts between 40 and 50°. Thus, the Fourier-transformed infrared scan shows a split in the CD2 peaks of the deuterated palmitic acid below 44°C. A similar split occurred for the CH2 methylene of ceramide. These findings suggest separate conformationally ordered phases or domains for the lipids. Thus, the most important result from this work is the detection of orthorhombic domains of palmitic acid and ceramide 3 at skin temperature. This was supported by the melt transition temperatures. The existence of more than a single lipid domain is thus supported by Moore's research. This work supports the fact that there may be distinct lipid domains in model stratum corneum, reinforcing the domain mosaic model of Forslind, discussed next.

A model proposed by Forslind called the domain mosaic model warrants some discussion.[72] It has been accepted that the lipids in the stratum are organized in some sort of multilayered structure. It has also been assumed that the lipids are at best randomly distributed in the bilayers. Forslind has hypothesized that this assumption is probably not the case as the lipids with very long chain fatty acids would tend to exist in the crystalline state. He feels that to satisfy all the functions of the stratum corneum, the lipids will have to be segregated into their own domains. Lipids with long-chain fatty acids segregate and exist in the gel or crystalline state, and this would provide the best barrier to water transport, but would also be a very rigid structure and would not address the mechanical requirements of the stratum corneum, i.e., flexibility. To provide this feature, lipids with shorter-chain fatty acids associate at the grain borders, where the lipid here is in the liquid crystalline state. These regions would allow some water to permeate the barrier and mix with the corneocytes to keep them pliable, as well as providing flexibility to the barrier, and allow hydrophobic substances to permeate into the barrier through this region. Some support for this model comes from the calorimetric data. The width of the transition peaks recorded by several authors can be related to the fact that the domains have a slightly different composition, which means that the calorimetric peak is actually a composite peak of overlapping transitions from different domains. Interestingly, the broad range of low-angle x-ray diffraction maxima have been interpreted to represent a whole range of repeat distances.[56] On the surface, the model seems very reasonable and accounts for the variety of functions the barrier must perform. The assumption of this model is that the lipids in the crystalline/gel state are completely resistant to water transport. If in fact this rigid domain cracks and produces holes whereby water has no barrier to transport from skin, this would present issues with the model and intact skin. Saturated fatty acid/soaps produce such a rigid structure, but their barrier to water transport is like that of pure water, i.e., they offer virtually no barrier to water transport because of the layer cracks. The future awaits further validation of the existence and function of the proposed lipid domains.

Moore et al. studied the role of ceramides 2 and 5 in the structure of the stratum corneum lipid[69]; ceramide 2 is a nonhydroxy sphingosine, and ceramide 5 is an alpha-hydroxy sphingosine. For ceramide 2 mixture with palmitic and cholesterol, a similar split in the CD2 and CH2 methylenes was found, supporting separate domains, and the different melt transition temperatures again support separate domains for ceramide 2 and palmitic acid. But for ceramide 5, the splitting of the stretches still exists, but palmitic and ceramide 5 phases collapse at 50°. These results support very different functions of ceramide 2 and ceramide 5 in the stratum corneum membrane, and this seems to be dictated by the different head groups. The results nonetheless support the domain mosaic model of Forslind for the stratum corneum lipid discussed above.

In Hou et al.'s review of stratum corneum lipid domains, he discusses another approach to determine the nature of the lipid domains in the stratum corneum — the use of electron paramagnetic resonance spectroscopy.[57] They used spin probes, and after their incorporation into the membrane or lipid, they examined their mobility. The probe, perdeuterated ditertbutyl nitroxide (pdDTBN) was selected because of its spherical shape and rapid isotropic motion. If the probe ends up in an anisotropic domain, it will be immobilized, but if it is incorporated into a fluid domain, the mobility can be tracked by spectroscopy. When the probe was placed in whole murine stratum corneum sheets, it was largely dissolved in isotropic domains with a thermal phase transition at 33°. This indicated that rapid isotropic motion of the probe is due to its presence in a fluid environment, as opposed to a crystalline environment. The probe's behavior in model lipids was very different. Thus, when working with model lipids, results from this and x-ray diffraction studies above must be considered with caution.

1.5.3 Summary Remarks about Lipid Macromolecular Structure

In conclusion for this section, there seems to be considerable evidence for the existence of polymorphism in the macromolecular structure of the stratum corneum lipid. Various authors have alluded to the origin and function or role of polymorphism in the stratum corneum. For example, Downing has suggested that it may be related to the assembly of stratum corneum lipid after extrusion and modification of the lipid. Other possible functions of polymorphic structures may relate to the maintenance of a certain amount of rigidity, and perhaps impenetrability, in the structure by the crystalline domains, yet maintaining some flexibility via the fluid domains to prevent skin cracking. Pilgrim has provided evidence that supports the existence of polymorphism that may originate from changes in the lipids at different layers of the epidermis and stratum corneum due to metabolic activity in the different layers. Studies combining individual components of the stratum corneum lipid seem to yield a variety of findings regarding the macromolecular structure of lipid, depending on the nature of the individual components used in the studies. Even a slight change in structure of the components used can alter the results and conclusions significantly. Transition temperatures that are in the region of skin temperature, which varies between 32° (outer skin layers) and 37° (inner skin layers), will also have a large effect on the macromolecular structure of the lipid *in situ*, as crystalline lipid will liquify above the transition temperature. Additionally, the actual components present will depend on the location in the stratum corneum, i.e., inner stratum corneum is enriched in phospholipids and glucoceramides vs. outer surface stratum corneum, which is enriched in free fatty acids and ceramides. The pH will also have a strong influence since at the layers closer to the living epidermis, the pH will be closer to neutral, as opposed to the acidic pH near the surface; this can alter the free fatty acids that are soaps near neutrality. There exists also a calcium gradient in the epidermis that could affect lipid structure, as discussed above. Even microorganisms on the skin surface, such as *P. acnes*, can alter the surface lipids, e.g., by converting triglycerides to free fatty acids. Other secretions of a specialized lipid form of sebaceous glands to the surface of skin may also affect the structure when they are present. Interpretations of actual structure and function of lipid domains will have to be considered with caution given the above influences, which can broadly change one's conclusions.

1.6 MANIPULATION OF LIPID STRUCTURE TO IMPROVE BARRIER FUNCTION

The final section of this chapter will review studies of the effects of moisturizing and barrier-enhancing ingredients on the Friberg model of the stratum corneum lipid. While this model may not incorporate all of the putative lipid domains suggested to be present, it does include both surface sebaceous lipid and epidermal lipid, along with 32% water, and is prepared at the acid pH of the skin surface; all of these parameters can affect lipid structure. It is felt that the Friberg model is a best estimate of the skin surface situation, and therefore a good tool to study effects of topical ingredients on lipid structure. We utilized differential scanning calorimetry to study the effects of the ingredients on lipid phase transitions and heats of fusion associated with the transitions (i.e., the enthalpy). We also studied the effect of low relative humidity conditions on the lipid transitions since low relative humidity has a dramatic effect on exacerbation of skin dryness and barrier damage.

Froebe et al.[73] prepared the model developed by Friberg (discussed earlier) and visually examined it using polarized light microscopy to assess changes at various relative humidity conditions.[74] Figure 1.9 shows the microscopic findings for the lipid samples maintained for up to 24 h at low relative humidity. First, the photographs show that at the initial mixing, the lipid exhibited reflectance properties of a liquid crystal under polarized light with intense color, birefringence, and presence of Maltese crosses at lower magnification (not shown). Over the 24-h period, the samples at low relative humidity tended to develop crystals, and thus changed to a crystalline state as they dehydrated. Therefore, removal of the water had quite a dramatic effect on the apparent macromolecular structure of the lipid, inducing crystallization of the lipid according to the microscopy. Crystallization of the lipid would seem at face value to be bad for the skin, as it would lead to breaks in the structure and would thus open up avenues for loss of water from the skin. We also tracked the glycerol effect on the model at low relative humidity conditions since such conditions typically lead to skin dryness and a damaged barrier. Glycerol is a well-established barrier enhancer/moisturizer/ humectant. We studied the effect of incorporating up to 15% glycerol in the model. The samples containing glycerol tended to remain longer in the apparent liquid crystalline state based on light reflectancy, even after 24 h at low relative humidity. Thus, glycerol seemed to prevent or slow down the transition of the model to solid crystals.

The author and colleagues studied this phenomenon in greater detail using differential scanning calorimetry (DSC) to assess phase transitions of the model at different temperatures at the various relative humidities and exposure times. They also tracked the water loss from the model during incubation at low relative humidity; moisture loss was measured gravimetrically.[74] DSC between 10 and 100°C revealed a broad endothermic transition between 30 and 70°C. This corresponds to the transition from a liquid crystalline phase observed by x-ray diffraction and microscopy at room temperature (discussed previously).[46,73] The transition maximum is centered around 52°C. This parallels the broad overlapping transition of intercellular lipids observed at 65°C for intact human and porcine stratum.[75–77] Upon dehydration over a 48-h period at 6% relative humidity (RH), DSC revealed a considerably sharper transition, shifted toward somewhat higher temperatures (60°C), suggesting an increase in cooperativity and a more ordered structure. This is consistent with the dehydration effect observed previously with phospholipids.[78] It is also consistent with the microscopic observations revealing the phase change to solid crystals in Figure 1.9 above. The effect was not as obvious at 92% RH because less dehydration is observed at this condition. Table 1.7 summarizes the corresponding enthalpy data for the transition from 52 to 60° in DSC of the model lipid and the model lipid containing cosmetic additives. It shows that enthalpy is greatest for the model lipid alone maintained at 6% RH for 48 h (52 J/g model

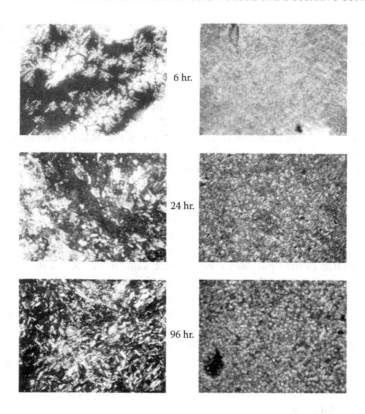

FIGURE 1.9 Photographs of model lipid systems exposed to low relative humidity (6%) conditions shown under light microscopy. The photograph shows the effect of lipid fluidizers on the structure. Note the appearance of crystals in the left figure without glycerol after incubation for 6 to 96 h at 6% relative humidity. When glycerol was present (right figure), there was a notable reduction in the extent of crystal formation during dehydration at low relative humidity. (Model lipid prepared with and without additives according to Froebe, C. et al., *J. Soc. Cosmet. Chem.*, 41, 51–65, 1990. With permission.)

lipid). This is consistent with the dehydration effect, leading to crystallization of the lipid; thus, it appears to take more heat to melt this phase. Table 1.8 shows the water loss from the model at each incubation time and relative humidity and verifies that the model lipid has lost most of its 32% water at 6% RH by 48 h. At 92% RH there was some dehydration and a slight increase in enthalpy to 24 J/g, model, but this is considered only a small change compared to the increase in enthalpy for the 6% RH sample at 48 h (52 J/g model).

Table 1.7 and Table 1.8 also show the effect of incorporation of cosmetic additives on the phase transition of the model. When glycerol was added to the model, it lowered the heat of fusion at all incubation times for both doses of glycerol, compared with the heat of fusion of the model without glycerol.

TABLE 1.7
Enthalpy Values for Model Lipid, Model Lipid + Glycerid Acid, and Model Lipid + Glycerol, Incubated for Different Times at 6 and 92% Relative Humidities

Incubation Time and Relative Humidity	Model Lipid Alone	Model Lipid + % Glycerid Acid			Model Lipid + % Glycerol	
		5%	10%	15%	5%	10%
0 h	15 ± 1	13	11	8	14	13
6 h at 6% RH	21 ± 1	15	15	12	17	20
24 h at 6% RH	43 ± 1	21	22	17	38	30
48 h at 6% RH	52 ± 1	35	28	23	45	35
6 h at 92% RH	20 ± 2	15	13	13	15	14
24 h at 92% RH	20 ± 1	17	15	15	—	15
48 h at 92% RH	24 ± 1	17	16	18	19	13

Enthalpy (J/g Lipid or J/g Lipid + Additive)

Source: Taken from Mattai, J. et al., *J. Soc. Cosmet. Chem.*, 44, 89–100, 1993. With permission.

TABLE 1.8
Percent Water Loss from Model Lipid, Model Lipid + Glycerid Acid, and Model Lipid + Glycerol, Incubated for Different Times at 6 and 92% Relative Humidities

Exposure Time and Relative Humidity	Model Lipid Alone %	Model Lipid + % Glycerid Acid			Model Lipid + % Glycerol	
		5%	10%	15%	5%	10%
0 h	—	—	—	—	—	—
6 h at 6% RH	18.2 ± 0.1	11.3	10.7	11.7	17.9	19.0
24 h at 6% RH	28.6 ± 0.5	25.8	19.9	20.8	29.0	27.8
48 h at 6% RH	29.5 ± 1.1	27.7	25.7	23.8	30.5	27.9
6 h at 92% RH	13.3 ± 0.5	6.3	6.0	6.1	8.9	1.3
24 h at 92% RH	21.6 ± 0.2	13.9	10.7	11.3	11.8	+1.8
48 h at 92% RH	24.9 ± 0.4	17.8	15.0	15.4	11.2	+1.5

% Water Loss

Source: Taken from Mattai, J. et al., *J. Soc. Cosmet. Chem.*, 44, 89–100, 1993. With permission.

For example, at the 48-h incubation time the enthalpy for the model alone at 6% RH was 52 J/g, and for the model with 10% glycerol it was 35 J/g. This was most apparent at the 6% RH conditions, but was even observed at 92% RH. Glycerol seemed to slow down the phase transition to solid crystals, consistent with the microscopy observations. Thus, glycerol seems to maintain fluidity of the lipid, and this provides an alternate reasonable mechanism for its well-known conditioning and moisturizing effects on skin. Interestingly, glycerol did not have an appreciable effect on the dehydration rate of the model at low relative humidity conditions. For example, the model with glycerol at 6% RH lost most of its water by the 48-h incubation time. Thus, glycerol is not very effective at slowing down moisture loss from the skin at low relative humidity, but in spite of this, it is a good dry skin treatment active. This is mostly due to glycerol's efficacy at fluidizing stratum corneum lipid, which leads to the beneficial effects on skin.

Another cosmetic additive was also studied — glycerid acid, a large bulky hydrophobic derivative of glycerol. This additive also delayed the appearance of crystals in the model lipid, as shown in Figure 1.9. Table 1.7 showed that the enthalpy of the transition was lower than the model lipid alone at all incubation times and relative humidities, and that this additive outperformed glycerol in reducing the heat of fusion of the model for all measurements. Additionally, Table 1.8 shows that glycerid acid was quite effective at reducing the water loss from the model at all conditions of relative humidity at the 10 and 15% doses. This additive seems to provide two functions that enhance skin condition: fluidization of the stratum corneum lipid and delay of water loss from the membrane. This additive was tested for its ability to prevent soap-induced dryness in human clinical trials (using the method of Highley et al.[79]) and was found to be more effective than glycerol (Rhein and Simion, unpublished data), supporting the dual mechanism proposed herein for glycerid acid-enhanced fluidization of the lipid and reduction in water loss from the lipid membrane.

1.6.1 SUMMARY REMARKS ABOUT THE ROLE OF LIPID FLUIDIZATION IN STRATUM CORNEUM FUNCTION

Thus, fluidization maintains the liquid crystalline structure, and this seems to be consistent with improvement of dry skin condition, since glycerol is amazingly good at improving dry skin and is perhaps the major ingredient used in formulations for this purpose. Fluidization is achieved by molecules that impart disorder to the membrane lipid chains, and glycerid acid, being such a large bulky hydrophobic molecule, would seem likely to impart such disorder when intercalated between the membrane lipid chains (see, for example, Figure 1.5 and Figure 1.7). Glycerol, on the other hand, would mostly intercalate between the polar head groups of the bilayer, in addition to its incorporation into the water layer. Intercalation between the head groups would most likely impart disorder to the membrane by perhaps interfering with the hydrogen bonding between the head groups and increasing water of hydration within the polar head groups. Golden et al.[78] has studied the disordering effect of penetration enhancers resulting in enhanced transdermal drug flux of salicylic acid into stratum corneum sheets. He examined a number of 18-carbon-chain-length fatty acids with varying degrees and types of unsaturation and found that the cis isomer (both the 9 and 11 isomers) was most effective at disordering the chains, resulting in lowering the thermal transition temperature of the lipid part. Trans fatty acids were somewhat effective, and saturated fatty acids were not effective. Using IR techniques, the IR antisymmetric stretch near 2920 cm^{-1} was also increased for the cis fatty acid, consistent with enhanced mobility of the hydrocarbon chains due to increased fluidity and disorder. The greater disorder also enhanced salicylic acid penetration. Thus, it seems that molecules that interfere with the tight structure of the native chains impart disorder and fluidity to the membrane.

It is felt that fluidity of the lipid is perhaps a double-edge sword, and that it is a matter of balancing the fluidity with the tight structure, as discussed previously. If the structure is too tightly packed, such as if the intercellular lipid is entirely in an orthorhombic structure, or as may happen if the lipids are too saturated, such as in essential fatty deficiency, cracks may occur in the structure and the barrier to water penetration becomes highly impaired and leaky. However, if the lipid is too fluid, water penetration is also enhanced and the skin is more vulnerable to penetration of foreign substances.[78] Pilgrim (thesis dissertation) has shown that in atopic skin the lipid at the skin surface is more fluid, i.e., contains more of the fluid phases vs. normal skin. Additionally, during barrier development the skin goes to a lot of trouble ridding itself of phospholipids, which would enhance the fluidity of the lipid, and in fact, authors have shown that in the lower layers of (living) epidermis the membrane is more fluid, likely due to the phospholipid enrichment there.[80] Also, in certain diseases such as X-linked ichthyosis, the accumulation of cholesterol sulfate leads to a more fluid membrane, as shown by Rehfeld et al.[84] In palmoplantar keratoderma (a scaly skin disorder), the free fatty acids exhibit a preponderance of short-chain monoenoic fatty acids, which would create a more fluid environment.[82] On the other hand, in lamellar ichthyosis, there is a shortage of free fatty acids and an accumulation of cholesterol in a crystalline form.[83] When the skin drys out, resulting in xerosis in low relative humidity conditions, the membrane structure crystallizes and is less fluid, as shown in the above model lipid studies. Clearly this impairs the barrier and has led to a plethora of products on the market, many of which contain glycerol to soften and moisten the dry, cracked skin. So it appears that it is the balance of fluidity and crystallinity or tightness that is important for healthy skin.

Several authors have applied stratum corneum lipid structures to enhance the barrier recovery after damage with surfactant, tape stripping, or acetone/ether treatment. Elias and colleagues[85,86] found that application of native stratum corneum lipids (glycosphingolipids, cholesterol, or saturated or unsaturated fatty acids or cholesterol palmitate) *individually* to acetone-damaged hairless mouse skin actually delayed barrier recovery, compared to vehicle alone (vehicle was propylene glycol and ethanol, 7:3). Even two-component mixtures of the lipid classes delayed barrier recovery. Only the three-component mixture of bovine ceramide/linoleic acid/cholesterol in equimolar amounts accelerated barrier recovery. Data also show that the lamellar body contents are abnormal, with numerous droplets, as opposed to lamellar sheets in the individual lipid treatments. Elias and colleagues went on to test the natural lipid mixtures in human skin — either tape stripped or acetone extracted — and in hairless mouse skin.[85,86] They tested a natural lipid mixture alone (3:1:1 fatty acids/ceramide mix/cholesterol) and a natural lipid mixture in about 20% phospholipid. The natural lipid with 20% phospholipid was significantly better than the vehicle at enhancing barrier recovery. The cholesterol alone decreased skin moisturization, assessed by a decrease in capacitance, while ceramides and palmitate increased capacitance. However, the natural lipid was more effective, and the natural lipid in 20% phospholipid was significantly better than any other sample tested, supporting the idea that the complete lipid mixture with the phospholipid is the best at fluidizing the lipid and enhancing barrier recovery. The phospholipid, while not a natural component of stratum corneum lipid, likely imparts some fluidity to the barrier lipid, and the other natural lipid provided the more rigid part of a layered structure to the deranged parts of the abrogated barrier.

However, the natural lipid mixture does not appear to promote faster barrier recovery from all insults. For example, barrier damaged by sodium lauryl sulfate (SLS) does not appear to recover faster than no treatment with the natural lipid, while barrier damaged by dodecyl benzene sulfonate or lauryl sarcosinate recovers faster with natural lipid treatment.[86] It is possible that the damage by SLS alternatively affects the keratin protein rather than impairing the lipid part of the stratum corneum; therefore, application of natural lipid will not accelerate repair in all instances. It depends on the nature of the damage.

We can conclude that this model is useful to the cosmetic chemist in identifying additives and formulations that fluidize skin lipids, leading to softening and conditioning of the skin. We conclude overall that sufficient fluidity must exist in the macromolecular lipid structure to keep the skin soft and supple. While polymorphism may exist in the stratum corneum lipid structure, an entirely rigid structure such as in orthorhombic phases will probably be too rigid, leading to cracking or openings in the (leaky) membrane and unprotected water loss. In the long run there needs to be a balance between these parameters — rigidity and fluidity. The polymorphism resulting in separate lipid domains in the structure may enable that balance.

REFERENCES

1. Odland GF. Structure of the skin. In *Physiology, Biochemistry and Molecular Biology of the Skin*, 2nd ed., Goldsmith LA (Ed.). Oxford University Press, Oxford, 1991.
2. Bennett JC, Plum F (Eds.). *Cecil Textbook of Medicine*, 20th ed. W.B. Saunders Company, Philadelphia, 1996.
3. Montagne W, Kligman AM, Carlisle KS. *Atlas of Normal Human Skin*. Springer-Verlag, New York, 1992.

4. Nelson W, Sun TT. The 50- and 58-kilodalton keratin classes as molecular markers for stratified squamous epithelia: cell culture studies. *J Cell Biol* 97, 244–251, 1983.

5. Eichner R, Bonitz P, Sun TT. Classification of epidermal keratins according to their immunoreactivity, isoelectric point and mode of expression. *J Cell Biol* 98, 1388–1396, 1998.

6. Fuchs E, Green H. Changes in keratin gene expression during terminal differentiation of the keratinocyte. *Cell* 19, 1033–1042, 1980.

7. Hitomi K. Transglutamases in skin epidermis. *Eur J Dermatol* 15, 313–319, 2005.

8. Dale B, Reising K. Proteins of keratohyalin. In *Biochemistry and Molecular Biology of the Skin*, Goldsmith LA (Ed.). Oxford University Press, New York, 1991, chap. 4.

9. Rawlings AV, Scott IR, Harding CR, et al. Stratum corneum moisturization at the molecular level. *J Invest Dermatol* 103, 731–740, 1994.

10. Schaefer HS (Ed.). *Skin Barrier: Principles of Percutaneous Absorption*, 1st ed. Karger AG, Basel, 1996.

11. Uitto J, Oikarinen A, Thody AJ. Mechanical and physical functions of the skin. In *Scientific Basis of Dermatology. A Physiological Approach*, Thody AJ, Friedman PS (Eds.). Churchill Livingstone, London, 1986.

12. Komuves LG, Hanley K, Lefebvre AM, Man MQ, Ng DC, Bikle DD, Williams ML, Elias PM, Auwerx J, Feingold KR. Stimulation of PPARalpha promotes epidermal keratinocyte differentiation *in vivo*. *J Invest Dermatol* 115, 353–360, 2000.

13. Friedmann PS, Cooper HL, Healy E. Peroxisome proliferator-activated receptors and their relevance to dermatology. *Acta Dermatol Venereol* 85, 194–202, 2005.

14. Kuenzli S, Saurat JH. Peroxisome proliferator-activated receptors in cutaneous biology. *Br J Dermatol* 149, 229–236, 2003.

15. Elias PM, Ahn SK, Denda M, Brown BE, Crumrine D, Kimutai LK, Komuves L, Lee SH, Feingold KR. Modulations in epidermal calcium regulate the expression of differentiation-specific markers. *J Invest Dermatol* 119, 1128–1136, 2002.

16. Bikle DD, Oda, Y, Xie Z. Calcium and 1,25(OH)2D: interacting drivers of epidermal differentiation. *J Steroid Biochem Mol Biol* 89/90, 355–360, 2004.

17. Zouboulis C. Retinoids: which dermatological indications will benefit in the near future? *Skin Pharmacol Appl Skin Physiol* 14, 303–315, 2001.

18. Lefebvre P, Martin PJ, Flajollet S, Dedieu S, Billaut X, Lefebvre B. Transcriptional activities of retinoic acid receptors. *Vitam Horm* 70, 199–264, 2005.

19. Kang S.The mechanism of action of topical retinoids. *Cutis* 75 (2 Suppl), 10–13, 2005.

20. Kligman A. Current status of topical tretinoin in the treatment of photoaged skin. *Drugs Aging* 2, 7–13, 1992.

21. Chivot M. Retinoid therapy for acne. A comparative review. *Am J Clin Dermatol* 6, 13–19, 2005.

22. Bikowski J. Mechanisms of the comedolytic and anti-inflammatory properties of topical retinoids. *J Drugs Dermatol* 4, 41–47, 2005.

23. Hönigsmann H, Thody AJ. Protection against ultraviolet radiation. In *Scientific Basis of Dermatology. A Physiological Approach*, Thody AJ, Friedman PS (Eds.). Churchill Livingstone, London, 1986.

24. Abraham W. Surfactant effects on skin barrier. In *Surfactants in Cosmetics*, Rieger M, Rhein L (Eds.). Marcel Dekker, New York, 1997, chap. 20.

25. Wertz P. Epidermal lipids. *Semin Dermatol* 11, 106–113, 1992.
26. Wertz PW, Downing ST. Ceramides of pig epidermis: structure determination. *J Lipid Res* 24, 759–765, 1983.
27. Greene SC, Stuart ME, Downing DT. Anatomical variation in the amount and composition of human skin surface lipids. *J Invest Dermatol* 54, 240–247, 1970.
28. Downing D. Variability on the chemical composition of human skin surface lipid. *J Invest Dermatol* 53, 322–327, 1969.
29. Nicolaidesa D, Wells A. On the biogenesis of free fatty acids in skin surface fat. *J Invest Dermatol* 29, 423–433, 1957.
30. Shalita A. Genesis of free fatty acids. *J Invest Dermatol* 62, 332–335, 1974.
31. Elias PM. Epidermal lipids, barrier function and desquamation. *J Invest Dermatol* 80, 44s–49s, 1983.
32. Werz P, Swartzendruber DS, Madison KD, Downing D. Composition and morphology of epidermal cyst lipids. *J Invest Dermatol* 89, 419–425, 1987.
33. Elias PM, Feingold K. Lipid related barrier and gradients in the epidermis. *Ann NY Acad Sci* 548, 4–13, 1988.
34. Michaels AS, Chandrasekaran SK, Shaw JE, Drug permeation through human skin: Theory and invitro experimental measurement. *J Am Inst Chem Eng* 21, 985–996, 1975.
35. Harris IR, Farrell AM, Holleran WM, Jackson S, Grunfield C, Elias PM, Feingold KR. Parallel regulation of sterol regulatory element binding protein-2 and the enzymes of cholesterol and fatty acid synthesis but not ceramide synthesis in cultured human keratinocytes and murine epidermis. *J Lipid Res* 39, 412–422, 1998.
36. Melton JL, Werz PW, Swartzendruber DC, and Downing D. Effects of essential fatty acid deficiency on epidermal o-acylsphingolipids and TEWL in young pigs. *Biochim Biophys Acta* 921, 191–197, 1987.
37. Nicollier M, Massengo T, Remy-Martin JP, Laurent R, Adessi GL. Free fatty acids and fatty acids of triacylglycerols in normal and hyperkeratotic human stratum corneum. *J Invest Dermatol* 87, 68–71, 1986.
38. Werz P, Swartzendruber DS, Madison KD, Downing D. Composition and morphology of epidermal cyst lipids. *J Invest Dermatol* 89, 419–425, 1987.
39. Harris IR, Farrell AM, Grunfield C, Holleran WM, Elias P, Feingold KR. Permeability barrier disruption coordinately regulates mRNA levels for key enzymes of cholesterol, fatty acid, and ceramide synthesis in the epidermis. *J Invest Dermatol* 109, 783–787, 1997.
40. Tanno O, Ota Y, Kitamura N, Katsube T, Inoue S. Nicotinamide increases biosynthesis of ceramides as well as other stratum corneum lipids to improve the epidermal permeability barrier. *Dermatology* 143: 524–531, 2000.
41. Smith WP, Christensen MS, Nacht S, Gans EH. Effect of lipids on the aggregation and permeability of human stratum corneum. *J Invest Dermatol* 78, 7–11, 1982.
42. Brysk MM, Rajaraman I, Penn P, Barlowe E. Cohesive properties of terminally differentiated keratinocytes. *Exp Cell Biol* 57, 60–66, 1989.
43. Imokawa G, Akaski S, Hattori M, Yoshizuka N. Selective recovery of deranged water-holding properties by stratum corneum lipids. *J Invest Dermatol* 87, 758–761, 1986.
44. Grubauer G, Feingold KR, Harris RM, Elias PM. Lipid content and lipid type as determinants of the epidermal permeability barrier. *J Lipid Res* 30, 89–96, 1989.
45. Imokawa G, Akasaki S, Kawamata A, Yano S, Takaishi N. Water retaining function in the stratum corneum and its recovery properties by synthetic ceramides. *J Soc Cosmet Chem* 40, 273–285, 1989.

46. Friberg SE, Osborne DW. Small angle x-ray diffraction patterns of stratum corneum and a model structure for its lipid. *J Dispersion Sci Technol* 6, 485–495, 1985.

47. Friberg SE, Suhaimi H, Goldsmith LB, Rhein LD. Stratum corneum lipids in a model structure. *J Dispersion Sci Technol* 9, 371–389, 1988.

48. Osborne DW, Friberg SE. Role of stratum corneum lipids as a moisture retaining agent. *J Dispersion Sci Technol* 7, 753–765, 1987.

49. Friberg SE, Kayali I, Rhein L, Hill R. A model for stratum corneum lipids and some implications. *Cosmet Toiletries* 102, 135–140, 1987.

50. White SH, Mirejovsky D, King GI. Structure of lamellar lipid domains and corneocyte envelopes of murine stratum corneum. An x-ray diffraction study. *Biochemistry* 27, 3725–3732, 1988.

51. Imokawa G, Hattori M. A possible function of structural lipids in the water-retaining properties of the stratum corneum. *J Invest Dermatol* 84, 282–284, 1985.

52. Kayali I, Suhery T, Friberg SE, Simion FA, Rhein LD. Lyotropic liquid crystals and the structural lipids of the stratum corneum. *J Pharm Sci* 80, 428–431, 1991.

53. Friberg SE, Kayali I, Beckerman W, Rhein LD, Simion FA. Water permeation of reaggregated stratum corneum with model lipid. *J Invest Dermatol* 94, 377–380, 1990.

54. Friberg SE, Kayali I. Water evaporation rates from model stratum corneum lipids. *J Pharm Sci* 78, 639–643, 1989.

55. Abraham W, Downing DT. Deuterium NMR investigation of polymorphism in stratum corneum lipids. *Biochim Biophys Acta* 1068, 189–194, 1991.

56. Bouwstra JA, DeVries MA, Gooris GS, Bras W, Brusse J, Ponec M. Thermodynamic and structural aspects of skin barrier. *J Controlled Release* 15, 209–220, 1991.

57. Hou SY, Rehfeld SJ, Plachy WZ. X-ray diffraction and paramagnetic resonance spectroscopy of mammalian stratum corneum lipid domains. *Adv Lipid Res* 24, 141–171, 1991.

58. Bouwstra J, Pilgram G, Gooris G, Koerten H, Ponec M. New aspects of the skin barrier organization. *Skin Pharmacol Appl Skin Physiol* 14 (Suppl 1), 52–62, 2001.

59. Bouwstra JA, Gooris GS, Bras W, Downing DT. Lipid organization in pig stratum corneum. *J Lipid Res* 36, 685–695, 1995.

60. Bouwstra JA, Gooris GS, van der Spek JA, Bras W. Structural investigations of human stratum corneum by small angle x-ray scattering. *J Invest Dermatol* 97, 1005–1013, 1991.

61. Bouwstra JA, Gooris GS, van der Spek JA, Lavrijsen S, Bras W. The lipid and protein structure of mouse stratum corneum: a wide and small angle diffraction study. *Biochim Biophys Acta* 1212, 183–192, 1994.

62. Pilgram SK, van Pelt AM, Spies JA, Bouwstra JA, Koerten HK. Cryoelectron diffraction as a tool to study local variations in the lipid organization of human stratum corneum. *J Microsc* 189, 71–78, 1998.

63. Bouwstra JA, Gooris GS, Salomons - de Vries MA, van der Spek JA, Bras W. Structure of Human stratum corneum as a function of temperature and hydration: a wide angle x-ray diffraction study. *Int J Pharm* 84, 205–216, 1992.

64. Garson J, Doucet J, Leveque J, Tsoucaris G. Oriented structure in human stratum corneum revealed by x-ray diffraction. *J Invest Dermatol* 96, 43–50, 1991.

65. Thewalt J, Kitson N, Araujo C, MacKay A, Bloom M. Models of stratum corneum intercellular membranes: the sphingolipid headgroups as the determiner of phase behavior in mixed lipid dispersions. *Biochem Biophys Res Commun* 188, 1247–1252, 1992.

66. Kitson N, Thewalt J, Lafteur M, Bloom M. A model membrane approach to the epithelial permeability barrier. *Biochemistry* 33, 6707–6715, 1994.

67. Pilgram GSK, Engelsma AM, Oostergetel GT, Koerten HK, Bouwstra JA. Study of the lipid organization of stratum corneum lipid models by cryoelectron diffraction. *J Lipid Res* 39, 1669–1676, 1998.

68. Pilgram GS, Engelsma-van Pelt AM, Bouwstra JA, Koerten HK. Electron diffraction provides new information on human stratum corneum lipid organization studied in relation to depth and temperature. *J Invest Dermatol* 113, 403–409, 1999.

69. Moore DJ, Rerek ME, Mendelsohn R. Role of ceramide 2 and 5 in the structure of the stratum corneum lipid barrier. *Int J Cosmet Sci* 21, 353–368, 1999.

70. Moore DJ, Rerek ME, Mendelsohn R. Lipid domains and orthorhombic phases in model stratum: evidence from Fourier transform infrared spectroscopy studies. *Biochem Biophys Res Commun* 231, 797–801, 1997.

71. Bouwstra JA, Cheng K, Gooris GS, Weerheim A, Ponec M. The role of ceramides 1 and 2 in the stratum corneum lipid organization. *Biochim Biophys Acta* 1300, 177–186, 1996.

72. Forslind B. A domain mosaic model of the skin barrier. *Acta Dermatol Venereol* 74, 1–6, 1994.

73. Froebe C, Simion FA, Ohlmeyer H, Rhein LD, Mattai J, Cagan RH, Friberg S. Prevention of stratum corneum lipid phase transitions *in-vitro* by glycerol: an alternate mechanism for skin moisturization. *J Soc Cosmet Chem* 41, 51–65, 1990.

74. Mattai J, Froebe CL, Rhein LD, Simion FA, Ohlmeyer H, Su D. Prevention of model stratum corneum lipid phase transitions *in vitro* by cosmetic additives: differential scanning calorimetry, optical microscopy, and water evaporation studies. *J Soc Cosmet Chem* 44, 89–100, 1993.

75. Van Duzee BF. Thermal analysis of human stratum corneum. *J Invest Dermatol* 65, 404–408, 1975.

76. Golden GM, Guzek DB, Harris RR, McKie JE, Potts RO. Lipid thermotropic transitions in human stratum corneum. *J Invest Dermatol* 86, 255–259, 1986.

77. Golden GM, Guzek DB, Kennedy AH, McKie JE, Potts RO. Stratum corneum lipid phase transitions and water barrier properties. *Biochemistry* 26, 2382–2388, 1987.

78. Golden GM, McKie JE, Potts RO. Role of stratum corneum lipid fluidity in transdermal drug flux. *J Pharm Sci* 76, 25–28, 1987.

79. Highley DR, Savoyka VO, O'Neill JJ, Ward JB. A stereomicroscopic method for the determination of moisturizing efficacy in humans. *J Soc Cosmet Chem* 27, 351–363, 1976.

80. Potts RO, Francoeur ML. Lipid biophysics of water loss through the skin. *Proc Natl Acad Sci USA* 87, 3871–3873, 1990.

81. Tanaka T, Sakanashi T, Kaneko N, Ogura R. Spin labeling study on membrane fluidity of epidermal cell (cow snout epidermis). *J Invest Dermatol* 87, 745–747, 1986.

82. Nicollier M, Massengo T, Martin J, Laurent R, Adessi G. Free fatty acids and fatty acids of triacylglycerols in normal and hyperkeratotic human stratum corneum. *J Invest Dermatol* 87, 68–71, 1986.

83. Lavrijsen AP, Bouwstra JA, Gooris GS, Weerheim A, Boddie HE, Ponec M. Reduced skin barrier function parallels abnormal stratum corneum lipid organization in patients with lamellar ichthyosis. *J Invest Dermatol* 105, 619–624, 1995.

84. Rehfeld SJ, Plachy WZ, Williams ML, Elias P. Calorimetric and electron spin resonance examination of lipid phase transitions in human stratum corneum: molecular basis for normal cohesion and abnormal desquamation in recessive X-linked ichthyosis, *J Invest Dermatol* 91, 499–505, 1988.
85. Mao-Quing M, Brown BE, Wu-Pong S, Feingold K, Elias PM. Exogenous nonphysiologic vs. physiologic lipids. *Arch Dermatol* 131, 809–816, 1995.
86. Yang L, Mao-Kang M, Taljebini M, Elias P, Feingold KR. Topical stratum corneum lipids accelerate barrier repair after tape stripping, solvent treatment, and some but not all types of detergent treatments. *Br J Dermatol* 133, 679–685, 1995.

2 Color Measurement Techniques

Nicholas Morante
Nick Morante Consultants

Makeup and color cosmetics are a unique staple in our society. They are products that, when applied, can make a person look better and, as a result, feel better about herself. In fact, if applied correctly, they can make a person feel very good about herself. There would be an outward glow on her face and her smile would be large, shiny, and bright. Color cosmetics have been a cornerstone of civilization for well over 1000 years. Yes, we are in the beauty business, the business of making women — and men for that matter — feel better about themselves. I say men because what actor does not go on stage without makeup? And that makeup better be applied correctly to make that actor look good under all those lights.

We are literally surrounded by color. Color influences our daily lives. The color of a person's skin can often be a health indicator. Color influences our choice of purchasing goods such as cars, clothes, food, and our favorite — cosmetics. We cannot get away from color. Many people are faithful to their favorite colors. It is really an emotional thing.

But as formulators and manufacturers, how can we guarantee that the shades we make for people are the same all the time? Our regular, brand-faithful customers are expecting to purchase the same exact shade of lipstick, makeup, or cheek blush every single time they go to a cosmetics counter — anywhere in the world. After all, if the shade is not the same, the customer may feel that the shade looks different, and possibly she will not look as good and, as a result, may not feel as good. That is our challenge every time we make a batch of product.

So what can we do, aside from the time-tested method of visual color matching, that will allow us to move into the age of higher technology? What happens when we try to make that same popular shade in production on a rainy day with poor sunlight, or on the night shift with no sunlight at all? We all must agree that the trained color eye is, and will always be, the final judge of color acceptability. Light boxes are good, but they are not that portable. However, there are some other methods that the formulator and production compounder can use to help him ensure that the shades he is making will be consistent color-wise batch after batch.

This chapter discusses such methods, and along the way, we will learn some basic principles of color.

The first thing one must do is to understand what color really is. Essentially, color is light — specifically visible light. Visible light occupies only a small range of wavelengths in the electromagnetic spectrum. This wavelength (λ) is measured in nanometers (nm). This spectrum includes x-rays, radio, television, ultraviolet, visible light, and infrared (or heat) radiation. Visible light has a wavelength range of 380 to 720 nm. For color measurement, we restrict this range from 400 to 700 nm. Radio and TV waves are useless unless we have receivers or receptors to pick up these waves. Our eyes are excellent receptors to pick up and evaluate the sensation of visible light as color. After all, sight is one of the five senses.

Color can be described in a number of ways. First, there is hue. Hue is the basic definition or description of a color — red, blue, green, yellow, etc. Chroma is the attribute of visual perception dealing with the intensity or saturation of a particular color or hue. Then we have lightness and darkness. Lightness deals with the amount of white there is in an observed object. Conversely, darkness deals with the amount of black in that object. A tomato has a red hue and is high in chroma. A pale pink flower is low in chroma, but both the flower and the tomato can have the same hue. The white in a red flower makes it look pink. Black and white have no chroma or hue. Spectral curves for white, black, and gray appear in Figure 2.1.

White is all color that is reflected. However, the amount of light that the white materials we know of can reflect is a maximum of approximately 75 to 85%. No white material really reflects 100% of the light that hits it. Black is all color that is absorbed. In fact, it absorbs most, but not all, of the light that hits it. Black does not absorb 100% of the light that hits it. Black can reflect light at 4% to 5%, but the lower that reflectance, the blacker it will look. That is why we look for that lowest reflectance in a black when we are formulating a mascara. The more light that is reflected off an observed object, the lighter it will appear. The more light that is absorbed by an observed object, the darker it will appear. Color cannot be seen in the dark. Light must be reflected off an object in order for its color to be seen. That is why it is not a good idea to get dressed in the dark.

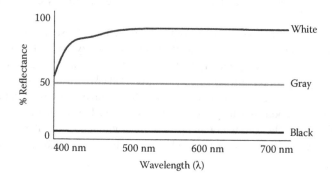

FIGURE 2.1

Materials that absorb most of the wavelengths of light below 400 nm (in the ultraviolet region 300 to 380 nm) make good sunscreens. The white curve shown in Figure 2.1 represents titanium dioxide, which starts to absorb light at low (blue) wavelengths and into the ultraviolet region. Hence, it is used as a sunscreen. Microfine varieties of titanium dioxide offer sunscreen protection factor (SPF) protection with minimal whitening or opacity.

Going back to our eyes being good receptors to see and evaluate color, our eyes contain three types of cones, each responsible for evaluating the visual stimuli for red, green, and blue, or R G B. The ability to visually evaluate the sensations of color varies from person to person, man to woman, young to old. Ninety-six percent of the population has normal color vision, while 4% has some form of abnormal color vision. This abnormality could involve one or more of the cones responsible for evaluating the R G B sensations — hence the term *color blindness*.

We technically can define color as the percent of visible light at specific wavelengths that is reflected back to our eyes. Short wavelengths are recognized as blue. As the wavelengths get longer, the sensations become green, then yellow, orange, and red. The total of all these color sensations is what we know as the visible light spectrum. It is evident when we view a rainbow in the sky, look at the colors on the surface of an oil slick, or look at the light transmitted through a prism. When white light passes through a prism, it is divided into single wavelengths. In the prism, the blue light is refracted more than the red light because the refractive index of the glass is a function of the wavelength. A blue object reflects blue light and absorbs all other wavelengths so we only see the blue color. Figure 2.2 represents the maximum reflectance of individual color at their visible wavelengths.

Spectral curves allow us to see a color numerically in terms of its wavelength and percent reflection. Knowing the percent reflectance at a given wavelength, any color can be identified.

Since reflection is the most important factor in observing light and color, one interesting effect can be shown by what is called retroreflection. Retroreflection is a pigment effect used mainly on street and highway signs where almost all the light is reflected back in the direction of illumination.

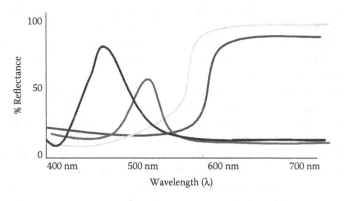

FIGURE 2.2

In combining colors, we know that certain primary colors, when mixed, yield secondary colors. This can be explained best by the terms *additive* and *subtractive mixtures*. Additive color mixtures are those that can be described as a superposition or other nondestructive combination of different colors. Subtractive color mixtures are absorbing color media or superposition of filters so that the spectral composition of light passing through the combination absorbs specific wavelengths and eliminates them from what we actually see.

Light scattering is caused by the optical properties and refractive index of a material or substrate. Materials such as skin and makeup can reflect, absorb, and scatter light differently and can affect color appearance. When light hits the skin, some is reflected back to our eyes, some is absorbed, and some is scattered and reflected back at a different angle from which it entered. Under certain lighting conditions, this will affect color and appearance. To evaluate color properly, so that all eyes see the same color under the same conditions, a standard light source must be used. This light source has been designated Northern Daylight, or D65. This designation is assigned to light that has a relative correlated color temperature of 6500K. The daylight wavelength range is 300 to 830 nm (the ultraviolet range 300 to 380 nm is necessary to characterize fluorescent colorants). There are other daylight sources: D50 (5000K) and D75 (7500K). Light source A is incandescent, a yellow-orange light with a wavelength range of 380 to 770 nm. Its color temperature is 2856K. Fluorescent lighting, or C, comes in various types and has a relative color temperature of 6774K, close to daylight temperature.

Color can look different depending on the light source used to evaluate the color. The same shade of makeup will look different on different skin under the same light. A makeup shade will look great on skin in a store under controlled fluorescent lighting but may look awful when you go outside in the sunlight or under incandescent lighting. When two shades match under various lighting conditions but have different color information or data, this is called metamerism. This phenomenon can best be demonstrated in lipsticks. Two shades can be made to match under various lighting conditions using totally different sets and quantities of colorants. The need to standardize a light source solves many problems when making visual color assessments.

Over the years, there have been a number of people who have set up systems for the easy evaluation of color difference. One of the first was A.H. Munsell, an American artist who in 1905 devised the Munsell Color System. He published an atlas where he had many different colored paper chips evenly spaced apart, and the difference between two colors could be determined from the book. This system is still in use today.

Later on, a group in Europe, the Commission Internationale de l'Eclairage (CIE), came up with another method of evaluating color. It has been developing methods for expressing color numerically since 1931. The CIE is now an internationally recognized standards organization dealing with light and color. In 1976, a three-dimensional plot known as the L a b color space was devised and adopted by CIE (Figure 2.3). This plot allows an observer to see where a particular color sits in color space when viewed under a standard light source. It is also called the CIELab coordinate system, and the three-color axes can be described as follows:

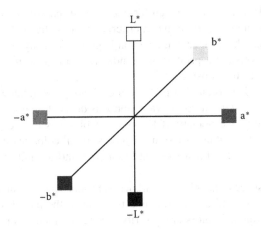

FIGURE 2.3

L* axis — lightness/darkness [+ L is whiter; –L is blacker]
a* axis — red/green [+ a is redder; –a is greener]
b* axis — yellow/blue [+ b is yellower; –b is bluer]

In all the systems of color evaluation in use today, color difference is represented by Delta E, ΔE, or DE. DE is a measure of the overall color difference between samples and is expressed as the square root of the sum of the squares of each color difference value. In CIELab color space, color difference can be expressed by the following equation. DE will have no units of measure.

$$DE = \sqrt{(dL^*)^2 + (da^*)^2 + (db^*)^2}$$

Shades A and B are makeup shades with medium color depth. Knowing the individual L, a, and b values, we can express their color difference numerically:

Calculating DE

	Shade A	Shade B
L* value	71.49	70.14
a* value	9.17	10.21
b* value	16.25	14.87
dL*	1.35	Lighter
da*	–1.04	Less Red (Greener)
db*	1.38	Yellower (Less Blue)

$$DE = \sqrt{(1.35)^2 + (-1.04)^2 + (1.38)^2}$$

$$DE = \sqrt{1.82 + 1.08 + 1.90}$$

$$DE = \sqrt{4.80}$$

$$DE = 2.19$$

A DE of 2.19 is not a bad match for makeup. DE pass/fail tolerances should be set up depending on specific match criteria. Historically, a DE of 1.00 represents the point at which the average person begins to visually see a color difference. The automotive and printing inks industries are much more critical with pass/fail tolerances than cosmetics.

Additionally, there is another method of evaluating color, known as the CMC color space. This system of color evaluation was devised by the Color Measurement Committee of the Society of Dyers and Colourists in Great Britain. This group was also responsible for issuing numbers for all colorants in use today, no matter what the industry. Each colorant has a color index number (CI#) for ease of identification.

CMC color space uses lightness/darkness, chroma, and hue values to calculate DE. Based on L, C, and h values, it is a function of the ratio L:Ch. The CMC believed that chromatic colors are described better by their saturation (chroma) C and color (hue) h than just by their a and b values. CMC can be used to show a specific numerical differentiation of colors, but the L, a, and b values in CIELab can show the direction and degree of the color shift. CMC color space has an elliptical shape that contains many smaller ellipses inside it. All the smaller internal ellipses are of varying size, depending on the human eye's sensitivity to a particular color. The larger the ellipse, the easier it is for the human eye to differentiate that particular family of colors. DE values for CMC are somewhat lower than those of CIELab.

Our eyes do a very good job of evaluating color and describing color difference, but they cannot quantify color differences. We can express color difference numerically, but what types of equipment are available to evaluate a numerical color difference electronically? We can do so with spectrophotometers. A spectrophotometer is an instrument that uses prisms or gratings to measure light transmittance or reflectance on the basis of emitted wavelengths to describe color. Spectrophotometers are extremely sensitive machines that can evaluate color as well as, if not better than, the human eye. They come in different types of geometry — the method by which samples are evaluated.

Most spectrophotometers are available with either of two different types of geometries. The geometries determine the angle of illumination of a sample being evaluated and the angle of observation of the instrument. The two types of geometries in wide use today are 45/0 and diffuse/8 (Figure 2.4).

Instruments with 45/0 geometry illuminate a sample at an angle of 45° and measure perpendicular to the surface of the sample. They observe under very similar conditions as the observation of color by the human eye. This instrument analyzes only the color of the sample, less the specular energy emitted by the sample. This specular energy is also referred to as gloss.

Instruments with diffuse/8 geometry use diffuse illumination and observe at 8° from perpendicular. Diffuse geometry instruments are usually referred to as spherical and use an integrated sphere as the main functional portion of the device. Using diffuse geometry, color measurement also incorporates the gloss of a sample. Spectrophotometers with diffuse geometry are usually equipped with devices to

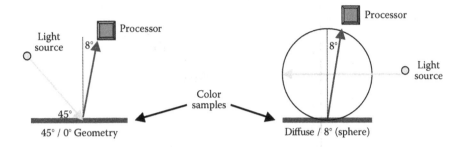

Color
samples

45° / 0° Geometry

Diffuse / 8° (sphere)

FIGURE 2.4

include or exclude specular energy, or gloss contribution, from the calculation. Glossy samples should be measured without the contribution of the gloss.

Color can also be evaluated by using a colorimeter. A colorimeter is an instrument that measures colorimetric data in terms of tristimulus (X Y Z) values using filters and light-emitting diodes (LEDs) to convert spectral information into a color description. In these types of color measurement instruments, R G B information is converted to X Y Z values. X is the red primary, Y is the green primary and Z is the blue primary. These tristimulus values are then calculated by the computer to numerically define a particular color. Both spectrophotometers and colorimeters can be either portable or bench-top models and are available from a number of reputable suppliers.

The Kubelka–Munk equation, which was first published in 1931, describes the reflectance (R) of a translucent sample as a function of light absorption (K) and light scattering (S) of the sample. It can also be stated that the absorption of light is proportional to the concentration of the colorants used in the sample. This equation is simplified from the original equation, which was calculated manually before the advent of computers, and is valid for all opaque samples.

$$\frac{K}{S} = \frac{(1 - R)^2}{2R}$$

The Kubelka–Munk equation is the numerical basis for all formulation and correction computer programs. The file structure is based on calculating white and black with mixtures of samples at various concentrations of each colorant used in the product. File accuracy and repeatability are dependent on sample preparation and presentation. Sample concentrations should be between the minimum and maximum used in a particular formulation. The equation assumes that all colorants have a linear build. This is true for inorganic colorants — iron oxides — but one must be very careful, as organic colorants can exhibit differences in color build. Additional concentrations may be necessary to establish linearity (Figure 2.5).

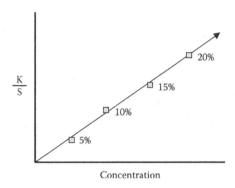

Concentration

FIGURE 2.5

A formulation system utilizing a calculating white and the base it is used in is called a two-constant system. A system that utilizes just the base (no white or titanium dioxide used) is called a one-constant system. An example of this would be an eye shadow or a blusher-type product using talc as the white.

A typical colorant set for a makeup usually takes 13 samples to build a working formulation or correction file. Titanium dioxide and iron oxides exhibit a good constant linear build so the concentrations can be fixed. Mixtures can be made using various monochromatic extenders of each colorant in a particular product. Titanium dioxide is the white of choice, and primary red, yellow, and black iron oxides are used as colorants. Mixtures are made using white and black, and the Kubelka–Munk equation calculates the numerical relationship of the colorants so it can recognize an unknown sample. Sample preparation and accuracy of mixtures dictate how well the file will work. Concentrations may vary depending on colorant use levels. One does not need a high percent mixture of a colorant if one only uses a small amount of that colorant in the formula. Examine the list of colorant mixtures shown below:

100% white (titanium dioxide)

100% black iron oxide
20%   black + 80% white
10%   black + 90% white
5%   black + 95% white

100% red iron oxide
20%   red + 80% white
10%   red + 90% white
95%   red + 5% black

100% yellow iron oxide
20%   yellow + 80% white
10%   yellow + 90% white
95%   yellow + 5% black

A set of mixtures such as the one above is fairly easy to assemble. Samples must be prepared and presented to any measurement device the same way every time. The method of sample preparation is dependent upon product type, and obviously the amount of sample to be presented is very critical. It is important to develop a procedure for product evaluation that can be followed and duplicated every time. This means film thickness and amount of sample must be the same every time a measurement is made. It is also important to note that when developing a procedure, you must take into account that you want the measurement device to see exactly what your eye sees in order for the data to be valid and meaningful. The accuracy of the sample concentrations and the method of preparation and presentation are key to having a valid working formulation and correction file.

For lipsticks, an optimum film thickness must be determined to guarantee repeatable results. It is very possible, especially when dealing with organic colorants, for a mass tone not to be the same as the write-off.

In the case of liquid makeups that contain titanium dioxide and iron oxide pigments, the mass tone usually does represent the skin tone. Where feasible, samples should be measured through optical glass. Optical glass is designed to eliminate deviations from reading to reading. For evaluating products such as clear shampoos, reading must be made with a bench-top spectrophotometer, as the reading now will become percent transmission rather than reflectance, and the sample gets placed inside the machine.

For powders, a paper press must be flat and level to prevent any deviations in the readings. Cracks will become a part of the reading and skew the data.

An accurate colorant file can save man-hours in the laboratory by allowing the formulator to spend more time on developmental work and less time on basic shade matching. It can also help in production by allowing fewer corrections and freeing up kettles for faster batch manufacturing and turnaround.

There are some limitations that the computer systems we have today may encounter:

- Most color measurement systems cannot solve for two variable whites. There must be one fixed white.
- It is difficult to measure pearlescent colors. A multiangle detector is required to observe and measure the colors that pearls exhibit at the various effect angles.
- A sufficient amount of sample is needed to present to the apparatus for measurement to fit the aperture size.
- The proper instrument is needed to evaluate certain types of samples. A bench-top instrument limits certain types of measurements and sample presentations.
- Portable units are not equipped to do transmission readings. Some instrument portability needs to accommodate certain types of measurements.

Even though these limitations make it seem like there are many negatives to the systems, one point must be made: these systems will be very successful when there are limitations in a person's visual color assessment capabilities. They are also very helpful when a formulator has numerous shades to develop in a very short amount of time, which seems to be the norm for most industries. The timesaving capabilities of color measurement systems are immeasurable in terms of cost savings and man-hours.

Color measurement devices can also be used when it becomes almost impossible to visually see minute changes in color or appearance. The spectral curves in Figure 2.6 represent female skin with medium tonality that is clean and undamaged. These curve deviations are normal and characteristic for any undamaged skin and can vary only slightly up or down. Readings were taken in five different positions just below the jawline.

These curve deviations are difficult to see visually, and only a measurement device can differentiate them to such a degree. The human eye is much too sensitive to see these deviations separately. The brain instantaneously averages the color of one's skin, and the eye cannot see the deviations.

A product was then applied to this same person on the same side of the face from which the original readings were taken. Five additional readings were then taken on this same side of the face. The spectral curves in Figure 2.7 represent the new readings in the same positions. Note that the curves now almost completely overlap. The uniqueness of this is that this product had no coverage and left behind a very thin, colorless, invisible film. The measurement device was able to pick up these minute changes and show the evenness of the skin after the

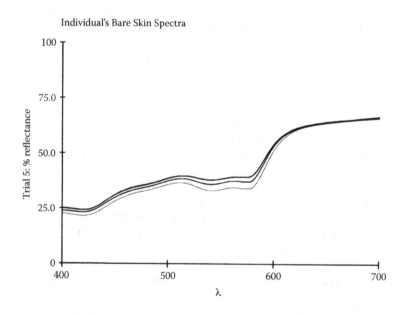

FIGURE 2.6

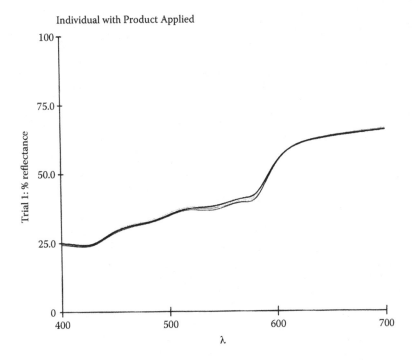

FIGURE 2.7

product was applied. This could never have been accomplished with just a visual observation.

Measurement devices such as spectrophotometers and colorimeters, in conjunction with software that can make color calculations, can become an important tool in the development of cosmetic products, in color evaluation, and in laboratory and production. Knowing the system's capabilities, new techniques can be developed to make the formulator's job just a little bit easier.

However, there is no substitute for the trained, experienced color eye, and the human eye should always be the final judge in any color evaluation.

3 Noninvasive Techniques to Measure Cutaneous Effects of Skin Care Products

Randall P. Wickett, Ph.D.,[1] Linda D. Rluein, Ph.D.,[2] and Svetlana Babajanyan, M.D.[2]
[1]University of Cincinnati
[2]Fairleigh Dickinson University

CONTENTS

3.1 INTRODUCTION

Noninvasive biophysical methods to investigate product effects on skin have advantages over clinical grading alone for both claim support and research guidance. Methods based on instrumental measurements are often considered more objective and quantitative than visual assessments and can provide more information about the details of product interactions with the skin. The desire for objective assessment of topical products has in part been driven by significant progress in the development of instruments and protocols for measurement of skin. It is now possible to objectively measure many skin parameters to supplement clinical grading. This chapter reviews some noninvasive methods and methods using living skin equivalents available to advance knowledge of skin physiology and assess efficacy of topical products. This review will only scratch the surface of a topic that has had several books devoted to it in recent years.[1-5] The European Expert Group on Efficacy Measurement of Cosmetics (EEMCO) has published guides for many categories of skin measurements, including most of those discussed in this chapter.[6-13]

3.2 THE EPIDERMIS

The vast majority of cosmetic products interact first and foremost with the top layer of the epidermis, the stratum corneum (SC). The epidermis has many vital protective functions.[14] It serves as a barrier to water loss from the skin and to entrance of toxic chemicals and microorganisms into the skin. Barrier function of the skin embodied primarily in the SC has been called the *la raison d'etre* of the epidermis.[15] The epidermis is itself divided into several layers, starting with the basal layer just above the dermis, proceeding upward through the prickle and the granular layers to the SC. Figure 3.1 represents the major layers of the epidermis. Barrier function resides primarily in the top layer of the epidermis, the stratum corneum (SC).

The cells of the SC are called corneocytes or squames. Corneocytes are flat cells that tend to be in the shape of either a hexagon or pentagon, about 25 μm on a side, with a surface area of about 1000 μm^2 and a thickness of about 0.5 to 1.0 μm.[16,17] On most body sites the SC is 12 to 16 cell layers thick, but it can

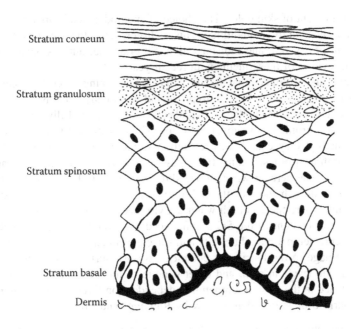

FIGURE 3.1 Diagram of epidermis.

vary from as little as 9 cell layers of the forehead or eyelids to as much as 25 on the dorsum of the hand and up to 50 or more on the palms or the soles of the feet.[18,19] SC squames are surrounded by a lamellar lipid matrix[20] that is the primary barrier to water loss and the ingress of toxic molecules.[21] This barrier can be disrupted by surfactants,[22-25] or even long exposure to water,[24] and is severely disrupted in soap-induced winter-dry skin.[26]

The SC barrier must be competent, but not perfect, as some water from the epidermis must be present to provide sufficient hydration for both SC flexibility and the functioning of enzymes that we now know are important to SC barrier function and desquamation. When the SC barrier function is perturbed, cell signaling molecules (cytokines) are released in the lower layers, leading to inflammation. This process will be discussed in more detail below.

3.3 SKIN HYDRATION AND MOISTURIZATION

3.3.1 DRY SKIN AND MOISTURIZERS

While assessment of dry skin by clinical grading is still important to both moisturizer and mildness studies, there are now many noninvasive methods to supplement and enhance the evaluation of dry skin, barrier function, and irritation. Available methods range from evaluation of barrier integrity to measurement of water loss, measurement of electrical properties, elasticity, infrared spectroscopy, magnetic resonance imaging, skin surface topography, scaling of the skin surface, and measurement of skin color. The choice of method depends upon the characteristics of the skin to be quantified. This section reviews the use of instrumental assessment of dry skin and moisturization. Several other authors have provided excellent reviews of these methods in recent years.[27–32]

Blank[33] first postulated that the SC of dry skin is lacking water. This seemingly obvious fact turned out to be hard to prove and was finally demonstrated conclusively about 40 years after Blank's hypothesis by Warner and Lilly,[34] who showed that the water profile of the upper SC of dry skin is different from normal skin, using a method they called high-resolution water imaging to determine water content profiles from scanning transmission microscopy images obtained on cryosections. The percent water in dry skin was found to be lower than that of normal skin through most of the SC, until just below the level of the stratum granulosum, where there is high water activity because the cells are viable.

The water content of the SC is influenced by several parameters, including environmental temperature, humidity and sun exposure, age, condition of the skin barrier, damage to the barrier by chemicals (drugs, surfactants), skin diseases, diet, hormone levels in skin, and other genetic factors. The maintenance of the water balance in the stratum corneum is dependent on three major mechanisms, as summarized in an excellent review by Rawlings and Matts:[35]

- The intercellar lamellar lipids whose physical conformation, predominantly an orthorhombic, laterally packed, 6.5-nm-long gel phase and a 13-nm-long periodicity lamellar phase, provides a tight and effective barrier to the passage of water through the tissue
- The presence of fully matured corneodesmosomes — desmosomal interconnections that link the corneocytes — which influences the tortuosity of the stratum corneum and thereby the diffusion path length of water
- The presence of the natural moisturizing factor, derived from filaggrin degradation

The conditions described above are thought to alter the water gradient in skin and induce dry skin. Once a state of dehydration has been provoked, an inevitable sequence of events — described by the authors as a "cycle of dry skin" — occurs. A mild inflammatory state ensues. This response is mediated via production and secretion of cytokines and growth factors such as IL-1α, TNF-α, KGF, and GMCSF, inducing a hyperproliferative state and aberrant differentiation. This leads to a rapid production of poor-quality barrier constituents as a rescue type of response to the insult (i.e., production of smaller immature corneocyte envelopes, reduced transglutaminase activity, and reduced filaggrin biosynthesis) it also leads to production of natural moisturizing factor derived from filaggrin degradation and changes in the epidermal lipid phase behavior because of changes in types of lipids produced, particularly ceramides. The role of these constituents in maintaining barrier function is further discussed in Chapter 1 of this edition. The main trigger in initiating this cycle is alteration in the water gradient in the stratum corneum, i.e., dehydration.

The goal of moisturizing products is to break the dry skin cycle. Moisturizing additives can be either occlusive to reduce water loss or humectants to hold water within the barrier by osmosis. Humectants like glycerol and urea may have actions in addition to humectancy. Glycerol may increase the fluidity of SC intercellular lipids[36,37] and has been reported to normalize degradation of SC desmosomes and sloughing of the corneocytes,[38] as well as speed barrier repair after disruption by tape stripping or surfactant damage.[39] Urea treatment has been shown to increase the resistance of the skin to surfactant treatment.[40] Moisturizers containing urea or glycerol have been shown to improve the elasticity of SC *in vivo*.[41–44] Bilayer-forming lipids such as ceramides have been used to replenish the barrier structure and normalize phase behavior. It has been reported that barrier lipids in combination with glycerol are more effective than petrolatum in relieving dry skin,[45] but Loden and Barany[46] reported that "skin identical lipids" were not more effective than petrolatum in enhancing barrier repair in detergent-damaged or tape-stripped skin. α-Hydroxyl acids can improve dry skin[47] and are well known as exfoliants that can remove dry skin scale, leaving smoother skin.[48] Berardesca has shown that they can also improve barrier function[49] in some cases. Nicotinamide has also been shown to provide benefits for dry skin in combination with glycerol.[50] Noninvasive biophysical methods for investigation of moisturizers are designed to detect and quantify these multifaceted qualities of effective moisturizing products.

3.3.2 TRANSEPIDERMAL WATER LOSS

Transepidermal water loss (TEWL) is defined as water transported *through* the skin by *passive* diffusion. If the subject is not sweating and the skin surface is free of exogenous water, then measurement of the rate of evaporation of water from the skin surface reveals the rate water is diffusing through the skin. An increase in TEWL may be caused by damage to the SC by acute or chronic exposure to irritants or by abnormal keratinization due to either a dry environment or a disease state. Dry skin associated with barrier damage generally leads to elevated TEWL,[51–56] but dry skin does not always have high TEWL. For example, senile dry skin[51] or dry skin induced by low humidity[57] may have lower than normal TEWL. Thus, care must be taken when interpreting TEWL measurements done in association with studies of moisturizing products. Typically dry skin along with increased TEWL is induced with several days of washing with soap. The efficacy of moisturizers is then measured after application onto the subject's dry skin.

Most current commercial instruments are based on the principle of measurement of the water vapor gradient above the skin surface[58–60] by two pairs of sensors (relative humidity (RH) and temperature) placed one pair above the other in a cylindrical probe. From the temperature and RH, the absolute humidity at each point can be calculated and Fick's first law of diffusion can be used to calculate the vapor transport rate. At least three different commercial instruments use this method.[59,61–62] Recently, a closed-chamber system for TEWL measurement was developed and published.[63,64]

TEWL depends on RH[65] and temperature,[66] so a climate-controlled room (20 to 22°C, 40 to 50% RH) is necessary with the open-chamber devices. If the subject is sweating, the measurements will increase dramatically. The test subject has to sit very quietly for at least 20 min (the temperature of 22° is below the sweat temperature), and the instrument has to be acclimated to the room prior to measurement. Guidelines have been published for the measurement of TEWL.[67,68]

TEWL measurements reflect the skin's function as a barrier to water moving through it. A decrease in TEWL can be seen with use of moisturizers such as petrolatum that attenuate water movement by covering the skin with an occlusive layer. This decrease may be accompanied by a slow increase in hydration within the skin.[69,70] Therefore, TEWL is occasionally used to document the short-term occlusive effects of moisturizing agents. However, the most common use of TEWL is to assess comparative effects of soaps or detergents on barrier integrity as a result of repeated cleansing. TEWL can be used to quantify the ability of moisturizers to protect the skin during repeated insults with cleansers in a multiple wash/treat protocol similar to Highhley's,[71] although the TEWL instrumentation was not commercially available when Highley first published the repeat-hand-wash method.

3.3.3 ELECTRICAL METHODS FOR ESTIMATING SKIN WATER CONTENT

Hydration has a major impact on the electrical properties of the skin. Dry stratum corneum has very low electrical conduction due to the low dielectric constants of its lipid constituents, and conduction increases dramatically with hydration. Tagami et al.[72] was a pioneer in the use of impedance to study skin hydration. The impedance, Z, is related to resistance (R) and capacitance (C) in a model that depicts the skin as a resistor and capacitor in parallel:[73–76]

$$Z = [R^2 + (1/2 \ \pi \ fC)^2]^{1/2}$$

where f is the frequency of the applied alternating current.

The conductance and capacitance of the skin of the forearm approximately double when the relative humidity increases from 66 to 86%.[29]

This chapter will review three of the most common devices used for assessing skin hydration through electrical measurements: the Corneometer® 825 (CM 825), the Nova™ Technologies DPM 9003, and the Skicon 200. These devices all report data proportional in some way to the relative hydration of the skin. The numbers should not be considered an absolute measurement of the percentage of water in the SC, as is sometimes done. For instance, a 50% increase in one of the electrical measurements on application of a moisturizer is sometimes reported as a 50% increase in hydration. In the opinion of this author, this is not correct. Hydration has almost certainly increased, but the percentage increase has not been exactly determined by the measurement. There is a published guidance for measuring stratum corneum hydration using electrical methods.[77]

3.3.3.1 Corneometer 825 (CM 825)

The Corneometer 825 (CM 825) (Courage + Khazaka, Köln, Germany) uses capacitance measurements to estimate hydration.[78–80] It operates around a mean frequency of 1 MHz. The measuring probe consists of fine gold wires with

75-μm spacing on a ceramic surface of 0.5 cm^2 (0.7 × 0.7 cm) covered by a thin glass plate to protect the probe.[79] There is no direct galvanic contact between the electrodes and the skin. The probe head is equipped with a spring mechanism that ensures the application of a constant pressure (1.6 N/m^2) when the probe is placed on the skin. Data are output in arbitrary units (ACU), ranging from less than 30 ACU in very dry skin[80] to about 100 ACU in well-hydrated skin.[81]

At lower levels of hydration, the sensitivity of the instrument is very good,[81] but it shows a decrease in sensitivity at the higher levels of hydration, compared to other instruments.[30] Different time frames of measurements are possible: consecutive measurements with up to 10 single measurements of 1.5 sec duration and calculation of a mean value or a continuous measurement over a duration of 3 sec, 70 sec, or 7 min. Measurements have been reported to correlate well to clinical grades of dry skin.[82] Our group has found the CM 825 useful for studies on very dry skin on the hands of health care workers.[83]

3.3.3.2 Nova DPM 9003

The Nova Dermal Phase Meter (DPM) 9003 (Nova™ Technologies Corporation, Portsmouth, NH U.S.) is a handheld device for evaluating skin hydration.[84,85] Interchangeable probes are available for the instrument. The standard probe that comes with the instrument has a flat circular surface with two concentric brass ring electrodes separated by a nonconducting polymer. The ring diameters are 8.76 and 4.34 mm and the probe is 113.41 mm long. The probe is applied to the skin with a constant application pressure of 0.6 N/m^2 with the aid of a spring system. Other probes of smaller diameters of 2, 4, and 6 mm are sold. The surface area of the standard electrode is 0.98 cm^2. The probe of the Nova DPM makes galvanic contact with the skin.

The DPM 9003 emits a 1-MHz span of simultaneously produced frequencies, producing a differential current source with a controlled rise time. Impedance is evaluated at several frequencies using a proprietary chip in the instrument. Values are reported as arbitrary units ranging from 90 to 999. The instrument is internally calibrated each time at start-up. There are different modes in which measurements can be taken either immediately, after 5 sec, or continuously.

Values from the Nova DPM typically range from 90 to 105 DPM units for dry skin to 130 to 400 DPM units for hydrated skin. The coefficient of variation has been reported to be 3.6%.[84] This lead author has extensive experience with the Nova DPM[42,86–88] and has found it to be very well suited to studies of moisturizer efficacy. Our group has also used it extensively in dynamic studies of SC water interaction, but they are beyond the scope of this review.[87,89–93] The Nova petite is a new instrument from Nova Technologies that interfaces directly to a personal data assistant. Data from the Nova petite correlate well with data from the DPM 9003.[85]

3.3.3.3 Skicon

The Skicon 200 (IBS Ltd., Tokyo, Japan) measures the conductance (reciprocal of impedance) of the skin at a single frequency of 3.5 MHz.[75,76] Data are reported in Siemens (S).[72–76] The Skicon has a circular probe of two concentric gold-covered ring electrodes separated by dielectric material with external diameters of 2.0 and 6.0 mm and a surface area of 0.28 mm. The probe makes direct galvanic contact with the skin and is applied with a constant pressure of 1.04 N/m^2. The range is 0 to 1999 μS. The instrument is calibrated with a standard external calibration device of 300 μS. Conductance values are measured after 3 sec application time. Skicon measurements have been reported to correlate well to dry skin clinical grades[82] and to *in vivo* measurements of water content by infrared spectroscopy.[94]

Skicon values typically range from 10 to 15 μS for very dry skin to more than 500 μS for well-hydrated skin. The Skicon has a lower sensitivity on very dry skin, with values from 0 to 15 μS. The MT-8C probe, with eight probe heads provided by Measurement Technologies (Cincinnati, OH), as an aftermarket add-on to the Skicon, has been shown to improve both the sensitivity in lower measurement ranges and the reproducibility of measurements.[82]

3.3.4 Correlations between Instruments

Several authors have investigated correlations between devices for measuring the electrical properties of the skin. Morrison and Scala[82] reported a correlation coefficient (r^2) of 0.689 ($r = 0.83$) between the Skicon 200 and the Corneometer 820 in a 14-person dry skin study. Clarys et al.,[78] Fluhr et al.[81] and Li et al.[86] compared the CM 825, Nova DPM 9003, and Skicon. The results of those three studies are summarized in Table 3.1.

Both Fluhr et al. and Li et al. found the best correlation to be between the Skicon and the Nova DPM. This agrees with the general observation that the Corneometer is relatively more sensitive in the lower end of the range of skin hydration and relatively less sensitive in the upper end than either the Skicon or the Nova DPM. This effect can be clearly seen in Figure 3.2 of Li et al.[86]

3.3.5 Short-Term Measurements and Clinical-Grade Reductions

Electrical measurements made from one to several hours after product application are often used to investigate the efficacy of moisturizers.[95–98] Li et al.[99] formulated moisturizing products with levels of glycerin, ranging from 0 to 15%, and investigated the correlation between readings made 1 h after application to

TABLE 3.1
Correlations between Electrical Instruments

Comparison	Clarys et al.	Fluhr et al.	Li et al.
Nova vs. Skicon	0.96	0.96	0.93
Nova vs. Corneometer	0.97	0.82	0.87
Skicon vs. Corneometer	0.89	0.83	0.89

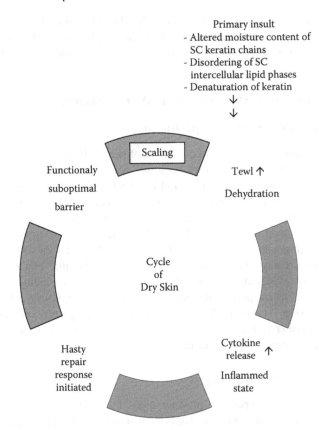

FIGURE 3.2 Dry skin cycle according to Rawlings.[36]

improvements in clinical grades. All three of the instruments discussed above were used. Table 3.2 shows the correlations found between 1-h device readings and improvements in clinical grade after 1 week of treatment.

Readings at 1 h were significantly correlated to improvements in clinical grades for the Nova DPM and Skicon 200, and the correlation with the CM 825

TABLE 3.2
Correlation between the 1-Hour Reading and the 2-Week Reduction in Skin Grade

Device	Regression Equation of Score Reduction (SR) on 1-h Reading	R^2	p Value
Nova DPM	SR = 0.0025X + 0.69	0.917	0.042
Skicon 200	SR = 0.0024X + 0.81	0.969	0.015
CM 825	SR = 0.0209X + 0.76	0.8427	0.082

was directional. The authors did not consider the differences between devices significant and concluded that readings 1 h after application with any of these instruments were predictive of clinical improvements with moisturizers based on glycerin.

3.3.6 Spectroscopic Measurement of Water Content

3.3.6.1 Magnetic Resonance Spectroscopy

Another method to quantify the water content of skin is the use of high-resolution proton magnetic resonance (MR) spectroscopy. MR spectroscopy is discussed in a previous review by Fischer et al.[30] and has been recently reviewed by Querleux.[100] The method involves noninvasive measurement of proton relaxation times and proton density in the human epidermis. Initial studies of the use of this technique were made by Hyde et al.[101] and Querleux.[102] In contrast to normal body MR imaging with a pixel size of 300 μm and a field of view of 8 cm, high-resolution MR creates a field of view measuring 18×50 mm^2 and a pixel size of 70×310 μm^2.[103] MR images can differentiate skin layers, including the dermis and epidermis. Further, proton density is directly proportional to the free water content of the skin. At present, MR is a research tool, though preliminary results indicate that further improvements may lead to a spectroscopic tool capable of imaging small-volume elements in the skin.[100]

3.3.6.2 Infrared Spectroscopy

The infrared absorbance spectrum of water in the skin can be obtained with appropriate instrumentation. It is possible that Fourier-transformed infrared spectroscopy (FTIR) can be used to assess skin hydration and the efficacy of moisturizers. Increased absorption at specific wavelengths after moisturizer application may reflect increased water content in the stratum corneum. FTIR is not yet optimized for widespread comparative moisturizer efficacy testing for several reasons, discussed by Bashir and Maibach.[28] First, interference from other absorbing compounds in the stratum corneum can occur. Also, the absorption bands of keratin proteins in the stratum corneum can change during hydration. A third problem is that the instrument measures only the outermost layers of the stratum corneum.

Near-infrared spectroscopy (NIR) of skin can differentiate types of water from the spectrum and has the potential to quantify product effects. Martin[104] showed that the diffuse NIR absorption spectra differentiated four types of water in skin: water associated with the lipid phase within the SC, bulk water in the SC, secondary water of hydration of SC keratin, and primary water of hydration of keratin. de Rigal et al.[105] reported a good linear correlation between global dry skin grades and NIR absorbance measured from 1936 to 1100 nm using an integration sphere to collect all reemitted radiation. The authors reported that the method was able to accurately rank the efficacy of moisturizing products.

One issue with NIR is the unknown depth of penetration of the light, complicating interpretation of the measurements. Arimoto et al. studied the NIR depth profile and showed that depth of the measurement is dependent on the geometry of the probe, the wavelength, and the hydration level of the SC.[106,107] The closer the separation distance between the source and the detector and the thinner the optical fiber, the shorter the penetration depth.

Zhang et al.[108] used NIR imaging to investigate the effects of a single application of water, a moisturizing lotion, a traditional body wash, and a moisturizing body wash 1 and 6 h after treatment. Results were compared to measurements with the CM 825 and the Skicon with the MT-8 probe attachment and visual evaluation. The electrical measurements and NIR imaging showed significant benefits for the moisturizing lotion at 1, 3, and 6 h. NIR and visual grading indicated some positive effect of the moisturizing body wash at 1 and 3 h that was not significant after 6 h. The traditional body wash and water showed decreases in conductance (Skicon) at all posttreatment time points and were mirrored by lower NIR water measurements at 3 and 6 h. The NIR scores showed a stronger correlation to visual grades than the electrical measurements. However, care must be taken in interpreting visual grades taken within a few hours of product application, as product constituents may alter the appearance of skin without significantly affecting the underlying physiology. This is one reason for the development of various regression test protocols, discussed below.

3.4 MEASUREMENT OF SKIN ELASTICITY

There are many reasons to investigate the mechanical properties of the skin *in vivo*. For a good overview of applications in both dermatology and cosmetic science, see the book *Bioengineering of the Skin: Skin Biomechanics*.[3] In cosmetic science we are often interested in the effects of moisturizers on SC elasticity, but we may also be interested in effects of aging, photoaging, or evaluation of conditions such as cellulite. Measurement of the viscoelastic properties of skin *in vivo* is complicated by the complex nature of the substrate. It is difficult to deform the SC without producing significant deformations in the underlying layers, and of course, it is not possible to deform the dermis without deforming the SC. The general principle is that smaller deformations (minimum strain) will help to localize the response to the SC, and larger deformation will reflect more on the properties of the underlying layers.

3.4.1 MOISTURIZER EFFECTS

Two of the most commonly used instruments for investigating the effects of moisturizers on skin elasticity are the Dermal Torque Meter® (DTM)[109–112] and Cutometer®.[113–115] These instruments can be used to study a variety of effects on skin elasticity.

When using the DTM, a constant torque is applied to the skin through an 18-mm-diameter disc that is fixed to the skin surface with double-sided tape. A guard ring is also taped to the skin surface to restrict the range of the deformation. The gap between the disc and guard ring is the operating gap and can be chosen to 1, 3, or 5 mm. For moisturizer studies, a 1-mm gap is used to limit the range of the deformation as much as possible.[112] The DTM can be used to investigate dermal effects such as skin pliability after healing of burns[116] or in studies of aging,[117] and in that case, a wider ring gap is appropriate.

The Cutometer relies on negative pressure to pull the skin vertically into the opening of the probe.[114,115] The height the skin rises into the probe is determined by an optical system. Probe sizes of 2, 4, 6, and 8 mm are available. The 2-mm-diameter probe is most suited to studies of moisturizers.[118,119] Negative pressures can be controlled between 20 and 500 mbar. Different modes are available, allowing either a stress–strain or a time–stress mode. The time–stress mode is comparable to the mode used by the DTM. With either instrument the stress (torque or vacuum) is applied quickly and held on for a set period of time while deformation is measured. Then the stress is released and the recovery of the skin's deformation is measured. This is illustrated in Figure 3.3. Parameters measured are detailed in Table 3.3.

Murray and Wickett investigated the sensitivity of the Cutometer to hydration by applying water for 10 min.[119] Measurements were made with the Cutometer at 200, 350 and 500 mbar in one acute hydration study and at 100 and 500 in another. Measurements of skin hydration were also made with the DPM 9003. A 2-week treatment with a glycerin-based moisturizer was also investigated. The most sensitive parameters seemed to be Uv and Uv/Ue. In agreement with our results, Dobrev[118] found Uv and Uv/Ue to be sensitive to a glycerin-based

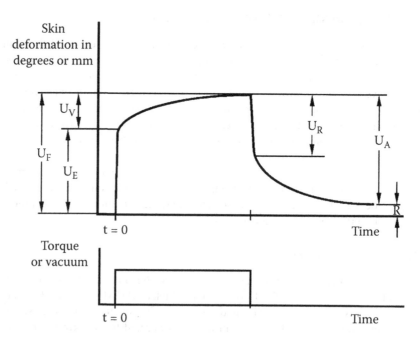

FIGURE 3.3 Typical (hypothetical) skin deformation curve as a function of time generated by a Dermal Torque Meter or Cutometer. Stress (torque or vacuum) is applied to the skin surface and deformation is measured. Following release of the stress, recovery (or hysteresis) is also measured.

TABLE 3.3
DTM® and Cutometer® Parameters from Figure 3.3

Ue	Elastic deformation of the skin due to the application of stress (vacuum or torque) by the instrument
Uv	Viscoelastic creep occurring after the elastic deformation
Uf	Total extensibility of the skin
Ur	Elastic deformation recovery due to stress removal
Ua	Total deformation recovery at the end of the stress-off period
R	Amount of deformation not recovered by the end of the stress-off period
Ua/Uf	Overall elasticity of the skin, including creep and creep recovery
Ur/Ue	Pure elasticity ignoring viscoelastic creep
Uv/Ue	Ratio of viscoelastic to elastic extension, called the viscoelastic ratio
Ur/Uf	Ratio of elastic recovery to total deformation

moisturizer 1 h after treatment. Neither study found good correlations between elasticity parameters and electrical measurements, and Wiechers and Barlow[120] concluded that moisturization and elasticity originate from different mechanisms.

We also investigated correlations between the Dermal Torque Meter, Cutometer, and DPM 9003 in a 2-week moisturizer study.[42] With the DTM, Ue, Uv, Uf, Ur, Ua, and R were all very sensitive to moisturizer and somewhat more sensitive to Cutometer parameters obtained at 500 mbar negative pressure. In another study, it was shown that reducing negative pressure to 200 mbar does increase the sensitivity of Cutometer parameters to moisturizer treatment.[88] In this study, a less effective moisturizer was used on dry legs for only 1 week by a nine-subject panel and measurements were made at 200 and 500 mbar (Table 3.4).

The 200-mbar vacuum level led to increased sensitivity. Ue and Ur increased significantly, even with this small base size, and Uv just missed significance, while none of the parameters reached significance at 500 mbar. From these data it appears that using a lower vacuum level may improve sensitivity to moisturizer-induced changes in elasticity. In this study, Ue and Ur appeared to be more sensitive to the moisturizer effect than Uv.

TABLE 3.4
Moisturizer Effect Measured at Two Different Vacuum Levels

Cutometer Parameter	Pretreatment	Posttreatment	p Value
Ue (200 mbar)	0.036	0.048	0.02
Ue (500 mbar)	0.068	0.079	0.46
Uv (200 mbar)	0.015	0.024	0.07
Uv (500 mbar)	0.025	0.029	0.60
Ur (200 mbar)	0.026	0.039	0.03
Ur (500 mbar)	0.050	0.061	0.26

3.4.2 Age and Body Site Variations

Cua et al.[121] used the Cutometer to evaluate age and regional differences in the viscoelastic properties of skin in a very thorough study with 33 subjects. Seventeen subjects were elderly, averaging about 75 years, and 16 were young, averaging about 28 years. Measurements were performed on 11 anatomical regions; three different loads were applied: 100, 200, and 500 mbar, and the 2-mm-diameter probe. The parameters reported were (Figure 3.3) Ue, delayed-distension Uv, immediate retraction (Ur), and final deformation (Uf) of the skin during perturbation with the device. To compare between subjects and anatomical regions, relative parameters independent of skin thickness were calculated: Uv/Ue, the ratio between the viscoelastic properties of skin and immediate distension, and Ur/Uf, which measures the ability of the skin to regain its initial position after deformation. Generally, Uv/Ue increased while Ur/Uf decreased with aging, but the difference was not significant for all body sites. Responses were variable with respect to load applied. Variability within anatomical regions was also noted. These findings are in agreement with earlier studies and suggest that the differences are mainly attributable to alterations in the elastic fiber network associated with aged skin.[122–124]

Our group[125] investigated the effects of age, body site, and skin thickness on mechanical properties of skin with the Cutometer using the 6-mm probe and the BTC-2000® (SRLI, Inc., Nashville, TN). The BTC-2000 is a suction device with probes available ranging up to 2 cm in diameter. Results with the two instruments were well correlated, and both showed significant effects of age. For example, Uf on the shoulder measured by the Cutometer was negatively correlated to age with $r = -0.75$ and $p < 0.001$.

We also used the BTC-2000 to characterize the biomechanical properties of skin with gynoid lipodistropy (cellulite)[126,127] in subjects undergoing weight loss using the 2-cm-diameter probe to sample the largest possible cross section of the collagen and elastin network in the dermis. We observed significant changes in the biomechanical properties with weight loss, including decreased stiffness, increased energy absorption (greater skin compliance,) and increased elastic deformation.

3.5 SKIN SURFACE ANALYSIS

Figure 3.4 depicts a scanning electron micrograph of a section of skin showing the challenge of measuring the surface properties of normal and damaged skin. The top figure is an ankle wrinkle with dry squames uplifted on the surface of the wrinkle. The bottom is a scanning micrograph of the surface under higher magnification depicting the dry squames. These two pictures require different techniques to quantify: (1) wrinkle characteristics or surface anisotropy, which is the density of the furrows as a function of depth and orientation, and (2) squame characteristics or surface topography indicative of roughness, peaks (bumps) and troughs (pores), dryness, and moisturizer efficacy. The next section focuses on measurements of skin surface topography and approaches to measuring microrelief and macrorelief.

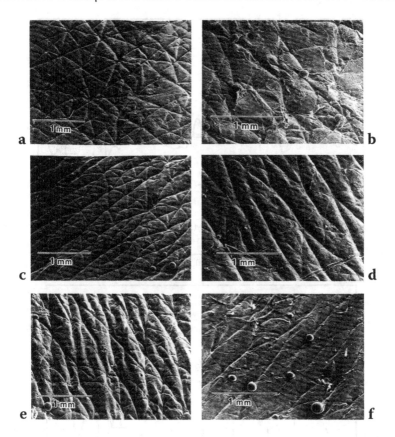

FIGURE 3.4 Scanning electron microscopy of ankle skin wrinkle. Note the dry skin squames. (From Murahata, et al. *J. Soc. Cosmet. Chem.* 35, 329, 1984. With permission.)

3.5.1 SKIN MICROTOPOGRAPHY

Images used to quantify the topography of human skin can be obtained either from silicone replicas or directly from the skin surface.[28,31,128–133] Replicas can be analyzed by stylus profilometry or by image analysis of the replica.

Replicas are typically obtained using a soft silicone such as Silflo® to make a negative replica of the skin surface. For stylus profilometry, a positive replica is made from the negative using a harder material, such as epoxy.[131,134–136] The positive replica is then scanned by a sensitive stylus moving in a direction perpendicular to the mean furrows in the replica, and displacement is measured electronically with a precision of 0.1 μm. The method is very time consuming, but also has high precision and reliability. Cook[134] provided a detailed review of the use of profilometry to measure cosmetic efficacy. He concluded that the roughness parameters burrowed from the metal industry by Hoppe[137] were likely to be the most useful for characterizing the skin surface. Figure 3.5 illustrates

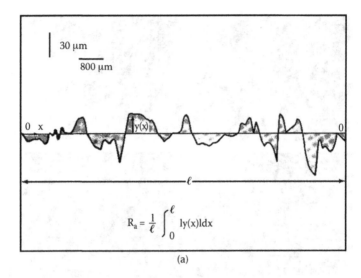

(a)

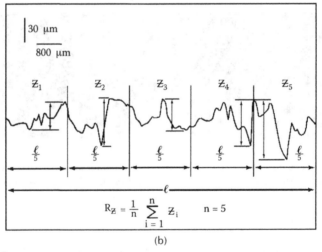

(b)

FIGURE 3.5 A and B: Skin surface profilometry scan depicting mean roughness parameters measured by Cook.[139]

the calculation of two of these parameters: the mean surface roughness, Ra, and the mean depth of roughness from the profile, Rz.

In a subsequent publication, Cook et al.[135] investigated the effect of hydration on roughness on the legs of 10 female subjects ranging in age from 24 to 38 years. All roughness parameters were decreased by a 30-min soak in a water bath, but the reduction in Ra was the only statistically significant change.

Another approach to analysis of replicas is to shine light on the negative replicas at various angles and generate a shadow. The width of the shadow reflects the depth of the furrow on the skin.[129,131] Corcuff et al. used this method to quantify the effects of age on the development of crow's-foot wrinkles in the periorbital area and to evaluate the effects of antiwrinkle products on human subjects.[138]

Robert et al.[139] studied the effect of 4 weeks of treatment with an antiwrinkle cream using skin replicas taken with Xanopren (Bayer, Puteaux, France). The replicas were observed on a Zeis photomicroscope (Zeis, Le Pecq, France) equipped with a black-and-white Sony video camera (Biocom, Les Ulis, France). The images taken by the video camera were introduced into the microcomputer, digitized, and evaluated by Visiolab 1000 software (Biocom, Les Ulis, France). The number, length, and average width of each wrinkle was measured. The wrinkle index (WI) is calculated for each treatment area, which is the total cumulative length of all wrinkles times the average width of all wrinkles in the area. The percent change in WI before/after treatment times 100. Twenty subjects used a wrinkle treatment for 4 weeks. In greater than 65% of the cases the treatment improved the WI.

De Paepe et al.[130] report the use of the Skin Visiometer (SV) 500 (Courage + Khazaka, Köln, Germany) to determine roughness profiles from silicon replicas. In this method replicas are dyed blue and optical absorbance is used to determine the profile. Rt, Rz, Rm, and Ra were determined. Reproducibility of the method was good for lines ranging in depth from 10 to 361 μ. A limitation is that lines deeper than 361 μ cannot be measured accurately. Application of a hydrating cream to the forearms of elderly female volunteers led to a positive trend toward reducing the roughness parameters, indicating better microrelief. Barel et al.[140] used this method to document the positive effect of 20 weeks of treatment with an oral supplement compared to placebo on the microrelief of forearms of Caucasian females with photodamaged skin.

Lagarde et al.[133] used a method of analysis of negative replicas based on the projection of interference fringes and image analysis to produce a three-dimensional image. They investigated both the roughness parameters of the surface and the anisotropy — the density of the furrows as a function of depth and orientation using sophisticated software that automatically determines all of these parameters. The anisotropy parameters supplemented the roughness parameters by providing more information on aging and young skin.

Zhouani and Vargiolu[128] describe detailed mathematical analysis of replica profiles in three dimensions. A major consequence of skin aging is loss of the isotropic crosshatched pattern of the skin surface and the appearance of anisotropic lines in the direction of skin tension. These lines can be ameliorated, at least to some extent, by effective moisturization. Zhouani and Vargiolu discuss the use of three-dimensional morphological "trees" to characterize skin line anisotropy and quantify the effects of treatments.

3.5.2 IMAGE ANALYSIS *In Vivo*

An alternative to skin replicas is image analysis of skin *in vivo*. Jaspers et al.[141] describe a method for *in vivo* determination of skin topography using image analysis of a pattern of parallel lines projected on the skin surface by a micromirror system. The line pattern is deflected by elevations of the skin surface, and software allows calculation of the roughness patterns from the magnitude of the deflections. This device is the PRIMOS (GFMesstechnik, Teltow, Germany). The parameter Rz (Figure 3.5) was found to be correlated to Rz, determined by profilometry of replicas with r = 0.97, and both Rz and Ra were found to be increased on subjects 55 to 60 years of age compared to subjects 20 to 30 years of age.

Friedman et al.[142] used the PRIMOS system to quantify the improvement in skin surface topology after laser treatment of acne scars. Reductions in Ra were dramatic and correlated well with clinical assessment. Jacobi et al.[132] reported more detailed analysis of the variation of roughness parameters from the PRIMOS with age and body site and used the device to quantify the reduction in the depth of wrinkles on the forehead after treatment with *botulinum toxin A*.

Image analysis from digital photographs was recently applied to assess lip wrinkles and the effect of lipsticks on lip wrinkle profile.[143] Results show that treatment with lipstick is able to significantly reduce appearance of wrinkles in digital images. This correlated with clinical assessment of severity of wrinkles.

3.5.3 Squamometry and Image Analysis

Image analysis of D-Squames® is a technique used regularly to assess skin surface scaliness. D-Squames are adhesive discs (Cuderm, Dallas TX) that are placed on the skin and then removed, bringing along the loose dry skin scales from the surface.[144] These discs can them be quantified using image analysis.[145,146] The extent of skin dryness due to cleansing effects of surfactants can be quantified.[54,145,147]

Squamometry is a combination of sampling corneocytes by adhesive coated discs (sometimes Scotch tape is used, but the round discs are better), followed by color measurements after staining the cells. D-Squame samples are stained with polychrome multiple stain (PMS). The stained samples can be quantified by computerized image analysis, or the color can be measured as the Chroma (C*) with the Minolta Chromameter® (see Section 3.8). De Paepe reports on this methodology and these limitations.[148]

Charbonnier et al.[149] demonstrated the utility of squamometry to differentiate the skin-drying potential of mild vs. irritating detergents. Compared to exaggerated hand-washing procedures, an open nonexaggerated assay better approximates consumer surfactant use. The goal was to observe skin surface damage induced by an open test with regard to discriminating between surfactant solutions. This human *in vivo* assay provided information about the effect of only three washes at the laboratory, each for 1 min, followed by rinsing and a 2-min rest between the washes, and then followed up with a week of at-home use. The dorsal hand and volar forearm were compared. Squamometry proved to be a sensitive assessment technique for detecting surfactant-induced subclinical skin surface alterations and for differentiating surfactant effects in this open-application assay, in as few as three washes, discriminating between the clinical effects of sodium lauryl sulfate (SLS) and sodium laureth sulfate (SLES).

3.6 MEASUREMENT OF SKIN GLOSS

Lentner and Wienert describe a method to determine the glossiness or shine of human skin *in vivo*.[150] Shiny skin is often considered undesirable, creating a demand for cosmetic additives that reduce skin shine. In this method, a tungsten filament light (2.5 V, 60 mA) is directed at the skin surface and light reflected at an angle of 60° is focused onto a photocell. The area of skin measured is 9×18 mm. The data are expressed in reflectance units (RU). The measuring range is 0.00 to 10.00 RU, at a resolution of 0.001 RU and an accuracy of <1 RU between 1 and 100 RU.

The difference in RU between forehead and forearm skin was assessed using a 30-person panel. Gloss on the forehead was significantly higher than on the forearm. No significant sex-related difference in RU on either the forehead or forearm was observed. A range of standard vehicle bases was tested on the forearm skin to determine gloss at various time points between 1 and 30 min. Significant differences in gloss between the cream bases at different time points were reported and profiled as a function of time. Bases with higher water content caused less increase in skin gloss. Pigmented cosmetics products — bases, blushes, powders, etc. — could also be also assessed with this technique.

3.7 SKIN SURFACE SEBUM

Measurement of skin surface sebum is desirable because it may provide an objective assessment of the "oiliness or greasiness" of the skin. This is important in the formulation of cosmetics tailored toward not causing oiliness or toward decreasing oiliness of the skin. Measurement of skin surface sebum also facilitates objective assessment of the efficacy of oil-control formulations and drug formulations that decrease sebum secretion. Using a variety of techniques, baseline measurements and treatment results can be monitored in an accurate and reproducible fashion.

Sebum is the oily secretion of the sebaceous gland. Sebum isolated from the skin surface is composed of triglycerides, wax esters, and free fatty acid. The fatty acids are present due to the action of the *Propionibacterium acnes* on the sebum. The fatty acid or fatty acyl group in the lipids is a mixture of both saturated and unsaturated chains; therefore, sebum exists as multiple phases, both solid and liquid.[151] The liquid phase helps dissolve the solid phase to maintain a constant flow of sebum from the pilosebaceous unit. If the balance between the solid and liquid phases is not appropriate and more of the solid sebum exists, the pores can become blocked and an inflammatory condition called acne results. Comedonal material has been shown to be enriched in saturated sebaceous material.[152]

There are two methods available for measuring sebum on the skin surface. The Sebutape® adhesive patch system (CuDerm Corp., Dallas, TX) can be applied to the skin to collect sebum.[153] After sebum absorbs onto the microporous opaque tape, the sebum-filled pores are no longer capable of scattering light and appear transparent. Placing these tapes against a black background allows image analysis to quantify the sebum on the tape.

The Sebumeter 810 PC® (Courage + Khazaka, Cologne, Germany) measures the amount of sebum absorbed onto an opaque tape. A cassette that can be advanced to expose fresh tape for each site/subject tested holds tape. The tape is applied to the skin for 30 sec and is then placed in the device for analysis by a photometer in the device holder. Serup[154] has compared the two methods for measuring sebum and suggests that "Sebutape is a specialized method for the determination of 'oiliness', the very last phase of sebum output, in which sebum droplets spread over the skin surface." In my experience, the Sebumeter is easy to use and gives accurate results quickly, but Sebutape can allow a count of active sebaceous glands and visualization of their distribution. Sebutape can also be extracted for analysis of the sebum[155] if desired, so each technique has its place. Rizer[156] has reviewed strategies for efficacy testing and claims support with regard to oily skin using surface sebum analysis in more detail.

3.8 SKIN COLOR

Measurement of the color of pigmented products is already covered in Chapter 2. This section will focus on color measurements to quantify erythema and natural skin pigmentation. Skin color is determined by a combination of the chromophores that absorb light and elements that scatter light.[157] Light is scattered by structures that have a different index of refraction than the medium in which they are embedded (e.g., cell membrane or stratum corneum–air interface). The concentration and distribution of these two components varies throughout the skin, leading to different optical properties at different sites. The major pigment contributing to basal skin tone is, of course, melanin. When capillaries are perfused with erythrocytes, they can contribute significant red color to the skin, leading to erythema.

Tristimulus colorimeters emit the wavelengths 700, 564.1, and 435.8 nm, corresponding to red (R), green (G), and blue (B) light.[158] While there are other color systems, the L a* b* system (Cielab) is most commonly used in the cosmetic industry, and the instrument most frequently employed is the Minolta Chromameter. In the L* a* b* systems a three-dimensional color space is defined by the three parameters. L* is lightness from 0 (black) to 100 (white), a* is the red-green scale, going from 60 for pure red to −60 for green, and b* is yellow-blue, going from 60 for yellow to −60 for blue.

A color change can be quantified by either the total color difference, ΔE, according to the equation

$$\Delta E = \{(\Delta L^*)^2 + (\Delta a^*)^2 + (\Delta b^*)^2\}^{1/2}$$

or the change in Chroma, ΔC, defined as

$$\Delta C = \{(\Delta a^*)^2 + (\Delta b^*)^2\}^{1/2}$$

In the evaluation of skin color, researchers may consider the overall color or focus on the parameter of interest. In studies of skin irritation, a* parallels erythema scores,[10,159–163] while studies of tanning or skin lightening may use L, ΔE, or ΔC.[160,161]

3.8.1 APPLICATIONS OF SKIN COLOR MEASUREMENT

Babulak et al.[159] used a Minolta Chromameter to assess the erythema produced by different soaps in a 24-h volar forearm patch test. Five percent solutions of different soaps were applied to demarcated sites on 21 subjects using a Duhring chamber. After 24 h the patches were removed, the sites rinsed and dried, and the color measured using a*. Skin color due to erythema resulting from irritancy of the soap and detergent bars paralleled TEWL as well as the Chromameter readings, that is, the most irritating bars also exhibited the highest color readings on the a* scale. Data are shown in Table 3.5.

When measuring erythema with any contact instrument, one must be careful to exert a constant and light pressure. The very definition of erythema is redness of the skin that is blanchable with contact pressure. There is a published guidance for the assessment of skin color.[10]

3.8.2 IMAGE ANALYSIS FOR SKIN COLOR MEASUREMENT

A disadvantage of the Chromameter is that it measures only a small spot. When analysis of large areas of skin is required, different methods must be employed. Miyamoto et al.[164] report development of a digital imaging system for the measurement of hyperpigmented spots on the face. Digital images were obtained under carefully controlled lighting conditions using a Sony DXC-537H 3-CCD camera at high resolution. Sophisticated software was developed to analyze the images picking out the spots and analyzing quasi-L* a* b* values. The same authors used this method to quantify the effects of six months of treatment with

TABLE 3.5
Comparative Assessment of Erythema Induced by Soaps Using the Chromameter[1]

Soap	Clinical Grade, Mean Rank[2]	TEWL (g/m²/h)		Chromameter Reading, a* Scale	
		Before	After	Before	After
Bar 1	4.2	5.1	11.4	7.5	9.8
Bar 2	2.5	4.8	9.3	7.8	8.9
Bar 3	3.7	4.5	13.5	7.0	9.9
Bar 4	2.1	4.4	8.9	7.1	8.8
Bar 5	4.8	4.8	13.2	7.5	10.1
Bar 6	3.8	4.8	11.2	7.4	9.5

[1] Rhein and Simion unpublished data.

[2] Lower the rank, the lower the invitation potential.

a skin-lightening moisturizer.[165] Both the image analysis method and visual grading showed significant improvements in hyperpigmented spots.

3.9 CLINICAL TRIAL DESIGNS FOR MEASURING MOISTURIZER EFFICACY AND MILDNESS OF SKIN CLEANSERS

3.9.1 MOISTURIZATION

Abrutyn et al.[166] have proposed the following sketch of study designs to investigate efficacy of moisturizing lotions (Table 3.6):

As an example protocol, De Paepe et al.[167] compared the effects of five body lotions and protective creams on water loss and electrical properties of skin. The lotions were applied to the inner forearm, and the transepidermal water loss was measured with a Tewameter® (Courage + Khazaka, Cologne, Germany) preapplication and 1-, 2-, and 3-h postapplication. Capacitance was measured with a Corneometer 820. Then the lotions were applied twice daily for 14 days. TEWL and capacitance measurements were made 12 h after the final application. Statistical differences were seen in the ability of each test product to reduce TEWL and increase capacitance. Some products were found to be more efficacious than others in both short-term and long-term studies, as assessed by the biophysical measurements.

Rawlings et al.[98] have reviewed protocols for moisturizer testing, including regression and mini-regression tests. In the classic regression test, 3 weeks of product application is followed by a 3-week regression phase in which no product is applied.[168] These tests are expensive and time-consuming. The development of noninvasive methods to assess moisturizers has led to the development of so-called mini-regression protocols where products are applied for 4 to 5 days followed by 3 days of regression.[169] In these protocols, panelists are usually treated with more than one product to allow within-subject comparisons. In this author's experience, electrical measurements with the instruments discussed above are a key part of most mini-regression protocols.

3.9.2 MILDNESS OF CLEANSERS

Barrier damage due to detergent cleansers can be assessed in several types of test methods. These include patch tests — the modified soap Chamber test[159] and the Kligman Frosch soap chamber test[170] — and use tests of various designs. Patch tests are excellent screening tools for safety testing because several products can be tested at once on either the backs or forearms, and irritation potential can be compared. However, for substantiation of claims, use tests are preferred. These tests usually employ some exaggerated method of exposure and instrumental assessments combined with visual grading (erythema and dryness). Kajs and Gartstein have reviewed the use of instrumental methods for assessing surfactant mildness.[54]

TABLE 3.6
Methods to Assess Moisturizer Efficacy

Test Method	Key Stressor	Parameters Measured	Treatment Modality and Evaluation Times	Measurable Benefit	References
Kligman leg regression test	Cold, dry weather	Clinical scoring Squamometry[a] Skin conductance or impedance (Novameter or Skicon)	Treat 14 or 21 days, then stop and track regression of skin Day 0 (baseline), (14), 21, 22, 23, 24, 25	Alleviation of dry skin and prevention of its return	Kligman (1978)[168] Boisits (1989), *J Cutan Aging Cosmet Dermatol* 1: 155–163
Mini-regression	Cold, dry weather	Skin conductance (Novameter or Skicon)	Treat forearms Daily for 4 days, measure conductance Day 0, 4, and regression on day 7	Moisturization	Grove (1992)[169]
Hand wash test	Repeated washing with soap	Clinical scoring Squamometry TEWL Corneometer (capacitance)	Wash, then treat with moisturizer, 5 times a day for 5 days; after last wash on day 5, do not treat Baseline and 1 h after final wash	Prevention of dryness induction, protection	Highley (1976)[71]
Reduction of preexisting irritation	Pretreat by patch testing with soap 1–2 days	Clinical scoring (erythema) TEWL	After soap patch, patch with lotion Baseline, 2 h after removing soap patch, 2 h after removing lotion patch test	Reduced irritation and skin water loss	Loden and Andersson (1996), *Br J Dermatol* 134: 215–220
Prevention of irritation	Patch testing with SLS after preapplication of lotion	Clinical scoring (erythema) TEWL	Pretreat with lotion a few days, then patch test 3 h with SLS Baseline and 3 h after SLS patch removed	Prevention of skin damage	Lachapelle (1996), *Curr Prob Dermatol* 25: 182–192

[a] Squamometry is discussed in a later section.

Obtaining objective data to discriminate between products in home-use testing is very difficult. Barel et al.[171] compared home-use testing to a modified soap chamber test[172] with a classic soap bar and a mild synthetic detergent bar. While subjects tended to perceive the soap bar to be harsher, neither grading nor instrumental methods distinguished the two products in the home-use test. Soap chamber testing clearly distinguished the synthetic detergent bar as milder in both instrumental (TEWL and Chromameter a*) measurements and visual grades.

The soap chamber test provides an exaggeration of use that aids in distinguishing between products, but it can be criticized because it is not representative of actual use conditions. This has led to the development of various tests that rely on exaggerated forearm washing.[172–176]

Simion et al.[177] used the arm wash method of Sharko et al.[175] to compare the effects of exaggerated washing of the forearms with a bar soap and a detergent bar. Thirty panelists who are prone to soap irritation participated. Each forearm was washed with its assigned bar for 2 min four times a day for up to 5 days. Subjects were equilibrated in a climate-controlled room for an hour before instrumental and clinical assessments. Baseline instrumental evaluations were taken along with baseline clinical scoring of erythema and flakiness/scaliness of the skin (each on a scale of 0 to 4, absent to severe) by an expert evaluator, and sensory attributes of redness, looks dry, feels dry, stinging/burning, tightness, and softness by the subjects themselves (each on an intensity scale of 0 to 6, none to extremely present). On the morning of each day of treatment, before each wash and 3 h after the final wash of the study, the subjects were equilibrated in the climate-controlled room and all evaluations were again taken.

Results are shown in Figure 3.6. After the third 2-min wash on day 1, the differences between the two cleansing products began to separate for both clinical assessments and self-perceived evaluations. The bar soap induced attributes consistent with a greater irritation potential than cleanser A. Panelists' self-assessments of intensity of flakiness, red, and looks dry were significantly different after the third wash, while clinically assessed erythema was significantly different before the first wash of day 2; clinical dryness was significantly different after the third wash on day 2. These and other self-perceived attributes, including tightness and burning, were also significantly different on day 2. The timing of the appearance of the emerging clinical and sensory attributes also varies.

The increased irritation potential of the soap bar vs. cleansing bar A was further substantiated by clinical and instrumental assessments forearm using washing methodology and patch testing (Table 3.7).

Currently, one of the most widely used methods for evaluating the mildness of cleansing products is the forearm-controlled application test (FCAT), first described by Lukacovic et al.[174] and modified by Ertel et al.[173] In the FCAT, circular sites on the volar forearms of panelists (typically 40 to 45) are washed using a standard procedure. Sites are randomized along the forearm and washed by technicians. Soap bars are rubbed with a wet Masslin® nonwoven towel for 6 sec to work up lather. The resulting lather is applied to the site, the site is lathered for 10 sec, and the lather is left standing for 90 sec. (Liquid products

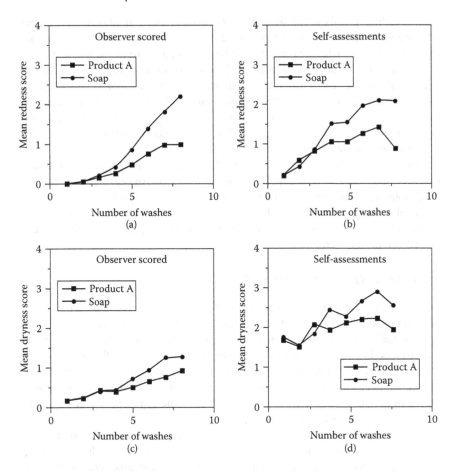

FIGURE 3.6 Measurement of clinical and self-perceived skin effects of bar soap.

TABLE 3.7
Comparison of the Irritancy of a Soap and Cleansing Bar Using Three Treatment Methods

	Forearm Wash Use Test — Sharko				Kligman Soap Chamber		Modified Soap Chamber — Rhein	
	Erythema	Scaling/ Dryness	Chroma Meter	TEWL, g/m²/h	Erythema	Scaling/ Dryness	Erythema	TEWL g/m²/h
Bar A	1.0	0.9	7.22	11.4	1.0	1.0	0.43	9.3
Soap	2.2	0.91.2	11.4	21.2	1.63	2.56	1.38	13.2

can be applied directly to the site.) While the product is standing on the site, other sites are washed. Finally, the site is rinsed with running water for 20 sec. A total of eight products (including controls) can be compared in one test with this method if the treatments are applied simultaneously to each arm. The procedure is repeated twice in the morning and twice in the afternoon, Monday through Thursday. On Friday, washings are carried out in the morning and final evaluations are made in the afternoon. Typically, TEWL, Chromameter, Corneometer, and Skicon measurements are made in addition to visual grading of dryness and erythema. The FCAT protocol can also be performed on dry legs (LCAT).

Ertel et al.[173] showed that consistent FCAT results can be obtained differentiating a mild synthetic detergent bar from a classic soap bar regardless of climatic conditions, but the experience of this author is that much better results can be obtained during cooler weather. Testing during winter conditions can distinguish between very mild products.[178] A number of clinical testing laboratories run FACT and LCAT protocols routinely.

3.10 *IN VITRO* ASSESSMENTS

In vitro skin equivalents are used successfully to assess effects of active compounds on skin. Two *in vitro* skin equivalent methods are compared in Table 3.8, and the findings and recommendations as to the advantages of these methods are discussed below. The effects of actives or treatments on cell viability using mitochondrial viability (MTT) dye assay; proliferation using 3-thymidine uptake (indicating DNA synthesis); differentiation measuring filaggrin, transglutaminase, involucrin, loricrin, etc.; and cytokine expression can be easily assessed to characterize the skin responses.

The Test Skin II method probably more closely typifies human skin, is an approved burn wound treatment, and is easier to handle, i.e., it is a dry sheet to be stored at room temperature until open. It also contains fibroblasts from which many of the growth factors originate. The SkinEthic is epidermal derived and lays on an inert polycarbonate filter rather than collagen. It arrives in a culture plate and must be kept cold until use. It lacks the dermal-derived and fibroblast-derived factors; these may want to be assessed for antiaging treatments such as matrix metalloproteinase inhibitors. It does have the advantage that there are many different skin versions available, such as oral and vaginal mucosal, tanned skin, and others. None have mast cells for looking at effects on histamine release, which is a marker for inflammation but is more representative of immune involvement.

Also, a third corporation, Matek Corporation, specializes in epidermal equivalents (www.mattek.com). It has epidermal models called EpiDerm, as well as other tissue organ cultures, like ocular, melanoderm, and Epi-airway. These cultures are also only epidermal in origin, but studies work very nicely with them if the epidermis is the target of interest. Some references comparing these models are provided.[179–182] Netzlaff et al. has compared three models for their suitability for testing phototoxicity, irritancy, and substance penetration. They have found that the barrier function in these models is much less developed than in native skin.[183]

TABLE 3.8

Comparison of Two *In Vitro* Human Skin Equivalents

Attribute	Test Skin II (Organogenesis, Inc.)	SkinEthic
(Contact)	www.testskinII.com	www.skinethic.com
Material	Full-thickness epidermal and dermal, human keratinocytes, biological active fibroblasts on bovine collagen type I	Epidermal on a polycarbonate filter, human keratinocytes
Storage and ease of use	Dry sheets, store at room temperature until open, then at 37°, use in 5 days	In culture plate of different sizes, store cold until use, use in 5 days
Epidermal markers	Involucrin, transglutaminase, filaggrin, desmoglein, desmoplakin	Filaggrin, transglutaminase, involucrin, loricrin, hemidesmosomes
Basement membrane markers	Laminin, integrin, type IV collagen, HS-proteoglycan	Type IV collagen, laminin, integrin -VI and -IV
Keratins	K1, K5, K6, K10, K16, K14 (suprabasal); AE1, AE3 (basal)	K1, K10 (suprabasal); K5, K14 (basal)
Fibroblasts	Secrete type IV collagen, fibronectin, GAGs, and growth factors described below	No fibroblasts
Cytokine/growth factor mRNA expression	FGF-1, FGF-2, FGF-7, ECGF, IGF-1, IGF-2, PDGF, TGF- and TGF- (1 and 3), IL-1, IL-6, IL-8, IL-11, VEGF, others as needed if derived from fibroblasts and kerats	IL-1, IL-6, IL-8, IL-11, others as needed that are derived from kerats
Lipids	Ceramides, cholesterol, cholesterol sulfate, FFA	Ceramides, lanosterol, triglyceride, cholesterol, FFA
Measurements	Cell viability (MTT), keratins, 3Hthymidine uptake, cytokine mRNA expression and protein, fatty acid	Cell viability (MTT), keratins, 3Hthymidine, cytokine mRNA expression and protein, fatty acid
Transit rates	11–14 days, similar to human epidermis/stratum corneum	Similar to human

3.11   CONCLUSIONS

Noninvasive methods for the measurement of skin have come a long way in the 30 years since the first meeting of the group that eventually became the International Society for Bioengineering and the Skin took place in Miami. Instruments that were then only "home built" are now widely available, and there has been a fantastic proliferation of new instruments and protocols for their use.

Hopefully, this review has given a flavor for some of the major instrumental methods and protocols employed for noninvasive quantification of cosmetic product effects. If your favorite measurement or protocol was omitted, I apologize but it was not possible to cover them all. Given the rate of current progress in the field, it seems certain that growth in this important area of skin research will continue, making the job of future reviewers even more difficult.

ACKNOWLEDGMENTS

The author thanks Linda Rhein for many valuable discussions on this work. Figure 3.1 was drawn by Robin M. Wickett.

REFERENCES

1. *Cutaneous Investigations in Health and Disease: Noninvasive Methods and Instrumentation.* New York: Marcel Dekker, 1989.
2. *Handbook of Non-invasive Methods and the Skin.* Ann Arbor, MI: CRC Press, 1995.
3. *Bioengineering of the Skin: Skin Biomechanics,* 1st ed. Boca Raton, FL: CRC Press, 2001.
4. *Measuring Skin.* Berlin: Springer-Verlag, 2004.
5. *Bioengineering of the Skin: Water and the Stratum Corneum,* 2nd ed. Boca Raton, FL: CRC Press, 2004.
6. Berardesca E. EEMCO guidance for the assessment of stratum corneum hydration: electrical methods. *Skin Res Technol* 1997; 3: 126–132.
7. Berardesca E, Leveque JL, Masson P. EEMCO guidance for the measurement of skin microcirculation. *Skin Pharmacol Appl Skin Physiol* 2002; 15: 442–456.
8. Leveque JL. EEMCO guidance for the assessment of skin topography. The European Expert Group on Efficacy Measurement of Cosmetics and Other Topical Products. *J Eur Acad Dermatol Venereol* 1999; 12: 103–114.
9. Parra JL, Paye M. EEMCO guidance for the *in vivo* assessment of skin surface pH. *Skin Pharmacol Appl Skin Physiol* 2003; 16: 188–202.
10. Pierard GE. EEMCO guidance for the assessment of skin colour. *J Eur Acad Dermatol Venereol* 1998; 10: 1–11.
11. Pierard GE. EEMCO guidance to the *in vivo* assessment of tensile functional properties of the skin. Part 1. Relevance to the structures and ageing of the skin and subcutaneous tissues. *Skin Pharmacol Appl Skin Physiol* 1999; 12: 352–362.
12. Rodrigues L. EEMCO guidance to the *in vivo* assessment of tensile functional properties of the skin. Part 2. Instrumentation and test modes. *Skin Pharmacol Appl Skin Physiol* 2001; 14: 52–67.

13. Rogiers V. EEMCO guidance for the assessment of transepidermal water loss in cosmetic sciences. *Skin Pharmacol Appl Skin Physiol* 2001; 14: 117–128.
14. Elias PM. Stratum corneum defensive functions: an integrated view. *J Invest Dermatol* 2005; 125: 183–200.
15. Madison KC. Barrier function of the skin: "la raison d'etre" of the epidermis. *J Invest Dermatol* 2003; 121: 231–241.
16. Marks R, Barton SP. The significance of the size and shape of corneocytes. In *Stratum Corneum*, Marks R, Plewig G, Eds. New York: Springer-Verlag, 1983, pp. 161–170.
17. Plewig G, Scheuber E, Reuter B, et al. Thickness of corneoctyes. In *Stratum Corneum*, Marks R, Plewig G, Eds. New York: Springer-Verlag, 1983, pp. 171–174.
18. Holbrook KA, Odland GF. Regional differences in the thickness (cell layers) of the human stratum corneum: an ultrastructural analysis. *J Invest Dermatol* 1974; 62: 415–422.
19. Ya-Xian Z, Suetake T, Tagami H. Number of cell layers of the stratum corneum in normal skin: relationship to the anatomical location on the body, age, sex and physical parameters. *Arch Dermatol Res* 1999; 291: 555–559.
20. Swartzendruber DC, Wertz PW, Kitko DJ, et al. Molecular models of the intercellular lipid lamellae in mammalian stratum corneum. *J Invest Dermatol* 1989; 92: 251–257.
21. Wertz PW. Lipids and barrier function of the skin. *Acta Dermatol Venereol Suppl (Stockh)* 2000; 208: 7–11.
22. Loden M. The simultaneous penetration of water and sodium lauryl sulfate through isolated human skin. *J Soc Cosmet Chem* 1990; 41: 227–233.
23. Scheuplein RJ, Ross L. Effects of surfactants and solvents on the permeability of the epidermis. *J Soc Cosmet Chem* 1970; 21: 853–873.
24. Warner RR, Boissy YL, Lilly NA, et al. Water disrupts stratum corneum lipid lamellae: damage is similar to surfactants. *J Invest Dermatol* 1999; 113: 960–966.
25. Fartasch M. Ultrastructure of the epidermal barrier after irritation. *Microsc Res Tech* 1997; 37: 193–199.
26. Rawlings AV, Watkinson A, Rogers J, et al. Abnormalities in stratum corneum structure, lipid composition, and desmosome degradation in soap-induced winter xerosis. *J Soc Cosmet Chem* 1994; 45: 203–220.
27. Barel AO, Clarys P, Gabard B. *In vivo* evaluation of the hydration state of the skin: measurements and methods for claim support. In *Cosmetics: Controlled Efficacy Studies and Regulations*, Elsner P, Merck HF, Maibach H, Eds. Berlin: Springer-Verlag, 1999, pp. 56–80.
28. Bashir SJ, Maibach HI. Cosmetic efficacy: an evidence oriented approach. In *The Chemistry and Manufacturing of Cosmetics*, Schlossman M, Ed. New York: Allured Publishing, 2000, pp. 163–182.
29. Bernengo J-C, Rigal J. Physical methods of measuring stratum corneum water content *in vivo*. In *Measuring the Skin*, Agache P, Humbert P, Eds. Berlin: Springer-Verlag, 2004, pp. 112–152.
30. Fischer TW, Wigger-Alberti W, Elsner P. Assessment of 'dry skin': current bioengineering methods and test designs. *Skin Pharmacol Appl Skin Physiol* 2001; 14: 183–195.
31. Hannon, W., Maibach H. Efficacy of moisturizers. In *Textbook of Cosmetic Dermatology*, 2nd ed., Baran R, Maibach H, Eds. London: Martin Dunitz, 1998, pp. 245–284.

32. Loden M, Lindberg M. Testing of moisturizers. In *Bioengineering of the Skin: Water and the Stratum Corneum*, 2nd ed., Fluhr J, Elsner P, Berardesca E, et al., Eds. Boca Raton, FL: CRC Press, 2004, pp. 387–406.

33. Blank IH. Further observations on factors which influence the water content of stratum corneum. *J Invest Dermatol* 1953; 21: 259–271.

34. Warner R, Lilly N. Correlation of water content with ultrastructure in the stratum corneum. In *Bioengineering of the Skin: Water and the Stratum Corneum*, Elsner P, Berardesca E, Maibach HI, Eds. Boca Raton, FL: CRC Press, 1994, pp. 3–22.

35. Rawlings AV, Matts PJ. Stratum corneum moisturization at the molecular level: an update in relation to the dry skin cycle. *J Invest Dermatol* 2005; 124: 1099–1110.

36. Frobe CF, Simion FA, Ohlmeyer H, et al. Prevention of stratum corneum lipid phase transitions *in-vitro* by glycerol: an alternate mechanism for skin moisturization. *J Soc Cosmet Chem* 1990; 41: 51–65.

37. Mattai J, Frobe CF, Rhein LD, et al. Prevention of stratum corneum lipid phase transitions *in-vitro* by cosmetic additives: differential scanning calorimetry, optical microscopy and water evaporation studies. *J Soc Cosmet Chem* 1993; 44: 89–100.

38. Rawlings A, Harding C, Watkinson A, et al. The effect of glycerol and humidity on desmosome degradation in stratum corneum. *Arch Dermatol Res* 1995; 287: 457–464.

39. Fluhr JW, Gloor M, Lehmann L, et al. Glycerol accelerates recovery of barrier function *in vivo*. *Acta Dermatol Venereol* 1999; 79: 418–421.

40. Loden M. Urea-containing moisturizers influence barrier properties of normal skin. *Arch Dermatol Res* 1996; 288: 103–107.

41. Aubert L, Anthoine P, de Rigal J, et al. An *in vivo* assessment of the biomechanical properties of human skin modifications under the influence of cosmetic products. *Int J Cosmet Sci* 1985; 7: 51–59.

42. Murray BC, Wickett RR. Correlations between Dermal Torque Meter, Cutometer and Dermal Phase Meter measurements of human skin. *Skin Res Technol* 1997; 3: 101–106.

43. Cooper ER, Missel PJ, Hannon DP, et al. Mechanical properties of dry, normal and glycerol-treated skin as measured by the gas-bearing electrodynamometer. *J Soc Cosmet Chem* 1985; 36: 335–348.

44. Batt MD, Davis WB, Fairhurst E, et al. Changes in the physical properties of the stratum corneum following treatment with glycerol. *J Soc Cosmet Chem* 1988; 39: 367–381.

45. Summers RS, Summers B, Chander P, et al. The effect of lipids with and without humectant on skin xerosis. *J Soc Cosmet Chem* 1996; 47: 27–39.

46. Loden M, Barany E. Skin-identical lipids versus petrolatum in the treatment of tape-stripped and detergent-perturbed human skin. *Acta Derm Venereol* 2000; 80: 412–415.

47. Middleton JD. Development of a skin cream designed to reduce dry and flaky skin. *J Soc Cosmet Chem* 1974; 25: 519–534.

48. Smith WP. Hydroxy acids and skin aging. *Cosmet Toiletries* 1994; 109: 41–48.

49. Berardesca E, Distante F, Vignoli GP, et al. Alpha hydroxyacids modulate stratum corneum barrier function. *Br J Dermatol* 1997; 137: 934–938.

50. Matts PJ, Oblong JE, Bissett D. A review of the range of effects of niacinamide in human skin. *IFSCC Mag* 2002; 5: 285–290.

51. Berardesca E, Maibach HI. Transepidermal water loss and skin surface hydration in the noninvasive assessment of stratum corneum function. *Derm Beruf Umwelt* 1990; 38: 50–53.

52. Fluhr JW, Praessler J, Akengin A, et al. Air flow at different temperatures increases sodium lauryl sulphate-induced barrier disruption and irritation *in vivo*. *Br J Dermatol* 2005; 152: 1228–1234.

53. Hachem JP, De Paepe K, Sterckx G, et al. Evaluation of biophysical and clinical parameters of skin barrier function among hospital workers. *Contact Derm* 2002; 46: 220–223.

54. Kajs TM, Gartstein V. Review of the instrumental assessment of skin: effects of cleansing products. *J Soc Cosmet Chem* 1991; 42: 249–272.

55. Treffel P, Gabard B. Measurement of sodium lauryl sulfate-induced skin irritation. *Acta Dermatol Venereol* 1996; 76: 341–343.

56. Loden M. Transepidermal water loss and dry skin. In *Bioengineering of the Skin: Water and the Stratum Corneum*, 2nd ed., Fluhr J, Elsner P, Berardesca E, et al., Eds. Boca Raton, FL: CRC Press, 2004, pp. 171–185.

57. Chou TC, Lin KH, Wang SM, et al. Transepidermal water loss and skin capacitance alterations among workers in an ultra-low humidity environment. *Arch Dermatol Res* 2005; 296: 489–495.

58. Nilsson GE. Measurement of water exchange through the skin. *Med Biol Eng Comput* 1977; 15: 209–218.

59. Pinnagoda J. Hardware and measuring principles: evaporimeter. In *Bioengineering of the Skin: Water and the Stratum Corneum*, Elsner P, Berardesca E, Maibach HI, Eds. Boca Raton, FL: CRC Press, 1994, pp. 51–56.

60. Gabard B, Treffel P. Transepidermal water loss. In *Measuring Skin*, Agache P, Humbert P, Eds. Berlin: Springer-Verlag, 2004, pp. 553–564.

61. Barel AO, Clarys P. Study of the stratum corneum barrier function by transepidermal water loss measurements: comparison between two commercial instruments: evaporimeter and Tewameter. *Skin Pharmacol* 1995; 8: 186–195.

62. Grove G, Grove M, Zerweck C, et al. Comparative metrology of the evaporimeter and the DermaLab TEWL probe. *Skin Res Technol* 1999; 5: 1–8.

63. De Paepe K, Houben E, Adam R, et al. Validation of the VapoMeter, a closed unventilated chamber system to assess transepidermal water loss vs. the open chamber Tewameter. *Skin Res Technol* 2005; 11: 61–69.

64. Nuutinen J, Alanen E, Autio P, et al. A closed unventilated chamber for the measurement of transepidermal water loss. *Skin Res Technol* 2003; 9: 85–89.

65. Hammarlund K, Nilsson GE, Oberg PA, et al. Transepidermal water loss in newborn infants. I. Relation to ambient humidity and site of measurement and estimation of total transepidermal water loss. *Acta Paediatr Scand* 1977; 66: 553–562.

66. Mathias CG, Wilson DM, Maibach HI. Transepidermal water loss as a function of skin surface temperature. *J Invest Dermatol* 1981; 77: 219–220.

67. Pinnagoda J, Tupker RA, Agner T, et al. Guidelines for transepidermal water loss (TEWL) measurement. A report from the Standardization Group of the European Society of Contact Dermatitis. *Contact Derm* 1990; 22: 164–178.

68. Rogiers V. EEMCO guidance for the assessment of transepidermal water loss in cosmetic sciences. *Skin Pharmacol Appl Skin Physiol* 2001; 14: 117–128.

69. Loden M, Lindberg M. Product testing of moisturizers. In *Bioengineering of the Skin: Water and the Stratum Corneum*, Elsner P, Berardesca E, Maibach HI, Eds. Boca Raton, FL: CRC Press, 1994, pp. 275–289.

70. Loden M. Biophysical methods of providing objective documentation of the effects of moisturizing creams. *Skin Res Technol* 1995; 1: 101–108.

71. Highley D. A stereomicroscopic method for determination of moisturizing efficacy in humans. *J Soc Cosmet Chem* 1976; 27: 351–363.

72. Tagami H, Ohi M, Iwatsuki K, et al. Evaluation of the skin surface hydration *in vivo* by electrical measurement. *J Invest Dermatol* 1980; 75: 500–507.

73. Tagami H, Ohi M, Iwatsuki K, et al. Electrical measurement of the hydration state of the skin surface *in vivo*. In *Stratum Corneum*, Marks R, Plewig G, Eds. Springer-Verlag, Berlin, 1983, pp. 251–256.

74. Tagami H, Yoshikuni K. Evaluation of the hydration state of the stratum corneum *in vitro* by electrical measurement. *Bioeng Skin* 1985; 1: 93–99.

75. Tagami H. Impedance measurements for evaluation of the hydration state of the skin surface. In *Cutaneous Investigations in Health and Disease*, Leveque JL, Ed. New York: Marcel Dekker, 1989, pp. 79–111.

76. Tagami H. Measurement of electrical conductance and impedance. In *Handbook of Non-invasive Methods and the Skin*, 1st ed., Serup J, Jemec GBE, Eds. Ann Arbor, MI: CRC Press, 1995, pp. 159–170.

77. Berardesca E, Distante F, Vignoli GP, et al. Alpha hydroxyacids modulate stratum corneum barrier function. *Br J Dermatol* 1997; 137: 934–938.

78. Clarys P, Barel AO, Gabard B. Non-invasive electrical measurements for the evaluation of the hydration state of the skin: comparison between three conventional instruments: the Corneometer, the Skicon and the Nova DPM. *Skin Res Technol* 1999; 5: 14–20.

79. Courage W. Hardware and measuring principle: Corneometer. In *Bioengineering of the Skin: Water and the Stratum Corneum*, Elsner P, Berardesca E, Maibach HI, Eds. Boca Raton, FL: CRC Press, 1994, pp. 171–175.

80. Khazaka G. Assessment of stratum corneum hydration: Corneometer CM 825. In *Bioengineering of the Skin: Water and the Stratum Corneum*, 2nd ed., Fluhr J, Elsner P, Berardesca E, et al., Eds. Boca Raton, FL: CRC Press, 2004, pp. 249–262.

81. Fluhr JW, Gloor M, Lazzerini S, et al. Comparative study of five instruments measuring stratum corneum hydration (Corneometer CM 820 and CM 825, Skicon 200, Nova DPM 9003, DermLab). Part I. *In vitro*. *Skin Res Technol* 1999; 5: 161–170.

82. Morrison BM, Scala D. Comparison of instrumental measurements of skin hydration. *J Toxicol Cut Ocular Toxicol* 1996; 15: 305–314.

83. Visscher MO, Wickett RR, Smith-Canning J. Effect of hand hygiene regimens on skin condition in health care workers (HCWs). *Am J Infect Control* 2006; accepted for publication.

84. Gabard B, Treffel P. Hardware and measuring principle: the NOVA DPM 9003. In *Bioengineering of the Skin: Water and the Stratum Corneum*, Elsner P, Berardesca E, Maibach H, Eds. Boca Raton, FL: CRC Press, 1994, pp. 177–195.

85. Wickett R. Hardware and measuring principle: the NOVA DPM. In *Bioengineering of the Skin: Water and the Stratum Corneum*, 2nd ed., Fluhr J, Elsner P, Berardesca E, et al., Eds. Boca Raton, FL: CRC Press, 2004, pp. 263–274.

86. Li F, Visscher M, Conroy E, et al. The ability of electrical measurements to predict skin moisturization. I. Effects of salt and glycerin on short-term measurements. *J Cosmet Sci* 2001; 52: 13–22.

87. Visscher MO, Tolia GT, Wickett RR, et al. Effect of soaking and natural moisturizing factor on stratum corneum water-handling properties. *J Cosmet Sci* 2003; 54: 289–300.

88. Wickett RR. Stretching the skin surface: skin elasticity. *Cosmet Toiletries* 2001; 116: 47–54.

89. Boyce ST, Supp AP, Harriger MD, et al. Surface electrical capacitance as a noninvasive index of epidermal barrier in cultured skin substitutes in athymic mice. *J Invest Dermatol* 1996; 107: 82–87.

90. Okah FA, Wickett RR, Pickens WL, et al. Surface electrical capacitance as a noninvasive bedside measure of epidermal barrier maturation in the newborn infant. *Pediatrics* 1995; 96: 688–692.

91. Visscher MO, Hoath SB, Conroy E, et al. Effect of semipermeable membranes on skin barrier repair following tape stripping. *Arch Dermatol Res* 2001; 293: 491–499.

92. Wickett RR, Mutschelknaus JL, Hoath SB. Ontogeny of water sorption-desorption in the perinatal rat. *J Invest Dermatol* 1993; 100: 407–411.

93. Wickett RR, Nath V, Tanaka R, et al. Use of continuous electrical capacitance and transepidermal water loss measurements for assessing barrier function in neonatal rat skin. *Skin Pharmacol* 1995; 8: 179–185.

94. Brancaleon L, Bamberg MP, Sakamaki T, et al. Attenuated total reflection-Fourier transform infrared spectroscopy as a possible method to investigate biophysical parameters of stratum corneum *in vivo*. *J Invest Dermatol* 2001; 116: 380–386.

95. Blichmann CW, Serup J, Winther A. Effects of single application of a moisturizer: evaporation of emulsion water, skin surface temperature, electrical conductance, electrical capacitance, and skin surface (emulsion) lipids. *Acta Dermatol Venereol* 1989; 69: 327–330.

96. Gabard B. Testing the efficacy of moisturizers. In *Bioengineering of the Skin: Water and the Stratum Corneum*, 2nd ed., Fluhr J, Elsner P, Berardesca E, et al., Eds. Boca Raton, FL: CRC Press, 2004, pp. 211–236.

97. Loden M, Lindberg M. The influence of a single application of different moisturizers on the skin capacitance. *Acta Dermatol Venereol* 1991; 71: 79–82.

98. Rawlings AV, Canestrari DA, Dobkowski B. Moisturizer technology versus clinical performance. *Dermatol Ther* 2004; 17 (Suppl 1): 49–56.

99. Li F, Visscher M, Conroy E, et al. The ability of electrical measurements to predict skin moisturization. II. Correlations between one hour measurements and long term results. *J Cosmet Sci* 2001; 52: 23–33.

100. Querleux B. *In vivo* skin magnetic resonance imaging and spectroscopy. In *Measuring the Skin*, Agache P, Humbert P, Eds. Berlin: Springer-Verlag, 2004, pp. 215–221.

101. Hyde JS, Jesmanowicz A, Kneeland JB. Surface coil for MR imaging of the skin. *Magn Reson Med* 1987; 5: 456–461.

102. Querleux B. Nuclear magnetic resonance (NMR) examination of the epidermis *in vivo*. In *Handbook of Non-invasive Methods and the Skin*, Serup J, Jemec BE, Eds. Boca Raton, FL: CRC Press, 1995, pp. 133–139.

103. Bittoun J, Saint-Jalmes H, Querleux BG, et al. *In vivo* high-resolution MR imaging of the skin in a whole-body system at 1.5 T. *Radiology* 1990; 176: 457–460.

104. Martin KA. Direct measurement of moisture in the skin by NIR spectroscopy. *J Soc Cosmet Chem* 1993; 44: 249–261.

105. de Rigal J, Losch MJ, Bazin R, et al. Near-infrared spectroscopy: a new approach to the characterization of dry skin. *J Soc Cosmet Chem* 1993; 44: 197–209.

106. Arimoto H, Egawa M. Non-contact skin moisture measurement based on near-infrared spectroscopy. *Appl Spectrosc* 2004; 58: 1439–1446.

107. Arimoto H, Egawa M, Yamada Y. Depth profile of diffuse reflectance near-infrared spectroscopy for measurement of water content in skin. *Skin Res Technol* 2005; 11: 27–35.

108. Zhang SL, Meyers CL, Subramanyan K, et al. Near infrared imaging for measuring and visualizing skin hydration. A comparison with visual assessment and electrical methods. *J Biomed Opt* 2005; 10: 031107.

109. Agache PG. Twistometry measurement of skin elasticity. In *Handbook of Non-invasive Methods and the Skin*, Serup J, Jemec GBE, Eds. Ann Arbor, MI: CRC Press, 1995, pp. 319–334.

110. Aubert L, Anthoine P, de Rigal J, et al. An *in vivo* assessment of the biomechanical properties of human skin modifications under the influence of cosmetic products. *Int J Cosmet Sci* 1985; 7: 51–59.

111. de Rigal J, Leveque JL. *In vivo* measurement of the stratum corneum elasticity. *Bioeng Skin* 1985; 1: 13–23.

112. de Rigal J. Hardware and basic principles of the Dermal Torque Meter. In *Bioengineering of the Skin: Skin Biomechanics*, 1st ed., Elsner P, Berardesca E, Wilhelm KP, et al., Eds. Boca Raton, FL: CRC Press, 2001, pp. 63–76.

113. Barel AO, Courage W, Clarys P. Suction method for measurement of skin mechanical properties: the Cutometer. In *Handbook of Non-invasive Methods and the Skin*, Serup J, Jemec GBE, Eds. Boca Raton, FL: CRC Press, 1995, pp. 335–340.

114. Berndt U, Elsner P. Hardware and measuring principle: the Cutometer. In *Bioengineering of the Skin: Skin Biomechanics*, 1st ed., Elsner P, Berardesca E, Wilhelm KP, et al., Eds. Boca Raton, FL: CRC Press, 2001, pp. 91–97.

115. Barel AO, Lambrecht R, Clarys P. Mechanical function of the skin: state of the art. In *Skin Bioengineering Techniques and Applications in Dermatology and Cosmetology*, Elsner P, Barel AO, Berardesca E, et al., Eds. Basel: Karger, 1998, pp. 69–83.

116. Boyce ST, Supp AP, Wickett RR, et al. Assessment with the Dermal Torque Meter of skin pliability after treatment of burns with cultured skin substitutes. *J Burn Care Rehab* 2000; 21: 55–63.

117. Escoffier C, de Rigal J, Rochefort A, et al. Age-related mechanical properties of human skin: an *in vivo* study. *J Invest Dermatol* 1989; 93: 353–357.

118. Dobrev H. Use of Cutometer to assess epidermal hydration. *Skin Res Technol* 2000; 6: 239–244.

119. Murray BC, Wickett RR. Sensitivity of Cutometer data to stratum corneum hydration level. *Skin Res Technol* 1996; 2: 167–172.

120. Wiechers JW, Barlow T. Skin moisturization and elasticity originates from at least two different mechanisms. *Int J Cosmet Sci* 1999; 21: 425–435.

121. Cua AB, Wilhelm KP, Maibach HI. Elastic properties of human skin: relation to age, sex, and anatomical region. *Arch Dermatol Res* 1990; 282: 283–288.

122. Balin AK, Pratt LA. Physiological consequences of human skin aging. *Cutis* 1989; 43: 431–436.

123. Bouissou H, Pieraggi M, Julian M, et al. The elastic tissue of the skin: a comparison of spontaneous and actinic (solar) aging. 1988. *Int J Dermatol* 1988; 27: 327–335.

124. Fazio MJ, Olsen DR, Uitto J. Skin aging: lessons from cutis laxa and elastoderma. *Cutis* 1989; 43: 437–444.

125. Smalls LK, Wickett R R, Visscher M. Effect of dermal thickness, tissue composition, and body site on skin biomechanical properties. *Skin Res Technol* 2006; in press.

126. Smalls LK, Hicks M, Passeretti D, et al. Effect of weight loss on cellulite (gynoid lipodystrophy). *Plast Reconstr Surg* 2006; accepted for publication.

127. Smalls LK, Lee CY, Whitestone J, et al. Quantitative model of cellulite: three-dimensional skin surface topography, biophysical characterization, and relationship to human perception. *J Cosmet Sci* 2005; 56: 105–120.

128. Zhouani H, Vargiolu R. Skin line morphology: trees and branches. In *Measuring Skin*, Agache P, Humbert P, Eds. Berlin: Springer-Verlag, 2004, pp. 40–59.

129. Corcuff P, Chatenay F, Leveque JL. A fully automated system to study skin surface patterns. *Int J Cosmet Sci* 1984; 6: 167–176.

130. De Paepe K, Lagarde JM, Gall Y, et al. Microrelief of the skin using a light transmission method. *Arch Dermatol Res* 2000; 292: 500–510.

131. Grove GL, Grove MJ. Objective methods for assessing skin surface topography noninvasively. In *Cutaneous Investigations in Health and Disease: Noninvasive Methods and Instrumentation*, Leveque JL, Ed. New York: Marcel Dekker, 1989, pp. 1–32.

132. Jacobi U, Chen M, Frankowski G, et al. *In vivo* determination of skin surface topography using an optical 3D device. *Skin Res Technol* 2004; 10: 207–214.

133. Lagarde JM, Rouvrais C, Black D. Topography and anisotropy of the skin surface with ageing. *Skin Res Technol* 2005; 11: 110–119.

134. Cook T. Profilometry of skin: a useful tool for the substantiation of cosmetic efficacy. *J Soc Cosmet Chem* 1980; 31: 339–359.

135. Cook T, Craft TJ, Brunelle RL, et al. Quantification of the skin's topography by skin profilometry. *Int J Cosmet Sci* 1982; 4: 195–205.

136. Makki S, Agache P, Mignot J, et al. Statistical analysis and three-dimensional representation of the human skin surface. *J Soc Cosmet Chem* 1984; 35: 311–325.

137. Hoppe U. Topologie der Hautoberfläche. *J Soc Cosmet Chem* 1979; 30: 213–239.

138. Corcuff P, Chatenay F, Brun A. Evaluation of anti-wrinkle effects on humans. *Int J Cosmet Sci* 1985; 7: 117–126.

139. Robert C, Robert AM, Robert L. Effect of a preparation containing a fucose-rich polysaccharide on periorbital wrinkles of human voluntaries. *Skin ResTechnol* 2005; 11: 47–52.

140. Barel A, Calomme M, Timchenko A, et al. Effect of oral intake of choline-stabilized orthosilicic acid on skin, nails and hair in women with photodamaged skin. *Arch Dermatol Res* 2005; 297: 147–153.

141. Jaspers S, Hopermann H, Sauerman G, et al. Rapid *in vivo* measurement of the topography of human skin by active image triangulation using a digital micromirror device. *Skin Res Technol* 1999; 5: 195–207.

142. Friedman PM, Skover GR, Payonk G, et al. Quantitative evaluation of nonablative laser technology. *Semin Cutan Med Surg* 2002; 21: 266–273.

143. Ryu JS, Park SG, Kwak TJ, et al. Improving lip wrinkles: lipstick-related image analysis. *Skin Res Technol* 2005; 11: 157–164.

144. Miller DL. Sticky slides and tape techniques to harvest stratum corneum material. In *Handbook of Non-invasive Methods and the Skin*, Serup J, Jemec GBE, Eds. Boca Raton, FL: CRC Press, 1996, pp. 149–151.

145. Schantz H, Kligman AM, Manning S, et al. Quantification of dry (xerotic) skin by image analysis of scales removed by adhesive discs. *J Soc Cosmet Chem* 1993; 44: 53–63.

146. Wilhelm KP, Kaspar K, Schumann F, et al. Development and validation of a semiautomatic image analysis system for measuring skin desquamation with D-Squames. *Skin Res Technol* 2002; 8: 98–105.

147. Schatz H, Altmeyer PJ, Kligman AM. Dry skin and scaling evaluated by D-Squames and image analysis. In *Handbook of Non-invasive Methods and the Skin*, Serup J, Jemec GBE, Eds. Boca Raton, FL: CRC Press, 1995, pp. 153–157.

148. De Paepe K, Janssens K, Hachem JP, et al. Squamometry as a screening method for the evaluation of hydrating products. *Skin Res Technol* 2001; 7: 184–192.

149. Charbonnier V, Morrison BM, Jr., Paye M, et al. Subclinical, non-erythematous irritation with an open assay model (washing): sodium lauryl sulfate (SLS) versus sodium laureth sulfate (SLES). *Food Chem Toxicol* 2001; 39: 279–286.

150. Lentner A, Wienert V. A new method for assessing the gloss of human skin. *Skin Pharmacol* 1996; 9: 184–189.

151. Motwani MR, Rhein LD, Zatz JL. Differential scanning calorimetry studies of sebum models. *J Cosmet Sci* 2001; 52: 211–224.

152. Nicolaides N, Ansari MN, Fu HC, et al. Lipid composition of comedones compared with that of human skin surface in acne patients. *J Invest Dermatol* 1970; 54: 487–495.

153. Kligman AM, Miller DL, McGinley Kj. Sebutape: a device for visualizing and measuring human sebaceous secretion. *J Soc Cosmet Chem* 1986; 37: 369–374.

154. Serup J. Formation of oiliness and sebum output: comparison of a lipid-absorbant and occlusive tape method with photometry. *Clin Exp Dermatol* 1991; 13: 369–373.

155. Mills JK, Vowels BR, Pagnoni A, et al. Comparison of image analysis of lipid absorbent tapes and thin layer chromatography (TLC) for determination of sebum excretion. *J Invest Dermatol* 1996; 106: 919.

156. Rizer RL. Oily skin: claim support strategies. In *Cosmetics: Controlled Efficacy Studies and Regulations*, Elsner P, Merck HF, Eds. Berlin: Springer-Verlag, 1999, pp. 81–91.

157. Kollias N. The physical basis of skin color and its evaluation. *Clin Dermatol* 1995; 13: 361–367.

158. Andreassi L, Flori L. Practical applications of cutaneous colorimetry. *Clin Dermatol* 1995; 13: 369–373.

159. Babulak S, Rhein LD, Scala D, et al. Quantitation of erythema in a soap chamber test using the Minolta Chroma (reflectance) meter: comparison of instrumental results with visual assessments. *J Soc Cosmet Chem* 1986; 37: 475–480.

160. Muizzuddin N, Marenus K, Maes D, et al. Use of a Chromameter in assessing the efficacy of anti-irritants and tanning accelerators. *J Soc Cosmet Chem* 1990; 41: 369–378.

161. Seitz JC, Whitmore CG. Measurement of erythema and tanning responses in human skin using a tri-stimulus colorimeter. *Dermatologica* 1988; 177: 70–75.

162. Serup J, Agner T. Colorimetric quantification of erythema: a comparison of two colorimeters (Lange Micro Color and Minolta Chroma Meter CR-200) with a clinical scoring scheme and laser-Doppler flowmetry. *Clin Exp Dermatol* 1990; 15: 267–272.

163. Wilhelm KP, Surber C, Maibach HI. Quantification of sodium lauryl sulfate irritant dermatitis in man: comparison of four techniques: skin color reflectance, transepidermal water loss, laser Doppler flow measurement and visual scores. *Arch Dermatol Res* 1989; 281: 293–295.

164. Miyamoto K, Takiwaki H, Hillebrand GG, et al. Development of a digital imaging system for objective measurement of hyperpigmented spots on the face. *Skin Res Technol* 2002; 8: 227–235.

165. Miyamoto K, Takiwaki H, Hillebrand GG, et al. Utilization of a high-resolution digital imaging system for the objective and quantitative assessment of hyperpigmented spots on the face. *Skin Res Technol* 2002; 8: 73–77.

166. Abrutyn A, Simion FA, Draelos Z. Ability of creams to reduce erythema, stratum corneum barrier damage and subjective itching. *J Cosmet Sci* 2000; 51: 85–88.

167. De Paepe K, Derde MP, Roseeuw D, et al. Claim substantiation and efficiency of hydrating body lotions and protective creams. *Contact Derm* 2000; 42: 227–234.

168. Kligman AM. Regression method for assessing the efficacy of moisturizers. *Cosmet Toiletries* 1978; 93: 27–30.

169. Grove GL. Skin surface hydration changes during a miniregression test as measured by *in vivo* electrical conductivity. *Curr Ther Res* 1992; 52: 556–561.

170. Frosch PJ, Kligman AM. The soap chamber test. A new method for assessing the irritancy of soaps. *J Am Acad Dermatol* 1979; 1: 35–41.

171. Barel AO, Lambrecht R, Clarys P, et al. A comparative study of the effects on the skin of a classical bar soap and a syndet cleansing bar in normal use conditions and in the soap chamber test. *Skin Res Technol* 2001; 7: 98–104.

172. Simion FA, Rhein LD, Grove GL, et al. Sequential order of skin responses to surfactants during a soap chamber test. *Contact Derm* 1991; 25: 242–249.

173. Ertel KD, Keswick BH, Bryant PB. A forearm controlled application technique for estimating the relative mildness of personal cleansing products. *J Soc Cosmet Chem* 1995; 46: 67–76.

174. Lukacovic MF, Dunlap FE, Michaels SE, et al. Forearm wash test to evaluate the clinical mildness of cleansing products. *J Soc Cosmet Chem* 1988; 39: 355–366.

175. Sharko P, Murahata RI, Leyden JJ, et al. Arm wash with instrumental evaluation: a sensitive technique for differentiating the irritation potential of personal washing products. *J Dermatol Clin Soc* 1991; 2: 19–27.

176. Strube DD, Koontz SW, Murahata RI, et al. The flex wash test: a method for evaluating the mildness of personal washing products. *J Soc Cosmet Chem* 1989; 40: 297–306.

177. Simion FA, Rhein LD, Morrison BM, Jr., et al. Self-perceived sensory responses to soap and synthetic detergent bars correlate with clinical signs of irritation. *J Am Acad Dermatol* 1995; 32: 205–211.

178. Wickett RR. Forearm wash testing of mild soap bars containing colloidal oatmeal. *Can Chem News* 1997; 49: 22–23.

179. Faller C, Bracher M. Reconstructed skin kits: reproducibility of cutaneous irritancy testing. *Skin Pharmacol Appl Skin Physiol* 2002; 15 (Suppl 1): 74–91.

180. Faller C, Bracher M, Dami N, et al. Predictive ability of reconstructed human epidermis equivalents for the assessment of skin irritation of cosmetics. *Toxicol In Vitro* 2002; 16: 557–572.

181. Netzlaff F, Lehr CM, Wertz PW, et al. The human epidermis models EpiSkin, SkinEthic and EpiDerm: an evaluation of morphology and their suitability for testing phototoxicity, irritancy, corrosivity, and substance transport. *Eur J Pharm Biopharm* 2005; 60: 167–178.

182. Tornier C, Rosdy M, Maibach HI. *In vitro* skin irritation testing on reconstituted human epidermis: reproducibility for 50 chemicals tested with two protocols. *Toxicol In Vitro* 2005.

183. Netzlaff F, Lehr CM, Werz PW, Schaefer UF. The human epidermis: an evaluation of morphology and their suitability for testing phototoxicity, irritancy, corrosivity, and substance transport. *Eur J Pharm Biopharm* 2005; 60: 167–178.

4 Using Consumer Research in the Development and Restaging of Personal Care Products

Donna C. Barson, M.B.A.
Barson Marketing Inc.

CONTENTS

4.1 INTRODUCTION

In the highly competitive personal care market, it is no longer effective just to push new products into the marketplace and hope that consumers will buy. Nor is it acceptable to spend vast amounts of money on marketing campaigns touting the differences between products, when in fact the differences between products are virtually nonexistent to consumers.

New products are very important to the lifeblood of a company, as consumers always flock to the newest and greatest. However, many more new products fail than succeed. Smart companies utilize consumer research as one of the bedrock principles of new product development. In contrast to the new development efforts of some of the grand titans of the beauty business in the middle of the last century, such as Charles Revson, Estee Lauder, Max Factor, and Helena Rubinstein, the days of developing a new product by hunches or feelings are over. Today, facts and statistical data are the engines that drive successful business decisions.

At one time, before the marketplace was as crowded with choices as it is today, new product decisions were often made by a more seat-of-the-pants approach, with grassroots consumer research playing a part. Charles Revson, who started Revlon, originally a nail polish company in the 1930s, was said to be inquisitive of his customers, mostly beauty salons, about what was right and what was wrong with his nail polishes, as well as those of competitors.

Bringing a product to market today is just too expensive to do without adequate consumer research. Over the past few decades it has been shown that problems with a product could be eliminated, minimized, or altered by some research *before* the product was brought to market. Instead of just tossing the product into the marketplace to sink or swim, it made sense to give it the best possible chance of success. Thus, research — consumer research — became more and more critical. Finding out what consumers think and what attributes are important to them before going ahead maximizes a product's chances of being a marketplace star.

Consumer research can unearth flaws in design, appearance, packaging, price — a whole host of factors that can lie like a lead weight on a product's chances of success. By understanding what consumers want, the benefits they would like to experience, and the attributes that are important, the marketer of new products has a better chance for success.

Today, with product development costs so high in the personal care industry and competition so fierce, it simply makes good economic sense to do everything possible to ensure that money is not wasted. Consumer research has the potential to save a company millions of dollars, along with saving a company's or brand's reputation. Consumer research can also point out the best way to position that product in the marketplace: What component of the product should be emphasized in marketing or advertising to appeal most to consumers? The personal care marketplace is extremely crowded; unless a company is very diligent about making a place for it, a product can come and go without notice.

Consumer research can also be used to expand opportunities. A new product that is developed and tested with consumers might yield product line extensions. For example, if a company develops a new moisturizer and then tests it with consumers, it might be possible for the company to get at the real purchase drivers, along with the added benefits that consumers would look for.

In summary, consumer research saves money, saves development time, points out possible flaws, and perhaps reveals new opportunities. There are no arguments against consumer research. But the ramifications of not doing market research are enormous.

4.2 THE BROAD CLASSES OF CONSUMER RESEARCH: PRIMARY AND SECONDARY

Now that the case has been made for consumer research, let us examine the different methodologies.

There are two broad categories of consumer research: primary and secondary. When combined, these methods are powerful tools for product development ideas, including the launch of new products, the repositioning of existing products, lines, and extensions, and so on.

4.2.1 PRIMARY RESEARCH

Primary research is conducted to collect new data to solve a marketing information need and to make an informed marketing decision. In contrast, secondary research is sifting through existing data gathered by prior research methods to find information that is applicable to your particular needs.

Primary research is used for a variety of important marketing functions, including attitude and usage studies, refocusing existing brands, new product assessments, and developing new product ideas. New product assessments are such things as idea/concept testing, product testing, package/advertising testing, market opportunity investigations, and trending.

Primary research is divided into two broad classes: qualitative and quantitative.

4.2.1.1 Qualitative Research

Qualitative research is mainly conducted through interviews and focus groups that make use of open-ended questions and loosely structured discussions. The major benefit to using primary research is that a company receives immediate consumer feedback. If a company has questions or concerns about a concept, product, or marketing strategy, qualitative research is used to obtain those answers immediately. Some examples of qualitative research methods include focus groups, one-on-one interviews, dyads, triads, quads, and mini-groups.

Qualitative research gives a company the opportunity for in-depth probing and diagnostic exploration, which enables it to understand the underlying attitudes, perceptions, and feelings about the concept, product, or marketing concern under examination. A company would use qualitative research to investigate product/brand/service positioning, identify the strengths and weaknesses of the product, position competitively (again from a strengths and weaknesses perspective), and brainstorm new ideas and concepts.

Qualitative research can be used in many different marketing scenarios, and certainly in the case of a personal care products company. It provides a "quick read" to see if the idea is worth pursuing. It is not too expensive to do quick focus groups, and the insights gleaned are invaluable for further development. The use of qualitative research can be critical in determining consumer attitudes. Let us consider some examples.

For the development of a new oral care product, some companies use focus groups to examine what consumers like and do not like about their present oral care regimen, along with a list of attributes that are important. Additionally, these consumers can also talk about the various brands that are currently in the marketplace. By using a focus group or other immediate attitudinal measuring stick, the company can incorporate what people like and what attributes are really important in its new oral care product. Then it can come up with a product, package, and marketing message that is appealing.

Qualitative research is also used to examine delivery systems — an increasingly important aspect in the new product development war. A wonderful product can be sunk by an awkward delivery system. A company interested in launching a new type of delivery system for an existing product could use qualitative research to set up mini-groups of consumers to assess what they liked and did not like from existing forms of this type of product. This will provide the company with valuable information *before* it expends a lot of time and money in developing a new delivery system.

While this might sound simple, there are pitfalls to be avoided if the data received are to be of any real use. The selection of a moderator is critical to the success of a focus or mini-group. The moderator *must* be unbiased and should not lead the respondents. This is a frequent problem when the moderator is an employee of the company commissioning the research. Instead, the moderator must be an unbiased person who gets honest answers, yet is strong enough to ensure that a dominant personality does not control the other members with his or her opinions. The moderator must put the consumers at ease by expressing neutrality. It should always be stressed to the respondents that there are no right or wrong answers — just opinions.

A good moderator knows how to avoid letting a single person control the opinions of a group. When members are unwilling to go against the group opinion, assessment groups can be used to create greater focus, with less bias and more evaluative power. For example, if there is a dominant person in a group, a good moderator could suggest obtaining initial, top-of-the-mind reactions through a private vote. People write their opinions on a pad, unseen by others, so there is no public pressure. Then a discussion could be held and a second private vote taken to see if peer pressure had changed any votes. This is a technique that is often used with good results.

When properly administered, qualitative research can be extremely insightful. However, users of this method should be aware of a few caveats. Qualitative research cannot quantify results or statistically project findings to the population as a whole. It also cannot be completely representative of the population under study.

However, with that in mind, qualitative research is a vital and extremely useful tool for the personal care industry, where competition is so keen and one little stumble can spell the difference between life and death for a product or line extension. Qualitative research can mean the difference between a product's acceptance or rejection when it enters the consumer marketplace.

4.2.1.2 Quantitative Research

Quantitative research, the second type of primary research, provides empirical evaluations of attitudes, behavior, and product performance. The advantage of this type of research is that enough response is obtained to be representative of the target audience. Quantitative research includes an in-depth analysis of numerous factors, including:

1. How consumers perceive the category under investigation
2. How consumers perceive current brands in the category
3. Assessing the needs of a target market
4. Analyzing the perceptions of a target market
5. Analyzing how well/badly competitors have met the needs of consumers

Types of quantitative research include attitude and usage (A&U) studies, brand positioning, purchase drivers, anticipatory testing, and assessment of consumer needs. The following is a noninclusive list of some of the different types of research.

Attitude and usage studies are a detailed investigation of how and why consumers are using current products in the category. A&U studies have numerous components, including:

1. Unaided/aided brand awareness — In unaided brand awareness, consumers are asked in an open-ended fashion which brands of a particular product category they are *aware* of. In contrast, in aided brand awareness consumers are presented with a list of brands from which to choose.
2. Unaided/aided brand usage — In unaided brand usage, consumers are asked which brands of hand cream they have *used* in a particular period, such as the past 6 months. For aided brand usage, they are presented with specific brand names of a product they may have used in the past 6 months.
3. Brand performance rating — This component rates products on a 5- or 10-point scale to indicate individual preferences. A consumer would typically be asked a series of brand-specific questions that rate the ability of specific products on a numeric scale.
4. Brand switching — In brand switching, consumers are asked how likely they would be to switch brands in the next 6 months (or some other predetermined period).
5. Purchase importance ratings — Purchase importance ratings use a numeric scale to rate various attributes of a product and discover their importance, such as fragrance, texture, absorbency speed, etc.
6. Frequency of use — Frequency of use asks very specific questions with very specific answers related to frequency of use of a product.
7. Usage occasions and patterns — usage occasions and patterns track the instances of when and why consumers use a certain product.
8. In-store purchase patterns — In-store purchase patterns examine the in-store purchasing habits of a consumer to determine at what point in his or her shopping experience he or she might be inclined to buy a particular product.
9. Intent to purchase — Intent to purchase utilizes a numeric scale for participants to indicate their likelihood for buying the product or brand in question.

Brand positioning, another part of quantitative research, rates specific brands on a list of product attributes, such as scent, appearance, texture, etc. Each brand's performance rating is compared to the overall rating of a particular attribute.

Anticipatory testing helps weed out ideas more likely to succeed from a whole batch of ideas or concepts presented to the test consumers. Diagnostic testing seeks to maximize consumer appeal and increase sales potential by honing in on those variables deemed most important and mostly likely to influence purchase decisions.

Purchase drivers are another key component of quantitative research. Here, consumers rate the importance of various product attributes in deciding whether or not to purchase a product in that category. From the resultant statistical analysis, the key drivers in the category can be determined, such as how important certain attributes of a product are in the purchasing decision.

As is likely obvious by now, the data gathered by quantitative research are much greater than those from qualitative research, because the sample size is so much larger. This makes data obtained through quantitative research methods much more statistically significant. Some of the survey methods used to conduct quantitative research include the following:

1. Mail surveys
2. Online surveys
3. Telephone surveys
4. In-home placement surveys
5. Mail intercepts
6. Central location testing

Market research firms often develop their own proprietary methods for conducting quantitative research.

An example of anticipatory testing would be if a company had various new product ideas and needed to determine which had greater consumer appeal at an early stage. After performing anticipatory testing, the client would receive a go/no go determination within a few weeks, which would allow it to take the next step in its product development efforts.

Diagnostic testing maximizes consumer appeal and increases sales potential. It features purchase interest, simulated shopping, and the testing of variables' benefits, delivery systems, etc. An example of diagnostic testing would be a concept assessment for a new form of a product or a new package design. A group of consumers is gathered and exposed to a mini-shelf set where the purchase decisions are made. Comprehensive diagnostic assessments of purchase decisions and further examinations of concept propositions are obtained.

4.2.2 SECONDARY RESEARCH

Secondary research is the other class of consumer research. Everything else discussed up to this point have been aspects of primary research.

Secondary research has numerous aspects. As can be discerned by its very name, secondary research is data gleaned from secondary sources, such as trade journals, advertising and promotional campaigns, etc. Secondary research looks at the past, present, and future. It is sometimes not as compelling or even as revealing as primary research, simply because a company is relying on already existing sources for data. Nevertheless, secondary research is an effective consumer research tool and should be viewed as a viable alternative to primary research.

Secondary research involves combing secondary, or already existing, sources, for data. A brief list of secondary research steps to follow might be:

- Compile a competitive advantage analysis (more about this below)
- Review trade journals, etc.
- Develop a competitive SWOT analysis, which looks at a product, brand, or company's strengths and weaknesses along with opportunities and threats that might impact the situation
- Examine demographic trends
- Examine product trends
- Examine marketing trends
- Examine merchandising/retail trends

How does a company go about examining the above-listed trends and developing a competitive analysis? They compile the information from already existing sources — hence the term *secondary research*. These sources can be anything from press releases and annual reports to advertising campaigns to talking to former employees. But what is critical here, and something many companies do not understand how to correctly initiate and use, is competitive intelligence. This is addressed below.

Let us examine some of the above-listed items in detail:

Demographic trends — This takes into account such factors as the aging of the population, more working women, more educated consumers, greater ethnic diversity, more affluent young adults, and changing consumer affluence.

Product trends — This considers such factors as new ingredients/technologies/ delivery systems, more value-added properties, more products targeted to the specific needs of diverse ethnic groups, more natural ingredients, more vitamins and enzymes, and longer-lasting and transfer-resistant products.

Marketing trends — This considers such factors as a younger market, the 45-year-old and older market, products that reverse and try to prevent aging, the changing world and its priorities, changing consumer spending patterns, the decline of brand loyalty, the appearance of more niche products, and the presence of men as skin care consumers.

Merchandising/retail trends — This examines more private label products, more products from doctors, open sell environments, Internet purchasing, cosmetic emporiums, and day spas and salons.

4.3 COMPETITIVE AND BUSINESS ANALYSIS

Another branch of market research that has become critical to the success of a product is competitive intelligence. Competitive intelligence does not simply mean "spying" on the competition. Rather, it is being aware of the environment in which businesses operate. In today's high-stakes business world, Company A simply must be aware of what Company B is doing. It makes good economic sense. An example of competitive intelligence would be when a company comes out with a firming moisturizer, a fruit-fragrance liquid soap, or some other product just prior to a competitor's launch of a similar product. This signifies that a company has its fingers on the pulse of the marketplace and knows what the competition is up to so a countermove can be prepared.

Competitive intelligence can help a business in numerous ways:

1. It can identify new markets, concepts, opportunities, or products.
2. It can aid in the relaunch or repositioning of existing products.
3. It can help generate ideas for new products, track trends, and help formulate business plans and strategies.
4. It can help identify attractive merger or acquisition targets.

Let us consider a general example of competitive intelligence. At one time, body washes were a big hit in Europe. However, they were virtually unknown in the U.S. Then a single company came out with a body wash product for the U.S. consumer. Before you could soap up a louffa, the American marketplace was flooded with numerous types of body washes. How was this done so fast? How were companies able to come out with competing products in record time to avoid ceding the marketplace to someone else? The answer is simple: competitive intelligence. American companies had studied the European market, knew that body washes were a big hit there, and knew it was only a matter of time until the product made the leap across the Atlantic to the U.S. So they conducted quantitative and qualitative research and knew that the American market was ready for this particular product. Thus, body washes were in the pipeline well before the first one was launched in America. When they became a big hit, all the other personal care companies were ready with their own product.

The next logical question is: Where does a company get competitive intelligence? Fortunately, as stated earlier, it does not require setting up some type of elaborate spying operation to obtain this data. Competitive intelligence is all around; one just has to know where to look. Here is a list of some places to obtain competitive intelligence:

- Company press releases
- Annual reports
- Trade publications
- Sales data
- New product alerts

- Federal statistics
- Websites
- Syndicated industry reports
- Personal contacts

Where most companies stumble with competitive intelligence gathering is in thinking that it is not that important, and therefore not assigning a very high priority to it. Competitive intelligence gathering is not a part-time job; it requires skill, ability, and savvy. Many companies assign a full-time staff member or even a whole department for competitive intelligence gathering. Others cannot because of budgetary considerations, but realize the importance of the function anyway and hire an outside firm or consultant with expertise in that area.

4.4 OUTSOURCING THE MARKET RESEARCH FUNCTION

While the term *outsourcing* is getting a bit of a bad name, companies turn to outside market research professionals for numerous reasons. Here are a few of the most common:

- There are no market research specialists within the company who can do the job adequately and professionally.
- The need exists to complement already existing in-house expertise.
- Simply put, too much to do and not enough time to do it.
- An outside perspective is necessary.
- The organization is deficient in keeping abreast of the industry and the marketplace and needs the expertise of professionals that continually monitor the field.

Companies that require market research gathering but feel they can do the job in-house should seriously and impartially evaluate whether they can truly accumulate the required data. For example, secondary research and competitive intelligence gathering are more than just clipping out articles about rival companies from the newspaper. It is a systemized, highly disciplined search for the type of data that a firm requires for its particular needs. Trying to accumulate everything you can find about a particular firm in the hopes of turning up one specific nugget of information is like trying to shoot a flea with a shotgun. Sure, you may possibly find what you are looking for — eventually — but you have to wade through so much extraneous material to find it that you squander significant time and money in the effort.

Similarly, some companies take a knee-jerk economic reaction to outsourcing these functions. They do not want to spend the money and figure that they are saving significant dollars by keeping everything in-house. But when considering the economic case for outside competitive intelligence gathering, companies should ask themselves one simple question: How much money will be lost if the proposed new product fails? This is truly one instance in which it pays to look long term, not short term, and in which being penny-wise can definitely result in being pound-foolish.

When outsourcing market research projects, a company should establish a strict set of guidelines to ensure that the process runs smoothly. After the initial meeting with the outside firm, the company should be able to develop a proposal that confirms project goals and outlines the methodology. Then the two groups — the outside firm and the company that initiated the project — should be in communication on a regular basis to focus the research and analyze the findings. It is a serious mistake to just assume that because an outside firm has been retained, the project can be forgotten about until the final report. Staying involved means maximizing the investment.

But if a company does have the resources and can do the job of competitive intelligence gathering in-house, then it is important to use that resource wisely. Before starting to accumulate intelligence on the competition, take some time to carefully plan the process: Exactly what type of information is needed? Once obtained, how is this information to be used? If the answers to these questions are not obvious and known to everyone involved in the process, then a lot of time, money, and effort will be wasted flailing about. The watchwords here are: *Think. Plan. Then go forward.*

Once the goals of the effort are determined, it is necessary to identify which competitors should be targeted. This is a critical step that some companies overlook. Sometimes companies who were assumed to be competitors are not. They could even be allies, supplying opportunities for networking and referral.

Once clear on the types of information needed and who the competition is, compile a list of competitors, along with their brands and individual products. Each brand should include the following information:

- Advertising position
- Benefits
- Distribution methods
- Features
- Fragrance
- Price and value
- Problems the products claim to solve and fail to solve
- Strengths and weaknesses
- Target customers
- Unique ingredients

Keep in mind that the above list is just preliminary. Categories can be added or subtracted depending on the specific needs of the project (another reason to have goals mapped out ahead of time). But the above represents a typical starting point for any competitive intelligence search.

4.5 CONCLUSION

In conclusion, using consumer research in the development and restaging of personal care products is an important, if not vital, component of a successful product launch or reposition. There are many ways to go about developing consumer research, as the above has just delineated. A company can pick and choose what methods it would like to implement. The important thing is to choose the research tools that obtain the desired information.

Part II

FUNDAMENTALS OF PERSONAL CARE AND DECORATIVE COSMETICS

5 Pigment Dispersions

Stéphane Nicolas
Sun Chemical Performance Pigments Group

CONTENTS

5.1 INTRODUCTION

In the manufacture of finished color cosmetics products, one of the largest challenges to the various modes of bulk product compounding operations is the dispersion of insoluble dry pigments into the many types of product media.[1]

Improper color dispersion can cause numerous problems that may impact different facets of the cosmetic industry, such as finished product instability and functionality, production delays, product losses and rework, waste of labor and material resources, and increases in related costs. Thus, the dispersion of pigments in desired media is of great technological importance to the decorative cosmetics manufacturers who deal with various pigmented systems.

Based on the previous chapters' review of the basic properties of cosmetic pigments and the mechanisms of the pigment dispersion process, whose basic aim is to change the physical state of pigments to achieve desired and optimum effects in specific applications systems, this chapter will emphasize the assets and advantages of using predispersed pigments to manufacture better quality cosmetic products at the least cost.[1]

5.2 A BRIEF INTRODUCTION TO PIGMENT

5.2.1 PIGMENT DEFINITION

Before embarking on a discussion of pigment dispersion, I will start with a review of the basic properties of color additives, which refer to the broad class of chemicals that are used to impart color effects to cosmetic and toiletry products.

The definition *pigment* proposed by the Color Pigment Manufacturers Association is:

Pigments are colored, black, white or fluorescent particulate organic and inorganic solids which usually are insoluble and essentially physically and chemically unaffected by the vehicle or substrate in which they are incorporated. They alter appearance by selective absorption and/or by scattering light. Pigments are usually dispersed in vehicle or substrates for application. Pigments retain a crystal or particulate structure throughout the coloration process.

As a result, pigments differ from another category of color additives: dyes. Dyes are those color additives that are soluble in the medium in which they are used. As a general rule in cosmetic products, the term *solubility* relates to water solubility.

The majority of the color additives used in toiletries are dyes, while the majority of those used in decorative cosmetics are pigments. All the color additives discussed in this chapter fall into the broad category of absorption pigments. That is, they produce color shades by selective absorption and reflection of visible light.

Pigments are divided into two broad categories: organic and inorganic (Figure 5.1). The organic pigments are generally brighter and more intense than the inorganic ones. On the other hand, the inorganic pigments exhibit better stability than organic ones.

5.2.2 PROPERTIES

Pigments supplied in the form of dry powders represent the traditional form of supply and use of pigments to the decorative cosmetics producers. They are composed of fine particles, normally in the submicrometer size range.

Pigments' color properties are generally influenced by particle size and distribution. Therefore, an assessment on the degree of dispersion must, above all, be considered in terms of these critical measurements.

Color Additives—Types

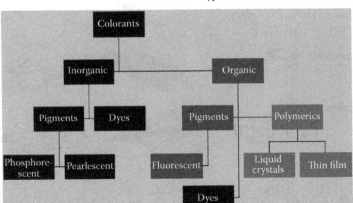

FIGURE 5.1 Color additive types and classification.

In general, the following color properties are affected to a greater or lesser extent by the size and distribution of the pigment particles in the vehicle in which they are embedded:

- Strength
- Transparency/opacity
- Glosses
- Shade
- Rheology
- Light stability/chemical stability

Pigment particles normally exist in the form of primary particle, aggregates, agglomerates, and flocculates.

Primary particles are individual crystals. As they are formed during the manufacturing process, they may vary in size, depending on the conditions of precipitation and growth, which are controlled by the pigment manufacturer (Figure 5.2). Usually, the size of primary particles is 50 to 500 mm, depending on the type of pigment.

Aggregates are collections of primary particles that are attached to each other at their surface or crystal faces and show a tightly packed structure. Agglomerates consist of primary particles and aggregates joined at the corners and edges in a looser type of arrangement. Flocculates consist of primary particle aggregates and agglomerates generally arranged in a fairly open structure. They may be broken down easily under shear, but will form again when such shear forces are removed and the dispersion is allowed to stand undisturbed.

As a general rule, large particles usually exhibit the following properties:

- Increased light fastness (light stability)
- Higher opacity

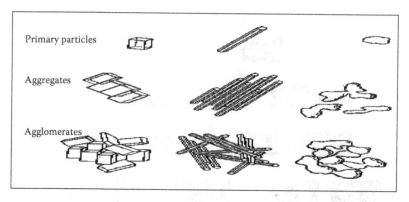

Primary particles

Aggregates

Agglomerates

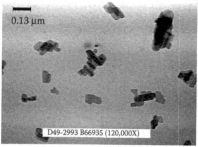

0.13 μm

D49-2993 B66935 (120,000X)

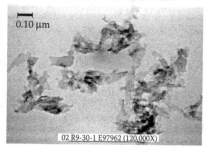

0.10 μm

02 R9-30-1 E97962 (120,000X)

FIGURE 5.2 Physical form of particles.

- Enhanced chemical resistance
- Better dispersibility
- Lower viscosity in fluid systems
- Lower color (tinctorial) strength (Figure 5.3)
- Lower surface area/surface energy

Small particles, on the other hand, exhibit the following properties:

- Reduced light fastness
- Maximum transparency
- Poorer chemical resistance
- Poorer dispersibility — prone to flocculation
- Higher viscosity in fluid system
- Higher color strength (Figure 5.3)
- Higher surface area/surface energy

The shade is another parameter that is influenced by the particle size (Figure 5.4). In the case of organic pigments, the following shade fluctuations are generally observed when the particle size of a selected pigment increases:

- Yellow pigments will undergo a red shift.
- Orange pigments will turn more reddish.

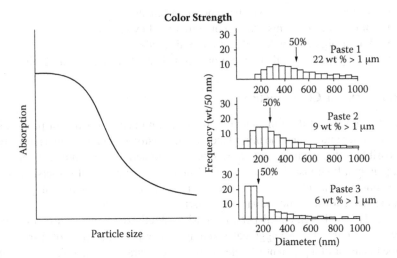

Color Strength

FIGURE 5.3 The color or tinctorial strength is the relationship between pigment particle size and the ability of a pigment vehicle system to absorb visible electromagnetic radiation. The ability of a given pigment to absorb light (tinctorial strength) increases with decreasing particle diameter and accordingly increased surface area, and this until it approaches the point at which the particles are entirely translucent. If we take Paste 2 as a reference, then it will have a lower tinctorial strength than Paste 3 (with the finest particles) and higher than Paste 1.

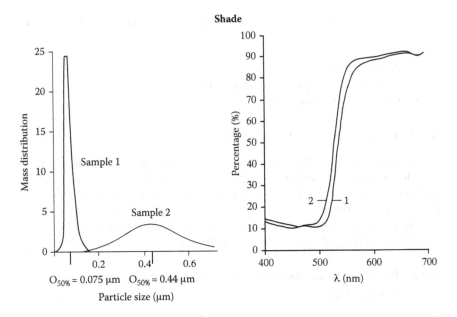

Shade

FIGURE 5.4 The shade is another parameter that is influenced by the particle size. At equal pigment concentration, remission curves 1 and 2 present, respectively, the behaviors of small particles and large particles of the same pigment.

- Yellowish pigments will become more bluish.
- Bluish red pigments will become more yellowish.
- Violet pigments will move to the bluish side.
- Blue pigments will show a more reddish shade (phtalocyanine blue).

5.2.3 GENERAL CONSIDERATION

After this review of the fundamental properties and characteristics of pigments, one can better understand the importance and necessity to obtain as full a reduction as possible to the primary particle size in order to achieve the optimum benefits of a pigment, both visual and economic. The primary purpose of dispersion is to break down pigment aggregates and agglomerates to their optimum primary particle size (down to individual single particles, if possible).

Ideally, good pigment dispersion consists chiefly of primary particles, with only a minimum of loose aggregates and agglomerates. The effect of dispersion on the behavior of a pigment vehicle system is comparable to the effect of simply reducing the average pigment particle size. The pigmented system will exhibit increased tinctorial strength, undergo a change of shade, be more transparent, provide enhanced gloss, increase in viscosity, and, finally, feature a reduced critical pigment volume concentration.

5.3 DISPERSION PROCESS

It is generally recognized that the dispersion process consists of three distinct stages:

- Pigment wetting
- Pigment de-aggregation/de-agglomeration
- Dispersion stabilization

5.3.1 PIGMENT WETTING (FIGURE 5.5)

The wetting stage involves the removal from the surface of the pigment particles of adsorbed molecules of gas, liquid, and other materials and their replacement with molecules of the vehicle. This is accomplished through preferential adsorption.

The efficiency of wetting depends primarily on the comparative surface tension properties of the pigment and the vehicle, as well as the viscosity of the resultant mix.

5.3.2 PARTICLE DE-AGGREGATION AND DE-AGGLOMERATION (FIGURE 5.6)

After the initial wetting stage, it is necessary to de-aggregate and de-agglomerate the pigment particles. This is usually accomplished by mechanical action provided by high-impact mill equipment. As the pigment powder is broken

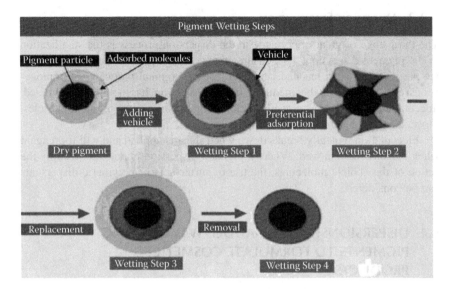

FIGURE 5.5 The process of pigment wetting.

down to the individual particles, higher surface areas become exposed to the vehicle and larger amounts of it are required to wet out newly formed surfaces.

During this stage of de-aggregation the amount of free vehicle diminishes and the viscosity of the dispersion increases. At higher viscosities, shear forces are more important and the breaking down and separation of the particles becomes more efficient.

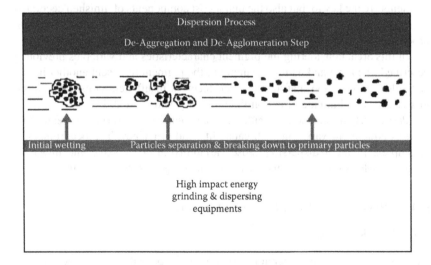

FIGURE 5.6 The process of pigment dispersion.

5.3.3 Dispersion Stabilization

The third stage of great importance in the dispersion process is the stabilization of the pigment dispersion. This ensures that complete wetting and separation of the particles has been reached, and also that the pigment particles are homogeneously distributed in the medium. If the dispersion has not been stabilized, flocculation may occur as a result of clumping together of the pigment particles. Flocculation is generally a reversible process.

Flocculation typically breaks down when shear is applied and will form again when the shear is removed. Where a pigment dispersion is not stabilized by the action of the vehicle molecules, the use of surfactants or polymeric dispersants can be considered.

5.4 DISPERSIONS: A VALUE-ADDED WAY OF USING PIGMENTS TO FORMULATE COSMETIC PRODUCTS

5.4.1 General Considerations

In the cosmetic arena, the decorative cosmetic market segment has grown exponentially over the past years and now represents a strategic and dynamic segment of the global cosmetic industry.

Thus, pressure increases on the target to more quickly release new and innovative finished products, and the need to reduce costs and improve efficiency to remain competitive grows. As the use of color has increased, so have the developments by pigment manufacturers.

Today's formulator has a tremendous choice of pigments to choose from. Pigments are the key to, but also the major cost components of, finished decorative cosmetic products; therefore, correct choices are essential to ensure that required product performance, customer satisfaction, and profit margins are achieved.

In this area, considering the pigment characteristics and variables previously described, the form and nature of supply of the pigment represent another important selection criterion that all too often receives insufficient consideration and that can have a dramatic effect on the efficiency and profitability.

Particularly for cosmetic manufacture in which formula variation is extensive, process equipment varies in both capability and efficiency. The occurrences of incomplete pigment dispersion cause variability in color value and unwanted ranges of color strength, and the basics of finished goods' shades are inconsistent.

5.4.2 Benefits of Using Pigment Dispersions

5.4.2.1 A Ready-to-Use

By definition, pigment dispersions are already dispersed and will require relatively simple incorporation into the suitable cosmetic medium. All requirements

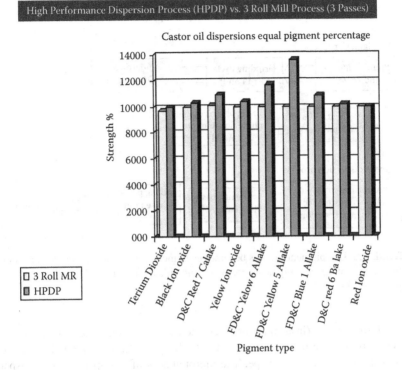

FIGURE 5.7 The effect of pigment processing on strength.

of manufacturers' product compounding processes to agitate, shear, mill, or grind formula for pigment dispersion are eliminated (Figure 5.7).

5.4.2.2 Quality Improvement, Process Control, and Color Value

There is evidence to support the view that pigment dispersions from specialist producers often offer quality benefits over in-house dispersions. They will have developed proprietary knowledge and expertise of dispersion techniques and will usually have available a range of advanced equipment and processing technologies not normally found in a color cosmetic factory, creating color blends that offer full-color extension unequaled by any of the pigment milling or grinding methods traditionally employed (Figure 5.8).

High-performance dispersion processes optimize particle size distribution to a very fine level (primary particle) as well as the stability of the pigment particles in the dispersion medium.

Higher levels of dispersion also lead to improvements in cleanliness of shade, giving the color formulator much more flexibility and versatility to optimize the color formulation. This is especially true for certain classes of pigment, such as

Manufacturing Process Comparison Dry
Pigment vs. Pigment Dispersion Example: Lipstick Formulation

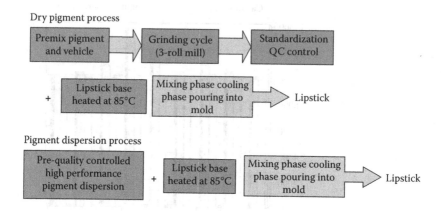

FIGURE 5.8 Dry pigment process becomes even more complicated and time consuming with the use of several pigments requiring individual pre-mix and grinding for each pigment considered.

ferric ferrocyanide (iron blue) or D&C Red 33 Al Lake, which are extremely difficult to disperse to full potential due to their very small crystal size, ease of aggregation, and acicular shape. The thoroughness of high-performance dispersions allows tighter color specifications than does the dry pigment alone.

Typical lot-to-lot color/shade variations noticeable with conventional dry pigment supplies are removed, reducing or eliminating drastically the need to make color adjustments in process. Shade matching to standard is achieved more readily and, in many cases, more closely, as the choice of ensuring full dispersion of dry color additions to batches is taken away.

5.4.2.3 Cost Control and Reduction

A key attribute of high-performance pigment dispersions is the amount of labor and production processing cost reduction they provide. Production output can be dramatically improved through the use of predispersed product; mixing only is much faster than full dispersion, and downtime for cleaning is greatly reduced.

In terms of efficiencies, due to the superior color strength and integrity of pre-quality-controlled high-performance pigment dispersions, savings will be realized by users by a reduction in their raw material inventories. Along with this reduction, users are offered an increase of cash flow, as dispersion programs include the procurement and maintenance of the cosmetic media (the cosmetic formula carrier vehicle) and pigment inventories. Such inventory management will assist cosmetic manufacturers in the reduction of their lead times. Batch size is also a key consideration; use of dry pigment will often be the best choice for large-batch regularly made products, but small series and infrequently made products are a different situation. Such products can have a big effect on cost through yield losses and production inefficiency. Yield losses from a 25-l bead mill, for example, will vary with batch size between 3 and 35%.

Along with the elimination of production steps and costs, increased color strength and consistency, and improved quality of finished products comes the elimination or reduction of capital outlay for processing equipment.

The use of dry powder pigment requires the cosmetic manufacturer to fully disperse the pigment using high-energy equipment, as opposed to the stir-in option provided by dispersions. Full-dispersion kits require a considerably higher capital investment than simple mixing equipment.

5.5 CONCLUSION

There is no question as to the desirability and effectiveness of a fully dispersed and stabilized pigmented system. Such a dispersion brings out the optimum color properties of the pigment in terms of color strength and consistency, gloss, transparency, and rheology. When a pigment is completely dispersed, it contains a larger number of primary particles; therefore, a smaller amount is required to produce the necessary coverage and color strength than would be necessary for a pigment that was not as well dispersed and contained a large number of aggregates, agglomerates, and flocculates.

Though today the main trend driving the decorative color cosmetic industry is innovation, in terms of new makeup concepts combined with new color effects, pressure increases on the need to produce more quickly, reduce costs, and improve efficiency to remain competitive and profitable in this global business arena. Production strategy is a major source for cost reduction and efficiency improvement.

With considerable cost savings that can be realized through their strategic uses, by reducing labor costs, minimizing capital expenditure on production kits, reducing inventory costs, easing capacity constraints, reducing yield losses, and streamlining production processes, high-performance pre-quality-controlled pigment dispersions definitely represent a value-added way of using pigments to formulate and manufacture cosmetic products.

REFERENCE

1. T.G. Vernardakis, *Coatings Technology Handbook*, D. Satas, Ed., Satas and Associates, Warwick, RI.

6 Contribution of Surfactants to Personal Care Products

P. Somasundaran, Soma Chakraborty, Puspendu Deo, Namita Deo, and Tamara Somasundaran
NSF Industry/University Cooperative Research Center for Advanced Studies in Novel Surfactants, Langmuir Center for Colloids and Interface, Columbia University

CONTENTS

6.1 INTRODUCTION

In recent years, the significance of polymers and surfactants has increased many-fold, as myriad applications are being found in the cosmetic industry. Personal care products such as shampoos, shower gels, and bath additives are mostly concentrated aqueous solutions of anionic surfactants in combination with salts. Additional additives used are nonionic and betaine-type surfactants, along with small amounts of dyes, perfumes, and preservatives. In cosmetics, surfactants are primarily used as wetting agents, cleansers, foaming agents, solubilizers, conditioners, thickeners, and to produce emollients. Apart from these functions, they are also used for creating a wide variety of dispersed systems, such as suspensions and emulsions, and for the synthesis of nanoparticles. Surfactants used for cosmetic formulations are expected to be safe and pure. Odoriferous and deeply

121

colored surfactants are also avoided for formulation, as they can affect the esthetics of a finished product. Since surfactants form an integral part of cosmetic formulations, their properties pertaining to cosmetic formulations have been widely studied; e.g., our group has described the mechanisms by which surfactants perform as cleaning agents,[1] whereas Balzer et al. have evaluated the effects of surfactants on the viscoelastic properties of personal care products.[2]

In addition to foaming, detergency, and mildness, rheological properties also have to be optimal in personal care product formulations. In use, the formulation fluids are expected to possess non-Newtonian flow, shear-thinning behavior characterized by slow flow from the container, absence of long threads, and easy distribution on the skin or hair. Such desirable properties are often obtained by including appropriate combinations of polymers and surfactants in formulations. It is highly beneficial if the formulations can also deliver sensory attributes at desired sites.

In this regard, hybrid polymers and nanoparticles designed to possess nanodomains can extract and deliver at will cosmetics or drugs or extract sebaceous or toxic materials by making use of possible perturbations in pH, temperature, or ionic strength of personal care systems. In this chapter, development of such systems based on polymer/surfactant colloid chemistry is explored for achieving transport and release of cosmetic and pharmaceutical molecules at desired rates at desired sites based on the above principles.

6.2 SOLUBILIZATION OF INSOLUBLE ATTRIBUTES

In cosmetic systems, including gels, ointments, creams, and lotions, the need for incorporation of water-incompatible attributes is met by using colloidal materials. Colloids in the form of emulsions, microemulsions, and micelles have been used for decades for drug delivery applications.[3]

Many colloidal systems, natural or man-made, are dynamic in nature and entertain many important interactions between their various components. Basic colloidal systems can be represented by the tetrahedron shown in Figure 6.1, with surfactants, polymers/proteins, solids, solvents, and gases/oils occupying different vertices, the behavior of the systems being determined by the interactions between various moieties. Future scientific and technological advances depend on fully understanding such interactions and utilizing them efficiently.

6.3 EMULSIONS AND MICROEMULSIONS

Emulsions and microemulsions are used in many cosmetic formulations. Emulsion is a two-phase colloidal system consisting of two immiscible liquids, one of which is dispersed as finite globules in the other. The most common type of emulsion has water as one of the phases and oil as the other. If the oil droplets are dispersed in a continuous aqueous phase, the emulsion is termed an oil-in-water (O/W) or inverse emulsion, whereas if oil forms the continuous phase, the emulsion is known as a water-in-oil (W/O) type system. The emulsion and inverse emulsion are

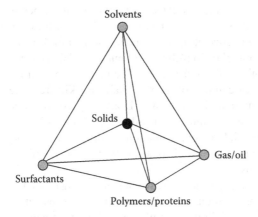

FIGURE 6.1 Diagram showing possible interactions among usual components in colloidal systems. (From Somasundaran, P., *J. Colloid Interface Sci.*, 256, 3–15, 2002. With permission.)

schematically shown in Figure 6.2a and b, respectively. Surfactants promote emulsion stability by reducing the interfacial tension between the oil and water phases. Microemulsions are specific systems in which the emulsifying agents are optimally adapted to the oil and water phase, and therefore show minimum interfacial tension. They commonly have droplet radii in the range of 25 to 500 Å.

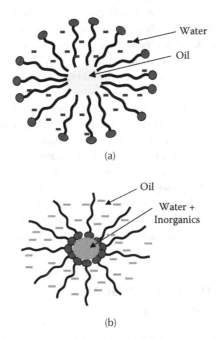

FIGURE 6.2 (a) Water-in-oil type emulsion. (b) Oil-in-water type emulsion (inverse emulsion).

Microemulsions can entrap flavors, fragrances, and other attributes or act as nanoreactors for the synthesis of nanoparticles that in turn can be used for the encapsulation of the attributes. In cosmetic formulations, O/W microemulsions find much broader applications than W/O microemulsions. One significant application of O/W microemulsion is for the solubilization of fragrances and flavor in products such as eau de cologne, aftershave, skin freshener, splash lotion, hair tonic, hair liquid, and mouthwash. Double microemulsions, which include oil–water–oil (O/W/O) and water–oil–water (W/O/W) systems, also hold considerable potential for encapsulation of drugs and sensory attributes. The mechanism by which microemulsions solubilize the insoluble attributes has been reviewed by Tadros.[5]

Though the surfactants are effective in solubilizing oily flavor and fragrances, it has been demonstrated that the odor intensity decreases with an increase in the surfactant concentration in the formulation.[6] Moreover, many surfactants associated with the microemulsion formulations have toxic and irritating effects on the skin. These adverse effects have been elaborated in the following section.

6.4 SOME ADVERSE EFFECTS OF SURFACTANTS

Surfactants can penetrate through the skin and interfere with the function of the cell membrane. It is known that long-chain, nitrogen-containing amphiphiles that are found in household and personal care products are potentially immunotoxic. To evaluate the potential risk associated with dermal exposure to nitrogen-containing amphiphiles commonly found in household and personal care products, the uptake of N,N-dimethyl-N-dodecylglycine and N,N-dimethyl-N-hexadecylglycine into human skin *in vivo* was measured in a study by Bucks et al.[7] During a 30-min contact period of the chemicals with the skin, about 45% of the compound penetrated the skin.

Disposal of surfactant-containing cosmetic products is also of major concern, as they have the potential to induce ecotoxicity. From the application pattern of surfactant-containing cosmetic products, it is inevitable that a part of the chemicals will be discharged into wastewater and will eventually enter the environment. Hence, there is a preference for using biodegradable and biocompatible surfactants for formulations. An ecological safety assessment to evaluate the biodegradability and ecotoxicological properties of the individual ingredients has been developed by Berger.[8] An alternative solution to avoid direct use of surfactants in cosmetic formulations is to encapsulate the attributes inside nanoparticles or liposomes.

6.5 ENCAPSULATION BY LIPOSOMES AND NANOPARTICLES

Encapsulation techniques are finding increasing use in the food and cosmetic industries to control the release of entrapped materials and to protect them against hostile surrounding environments. Fragrance encapsulation and their controlled release play an increasing role in fragrance marketing and cost savings. Also, fragrance samples attached to magazines and fliers as films or fine powders give consumers an opportunity to try the fragrance, which enhances its marketability. Encapsulation stabilizes the fragrance and controlled release prolongs the lifetime of the fragrance, and these factors result in economic benefits. The importance of encapsulation in food and cosmetic industries and various mechanisms of controlled release have been discussed in detail by Peppas et al.[9]

6.6 LIPOSOMES IN COSMETIC INDUSTRY

Liposomes, or (phospho)lipid vesicles, are self-assembled colloidal particles. They are vehicles of phospholipids with an aqueous cavity, which engulfs the water-soluble actives (Figure 6.3). Liposomes, introduced as drug delivery vehicles in the 1970s, have been most widely investigated and used in several hundred products in the market, including sunscreen lotions, skin creams, and perfumes. One of the first cosmetic applications of liposomes was in skin-moisturizing agents (humectants). Cosmetic applications of liposomes have been discussed in detail by Seiller et al.[10] These applications depend on the ability of liposomes to solubilize hydrophobic molecules in natural lipid–water systems; they act as a slow-release reservoir and perhaps enhance penetration through mucosal membranes and also reduce the skin toxicity and irritation.

We have recently evaluated the potential of liposomes to extract the drug amitriptyline. The liposomes used for the study were made of 1:1 phosphatidyl choline and phosphatic acid. The drug concentration in the lipid bilayers after interaction of the liposomes with amitriptyline was determined, and the results obtained are shown in Figure 6.4.

In the absence of any added salt, the drug concentration in the lipid bilayers increased linearly with the increase in drug concentration. In water, the surface charge of the liposomes is highly negative due to the presence of the anionic groups on both the phosphatidic acid and phosphatidyl choline. This favors electrostatic interactions between the liposomes and the cationic drug molecule, as shown in Figure 6.5.

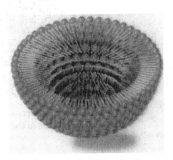

FIGURE 6.3 Spherical liposome formed by the lipid bilayer. (From http://saints. css. edu/ bio/schroeder/liposome.gif. With permission.)

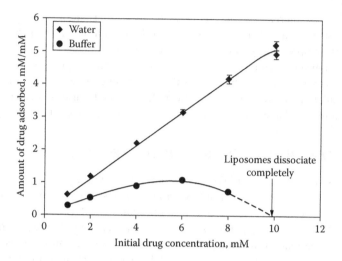

FIGURE 6.4 Adsorption of drug onto 1 m*M* liposome. (From *N. Deo et al., Collides and Surfaces B: Biolnter faces,* 2004. With permission.)

To evaluate alterations that are caused by the drugs on the lipid bilayers, an effective drug/liposome molar ratio in the aggregate is defined as follows:

$$Re = \frac{(total\ drug) - (drug\ monomer)}{(total\ liposome) - (Phospholipidmonomer)} \qquad (6.1)$$

The amount of phospholipid monomer is negligible in water due to its poor solubility. Hence, Equation 6.1 reduces to

$$Re = \frac{(total\ drug) - (drug\ monomer)}{(total\ liposome)} \qquad (6.2)$$

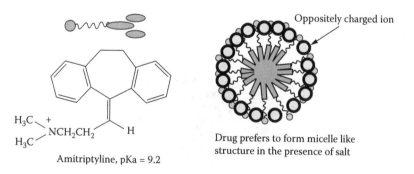

Amitriptyline, pKa = 9.2

Drug prefers to form micelle like structure in the presence of salt

FIGURE 6.5 Schematic representation of the effects of oppositely charged ions in micelle formation of amitriptyline. (From N. Deo et al., *Collides and Surfaces B: Biointerfaces,* 2004. With permission.)

This indicates that partitioning of drugs between the bilayers and the aqueous medium governs the incorporation of drugs into the liposomes, thereby producing saturation and solubilization of these structures.

A partition coefficient K (mM^{-1}) is defined as

$$K = \frac{S_p}{(P + S_p)\, S_w} \tag{6.3}$$

where P is the total phospholipid concentration, S_p is the concentration of the drug in the bilayer (mM), and S_w is the concentration of the drug in the aqueous medium (mM). For P $\gg S_P$, Equation 6.3 reduces to

$$K = \frac{S_p}{(PS_w)} = \frac{Re}{S_w} \tag{6.4}$$

where Re is the ratio of the drug to the phospholipid in the vesicle bilayer.

The partition coefficients of the drug have been determined by applying Equation 6.3 and plotted as a function of a drug concentration (Figure 6.6). The K-value decreased significantly in the phosphate buffer due to electrostatic effects. The K-value also decreased with an increase in drug concentration and remained constant above 6 mM, indicative of saturation of the bilayer with the drug molecules.

Complete destruction of the liposome structure was detected upon further increase in the drug dosage above 6 mM due to the decrease in the electrostatic effects. It is clear that the structure of the liposome can be designed and modified for extracting attributes.

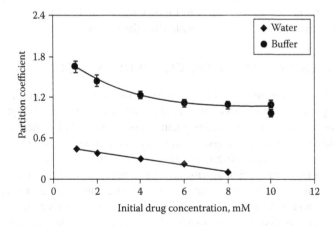

FIGURE 6.6 Effects of ionic strength on the partition coefficient (K). (From N. Deo et al., *Collides and Surfaces B: Biointerfaces*, 2004. With permission.)

Surfactants can interact with skin in several ways. They first interact with the surface of the stratum corneum, then penetrate this layer and perhaps beyond it. One of their potential sites of action within the stratum corneum is the intercellular lipid. In this regard, the interaction of surfactants with liposomes represents a good model for studying the effect of surfactants on biological membranes. López et al.[12] have studied the solubilization effect of sodium dodecyl sulfate on phosphatidyl choline liposomes. They observed an initial contraction of the vesicles, followed by relaxation and formation of the mixed micelles.

We monitored the interaction of phosphatidyl choline liposomes with dodecyl sulfonate surfactant. Even simple combinations of the relevant species in liposomes and the above components show some interesting effects. Thus, when a surfactant such as dodecyl sulfonate is added to a liposome made up of phosphatidyl choline and phosphatidic acid, initially the size of the liposome increases and subsequently it is solubilized. Furthermore, while the addition of cholesterol stabilizes liposomes, proteins destabilize them; the reasons for this effect are still far from evident. Electron spin resonance studies have shown the polarity and viscosity of liposomes to change to those of micelles of dodecyl sulfonate at sufficiently high concentrations of the surfactant (Figure 6.7a).

These results suggest that liposome stabilization by dodecyl sulfonate involves the adsorption of sulfonate on them, leading to an increase in size, and their subsequent disintegration into mixed micelles composed of liposome components and dodecyl sulfonate, resulting in a drastic decrease in size (Figure 6.7b).

The actual processes by which such disintegration takes place are not known. Some preliminary results suggest that phosphatidic acid would exit first, leading to the weakening of the liposome structure and its dissolution. Similarly, the mechanisms by which species such as cholesterol stabilize liposomes and proteins destabilize them are also not known. Liposomes are highly biocompatible and reduce irritation, but they are less stable than the nanoparticles.

6.7 NANOPARTICLES IN THE COSMETIC INDUSTRY

The polymeric nanoparticle is also a reservoir that can encapsulate active substances to protect them from the surrounding environment and adjust its properties in response to the requirements. Such nanoparticles are used for the preparation of formulations containing drugs, vitamins, steroids, proteins, enzymes, flavors, and fragrances. The main objectives are the development of formulations with prolonged activity, protection against adverse conditions, and controlled release of active ingredients. The nanoparticles are divided into two main categories: nanospheres and nanocapsules. Nanospheres are polymer matrices in which the active material is dissolved or dispersed. In the case of the nanocapsules, a polymer wall entraps an oily reservoir in which the active material is dissolved. In general, nanoparticles refer mainly to nanospheres in the literature.

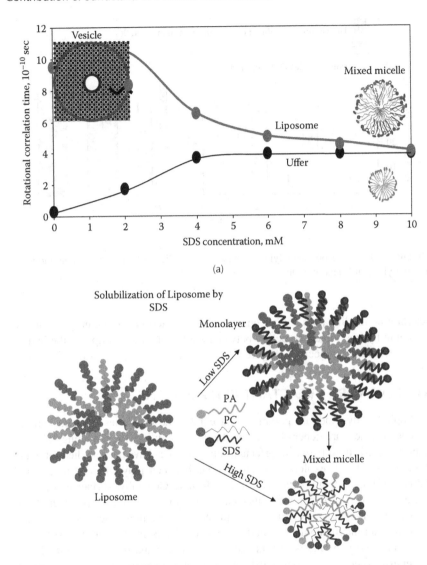

(a)

(b)

FIGURE 6.7 (a) Change in rotational correlation time of 5-doxyl stearic acid due to interactions with SDS. Buffer: increased correlation time (T) – transfer into SDS micelle. Liposome: decreased T – transfer into less rigid mixed micelle. (b) Depiction of solubilization of liposomes under low and high SDS concentrations. (From P. Deo et al., *Langmuir*, 2003, vol. 19, page 7271. With permission.)

Nanoparticles, owing to their submicron size, get well dispersed in cosmetic products. They can encapsulate a large amount of fragrance due to their large surface area.

Poly(acrylic acid) nanopaticles synthesized by the inverse microemulsion technique have been found to be able to extract the linalyl acetate fragrance, and

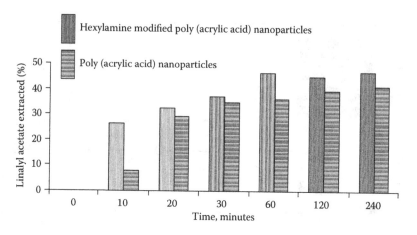

FIGURE 6.8 Extraction of linalyl acetate by poly(acrylic acid) and hexylamine modified poly(acrylic acid) nanoparticles.

hexylamine modification further enhanced the extraction significantly due to the favorable hydrophobic interaction between the hexylamine group and the hydrophobic fragrance molecules (Figure 6.8).

6.8 POLYMER SURFACTANT INTERACTIONS

Hydrophobically modified polymers that exhibit the properties of surfactants as well as polymers are generally used as rheology modifiers for providing colloidal stability. Interactions between surfactants and polymers have been studied for many years. Caria et al.[13] explored the interactions between poly(ethylene oxide) and didodecyl dimethylammonium bromide surfactant. Generally, surfactant–polymer interactions occur between individual surfactant molecules and the polymer chain, or as polymer–aggregate complexes of micelles and hemimicelles. These interactions can alter the rheological properties markedly. Thus, interactions between ionic surfactants and nonionic polymers can uncoil and expand polymer chains due to the repulsion between the ionic head groups of the surfactants bound to the polymer. Such unfolding will result in the release of the attributes trapped inside the hydrophobic nanodomain of the coiled polymer.

The rheological effect of hydrophobic modification of the polymer is clearly shown in Figure 6.9 for the case of hydroxy ethyl cellulose (HEC) and its hydrophobically modified analogue (HMHEC). The reduced viscosity of HMHEC gradually increases with surfactant concentration and then decreases in the vicinity of the critical micelle concentration. Minimum viscosity is observed at a surfactant concentration of $3.26*10^{-4}$ mol/l. Above this concentration, the viscosity again increases and approaches the value of aqueous solution. Since the solvent power of the water is not greatly affected by the presence of the surfactant,

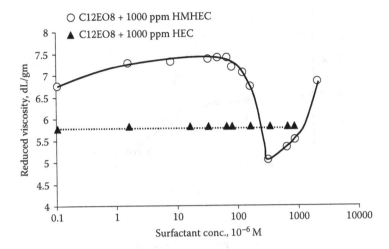

FIGURE 6.9 The reduced viscosity of HEC and HMHEC solutions (1000 ppm) as a function of added $C_{12}EO_8$.

the changes in the reduced viscosity can be considered to be due to the changes in the hydrodynamic volume of the polymer molecule and the polymer–polymer interactions. In the dilute polymer concentration region, the changes in the hydrodynamic volume are more significant than interpolymer interactions, and the variation in viscosity reflects the structural changes of the polymer. The low viscosity is the result of the compact polymer structure stabilized through the intramolecular association of the hydrophobic groups on the polymer. Hence, the initial increase in viscosity can be attributed mainly to chain expansion due to the surfactant binding on the polymer, resulting in a less compact structure. In the region of the critical micelle concentration (c.m.c.) of the surfactant, the bound surfactant molecules on the same chain associate to form a highly compact structure. The minimum obtained in Figure 6.9 is the result of this intramolecular (associated) polymer structure, and the surfactant concentration ($3.26*10^{-4}$ mol/l, $C_{12}EO_8$) corresponds to the onset of free micelles in the system. A further increase in the viscosity in the micellar range is possible due to the solubilization of the hydrophobic groups in micelles, which reduce their association, or the bridging of the polymer chain through micelles. The constant viscosity observed for the HEC–$C_{12}EO_8$ system implies a low degree of binding of the polymer with the individual surfactant molecules or its micelles.

Similarly, poly(maleic acid/octyl vinyl ether) (PMAOVE) was found to interact with sodium dodecyl sulfate (SDS) by Deo et al.[14] to yield enhanced viscosity and reduced surface tension. This is attributed to the coexistence of the mixed micelles of PMAOVE and SDS. This behavior of PMAOVE, as shown in Figure 6.10A and B, is noteworthy for its potential as a thickener in hair-styling gels.

The ability of the hydrophobically modified polymers to form nanodomains can also be utilized for the release of organic sensory attributes. Thus, the

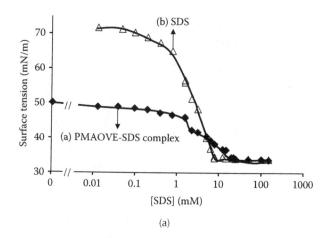

(a)

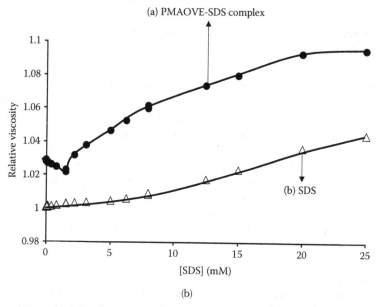

(b)

FIGURE 6.10 (A) Surface tension of aqueous solutions of sodium dodecyl sulfate in the absence (b) and presence (a) of 0.1% (wt/wt) PMAOVE as a function of SDS concentration. S.D. = ±2%. (B) Relative viscosity of aqueous solutions of sodium dodecyl sulfate in the absence (b) and presence (a) of 0.1 % (wt/wt) PMAOVE as a function of SDS concentration. S.D. = ±2%.

PMAOVE system forms hydrophobic nanodomains that can solubilize and release organic molecules by dilution or changes in pH or salinity. The effect of dilution and pH on such a release is shown in Figure 6.11A and B. These show that hydrophobically modified polymers uncoil on dilution or on increase in the pH of the medium and release the trapped hydrophobes.

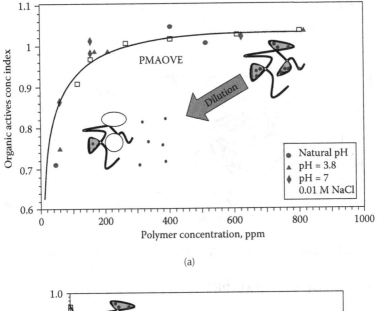

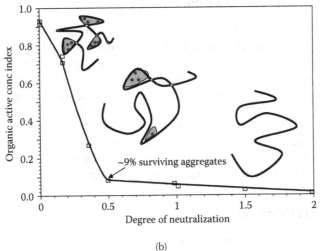

FIGURE 6.11 (A) Effect of dilution on the uncoiling of PMAOVE for the release of organic actives. (B) Effect of pH of the medium on the uncoiling of PMAOVE for the release of organic actives.

Interestingly, such polymers can also release entrapped material upon deposition on solids. Figure 6.12 shows the results obtained when PMAOVE is deposited on alumina particles. It can be seen that organics entrapped are less when the PMAOVE is in contact with the solid than when it is in micelles above 200 ppm. Evidently, the hydrophobic polymeric entanglements loosen up on coming in contact with a surface and facilitate the release of entrapped moieties.

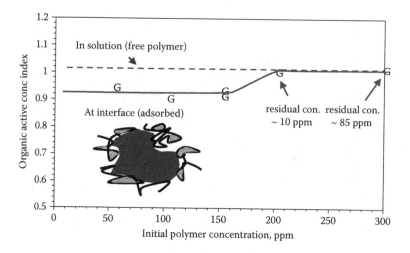

FIGURE 6.12 Uncoiling of hydrophobic domain in contact with a surface.

6.9 CONCLUDING REMARKS

Surfactants as such or in the form of colloids and emulsions play a major role in cosmetic formulations. Their interaction with liposomes and polymers, as well as their participation in the synthesis of micro- and nanoparticles, has significant impacts in the cosmetic industry. We have demonstrated that due to the interaction of the surfactants with liposomes, liposomes initially increase in size and subsequently get solubilized. Surfactants also caused unfolding of the nanodomains formed by the hydrophobically modified polymers. When the potential of the poly(acrylic acid) nanoparticles to extract fragrances was evaluated, it was observed that around 40% of the fragrance linalyl acetate was extracted in 6 h. The ability of the liposomes to extract organic attributes was also studied.

ACKNOWLEDGMENTS

The authors acknowledge financial support from the National Science Foundation, the Industrial/University Cooperative Research Center (IUCR) at Columbia University and University of Florida Engineering Research Center, and the industrial sponsors of the IUCR Center.

REFERENCES

1. P. Somasundaran, L. Zhang, and A. Lou, *Cosmetics & Toiletries* 116: 53–58 (2001).
2. D. Balzer, S. Varwig, and M. Weihrauch, *Colloids and Surfaces A: Physicochemicals and Engineering Aspect* 99: 233–246 (1995).
3. K. Kostarelos, *Advances in Colloids and Interface Science* 106: 147–168 (2003).

4. P. Somasundaran, *Journal of Colloid and Interface Science* 256: 3–15 (2002).
5. Th. F. Tadros, *Advances in Colloid and Interface Science* 46: 1-47 (1993).
6. J.M. Blakeway, P. Bourdon, and M. Seu, *International Journal of Cosmetic Science* 1: 1 (1979).
7. D.A.W. Bucks, J.J. Hostynek, R.S. Hinz, and R.H. Guy, *Toxicology and Applied Pharmacology* 120: 224–227 (1993).
8. H. Berger, *International Journal of Cosmetic Science* 19: 227–237 (1997).
9. L.B. Peppas, M.A. El-Nakoly, D.M. Piatt, and B.A. Charpentier, Eds., *ACS Symposium Series 520*, p. 45 (1996).
10. M. Seiller, M.-C. Martini, S. Benita, and S. Benita, Eds., New York: Marcel Dekker, p. 587 (1996).
11. http://saints.css.edu/bio/schroeder/liposome.gif.
12. O. López, M. Cócera, E. Wehrli, J.L. Parra, and A. de la Maza, *Archives of Biochemistry and Biophysics* 367: 153–160 (1967).
13. A. Caria, O. Regev, and A. Khan, *Journal of Colloid and Interface Science* 200: 19–30 (1998).
14. P. Deo, S. Jockusch, M.F. Ottaviani, A. Moscatelli, N.J. Turro, and P. Somasundaran, *Langmuir* 19: 10747–10752 (2003).
15. N. Deo, T. Somasundaran, P. Somasundaran, Solution properties of amitriptyline and its partitioning into lipid bilayers, *Colloids and Surfaces B: Biointerfaces* 34: 155–159 (2004).

7 Cleaner/Conditioner Systems: Surface Chemical Aspects

E.D. Goddard
Cambridge, Maryland

CONTENTS

7.1 INTRODUCTION

The traditional process of washing and conditioning, by surfactants, of the keratinous substrates, hair, and skin is quite well understood in terms of the surface chemistry of these agents and substrates.[1,2] In the case of one-shot cleaner/conditioner systems, for which the technology is still evolving, the state of knowledge of mechanisms is far less complete. This is especially true when conditioning oils are incorporated in the formulations. In attempting to shed light on mechanisms in the latter systems, it has seemed appropriate to briefly outline surface chemistry elements of the single processes of detergency and conditioning, as well as the nature of keratin substrates themselves. While some of the information on the former processes is simple to apply, one-shot cleaner/conditioner systems — in which both oil removal and oil deposition can be involved — are much more complex. Highlights of recent work in this area will be presented and analyzed. Finally, suggestions are made for the design of a simple apparatus that will allow observations of the fate (spreadability, etc.) of oils, incorporated in conditioning/washing formulations, with respect to their capture and spreading on keratin model substrates submerged in detergent solutions.

7.2 DETERGENCY: ADHESION AND CONTACT ANGLE

Detergency is basically concerned with the phenomenon, and the overcoming, of adhesion between two contacting phases, viz., a soiling material and a substrate material. Adhesion is defined in terms of the work or energy required to separate unit area of the interface between the two phases to create two separate interfaces of each of the phases with a common external medium, e.g., water or air. Mathematically, this is expressed in terms of the work of adhesion, W_A, where $W_A = \gamma_1 + \gamma_2 - \gamma_{12}$ and γ; represents the relevant surface or interfacial tension.

If one of the two contacting phases, say 2, is a liquid, the physical picture becomes much simpler to visualize and evaluate (Figure 7.1). Resolving horizontal forces (at equilibrium), one has $\gamma_1 = \gamma_{12} + \gamma_2 \cos \theta$. Hence, $W_A = \gamma_2 (1 + \cos \theta)$, where θ is the contact angle the liquid makes with the solid.

This is known as the Young equation, formulated by Thomas Young over 200 years ago. It is of fundamental significance, as it allows evaluation of the degree of adhesion in terms of readily measurable parameters, γ_2 and θ.

In practical terms, if it is desired to reduce W_A, i.e., facilitate the removal of oil, one should try to reduce γ_2 and increase θ, i.e., cause roll-up (dewetting) of the oily phase. This action, together with emulsification of the displaced oil, represents the well-known role of a surfactant (Figure 7.2). For simplicity, the surfactant adsorbed on the solid surface is omitted from Figure 7.2.

Hair and skin surfaces are naturally hydrophobic; keratin has a surface energy approximating that of polyethylene and, like it, is wettable by oils in air.[3] But keratins have a dual nature: on immersion in water they display evidence of hydration and are no longer readily wettable by mineral oil.[4] In consequence, they are protected against (re)deposition of any such oil particles that may be suspended in a contacting aqueous medium. On the other hand, preapplied oil tends to adhere to a keratin surface when it is subsequently immersed in water unless surfactant is added to the system. This latter manifestation is the essence of the detergency (oil removal) process depicted in Figure 7.2. Elegant microscopic studies of the roll-up and removal of mineral oil droplets from keratin (wool) fibers by Stevenson some 40 years ago[5] clearly show the efficiency of anionic surfactant (sodium oleate) in this respect.

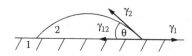

FIGURE 7.1 Sessile drop.

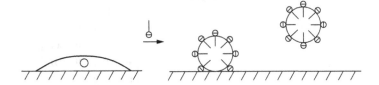

FIGURE 7.2 Action of surfactant in causing roll-up and removal of oil from a solid surface.

The adsorption of anionic surfactant that occurs on keratin fibers can be regarded as nonspecific "physisorption"; it takes place against an unfavorable electrical gradient at the pH of washing (see below). These surfactants are largely removed on decreasing their concentration (as in rinsing). This behavior contrasts with that of cationic surfactants, which tend to be retained, as discussed below.

7.3 ELECTRIC FORCES AND ADSORPTION IN CONDITIONING

The second important surface property of hair and skin concerns their electrical charge, just referred to. Here the characterizing parameter is the isoelectric point. Though somewhat dependent on the ionic strength of the bathing solution, the isoelectric point of hair fibers is rather low, viz., pH 3.2 in 10^{-4} M KCl solution.[6] This means that over most of the pH range, hair fibers in contact with water will be strongly attractive to positively charged entities, such as cationic surfactants and cationic polyelectrolytes. (The behavior of the other important substrate, viz., skin, is similar, although its isoelectric point is about 1 pH unit higher.[6]) Evidence of strong adsorption of cationic agents has been shown by many techniques, for example, by streaming potential measurements on hair.[6] This technique also allows ready determination of the desorption characteristics of such agents. Figure 7.3 shows that adsorbed cationic agents are slowly released on rinsing the hair after preexposure to the agent. While this gradual release is evident from the start of rinsing in the case of the cationic polyelectrolyte Polyquaternium-10, a two-stage process (rapid and then gradual decay) is obtained with a typical cationic surfactant, cetyl trimethyl ammonium bromide (CTAB). The long accepted view of this latter phenomenon is that the outer part of the adsorbed double layer is readily stripped during rinsing (Figure 7.4). On the other hand, the strongly (electrostaticly) bound primary layer survives rinsing and provides the boundary layer lubrication associated with softening and manageability — and also a reduction of electrostatic charging of separating surfaces (Figure 7.5) by matching of the dielectric constant of such surfaces (Cohen's rule). While polyelectrolyte (polycationic) materials are also effective as antistatic agents, they are seldom used alone for conditioning, mainly as a result of the limited boundary lubrication they confer.

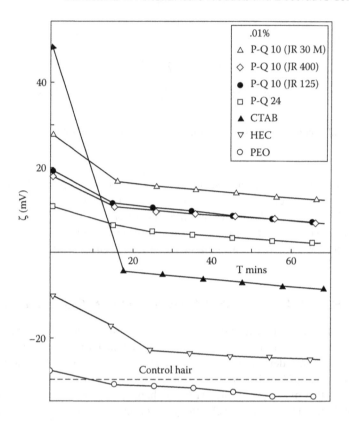

FIGURE 7.3 Decay of zeta potential of hair during a 1-h rinse (10^{-4} M KNO$_3$) after exposure to various treating solutions (0.01%). (From Goddard, E.D., *Cosmet. Toilet.*, 102, 71, 1987. With permission.)

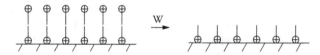

FIGURE 7.4 Stripping of outer portion of adsorbed double layer of cationic surfactant on rinsing with water (W).

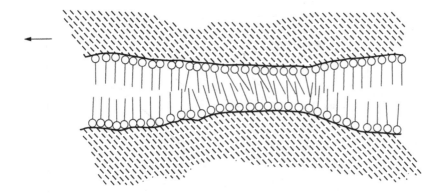

FIGURE 7.5 Nature of contact region in boundary lubrication and static control.

7.4 ONE-SHOT CLEANERS/CONDITIONERS

This category of shampoo, containing a conditioning polycation in a surfactant base formulation, became established some 30 years ago. While not as efficient as systems with a separate conditioning step, the convenience factor ensured its success.

Direct adsorption studies (radiotracer) showed finite levels of polycation adsorption from these systems.[7] The inference is that an adsorbed double layer composed of polymer/surfactant complexes constitutes the effective lubrication entity (Figure 7.6).

A totally different mechanism, known as the Goddard–Lochhead effect, has also been proposed to explain the conditioning provided by such systems, e.g., ease of combing, overall manageability, etc. It is best explained in terms of the formation of slippery insoluble polycation/anionic complexes at a certain dilution level. These become entrained in and lubricate the hair mass.[8-10] A solubility diagram illustrates the effect (Figure 7.7). The suggested mechanism, while plausible, needs further evaluation.

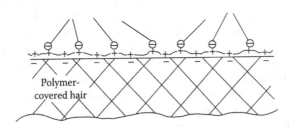

FIGURE 7.6 Adsorbed layer of polycation attracts lubricating layer of anionic surfactant.

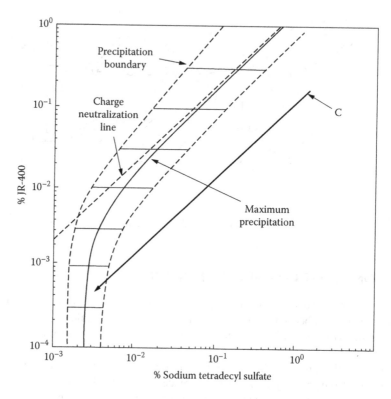

FIGURE 7.7 Conditioning via a precipitation mechanism. Following the heavy line, an initially clear solution (C, shampoo strength) can, on dilution (the rinse), pass into the precipitation zone. (From Goddard, E.D., in *Principles of Polymer Science and Technology in Cosmetics and Personal Care*, Goddard, E.D. and Gruber, J.V., Eds., Marcel Dekker, New York, 1999, chap. 5. With permission.)

7.5 INCORPORATION OF OIL

A new, and apparently self-contradictory, approach to formulating a conditioning shampoo was introduced by Lever Brothers Company in the 1960s: mineral oil was incorporated in the formulation.[11] The implicit mechanism requires deposition of oil droplets (formed and dispersed by mechanical shaking of the formulation prior to use), followed by spreading on the hair fibers — the exact opposite of the detergency process (Figure 7.2). The rationale, of course, concerns the fact that shampooing of hair is a multistage process, comprising washing, rinsing, drying, and combing. Conditions during washing, which favor oil removal and stabilization of suspended oil droplets, change markedly during rinsing when, mainly due to depletion of surfactant, the suspended oil droplets become destabilized and then, in a reversal of the process shown in Figure 7.2, tend to deposit on exposed surfaces — the fibers of hair in our case. The implied expectation is that added conditioning oil will deposit while removed oily soil will not.

In general terms, this expectation of (added) oil particle deposition has evidently been realized in practice. Theoretical aspects of the former processes are presented below. In formulations developed later by Lever Brothers[12] and other companies,[10,13–15] the oil was preemulsified for greater efficiency. Also, silicone oil has become the oil of preference because of its greater spreading efficiency.

7.6 DEPOSITION: THE DLVO THEORY AND KINETIC EFFECTS

A critical step in the conditioning process with oil-containing shampoos concerns the attraction force between the dispersed oil particles and the keratin substrate, followed by attachment and finally spreading. The fundamental theory governing interaction between particles immersed in a liquid medium was formulated by Derjaguin, Landau, Verwey, and Overbeek (DLVO). A modification of the theory by Hogg, Healy, and Fuerstenau[16] treats the case of interaction of colloid particles with a macrosurface. The theory allows the calculation of force/distance profiles representing the summation of (longer-range) electrical interaction and (shorter-range) van der Waals interaction forces. A recent paper by Somasundaran et al.[17] illustrates the interplay of such forces for the case of aqueous latex particles, charged positively or negatively, interacting with a negatively charged glass plate. Calculations showed that for particle/plate systems of like sign of charge, long-range repulsive electrical forces would lead to a considerable energy barrier opposing the deposition of particles (Figure 7.8b). In the other case, i.e., pairs of opposite sign of charge, attractive forces would prevail over the entire force/distance profile, thus favoring deposition of particles on the plate (Figure 7.8a). These predictions were in harmony with the actual deposition densities that were observed.

Jachowicz and Berthiaume have carried out extensive studies, both theoretical and experimental, on the interaction patterns and deposition of emulsified silicone droplets on hair. In their first paper,[18] which studies the deposition of various emulsified silicones (amino-, carboxy-, and nonfunctionalized), the importance of attractive electric forces in promoting deposition of the silicone droplets was clearly shown. Indeed, in some cases exposure of the hair to oppositely charged silicone emulsion particles led to gross deposition, which indicates the high probability of secondary processes occurring, such as spreading. Heavy deposition of emulsified aminosilicones has also been demonstrated by other workers using scanning electron microscopy.[19,20] Conditions favorable for such deposition can also be achieved by pretreatment of hair fibers with a cationic polymer prior to exposure to emulsions of silicone oil modified with anionic or nonionic groups.[18]

Another fundamental in colloid science as it applies to particle/substrate interactions concerns the *rate* of deposition of the particles onto the substrate. This aspect has been discussed by many investigators, including Kitchener,[21] van de Ven,[22] and Spielman and Friedlander.[23] Jachowicz and Berthiaume have used their experimental data,[18] on the deposition of particles of an aminosilicone emulsion onto hair, to assess adherence to the predictions of the theory of Spielman

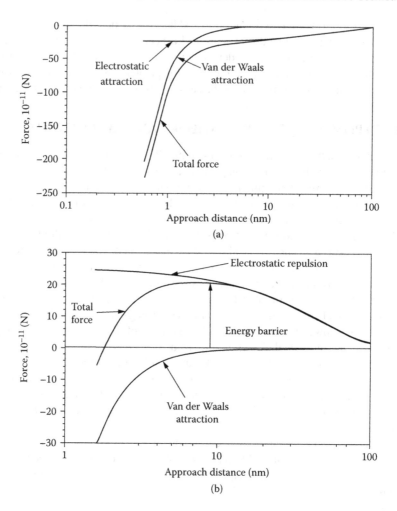

FIGURE 7.8 Interaction force/distance profile for plate/particle systems of (a) unlike charge and (b) like charge. (From Somasundaran, P. et al., *Colloids Surf A*, 142, 83, 1998. With permission.)

and Friedlander,[23] for spherical particles onto a smooth cylinder. Very good agreement between theory and the initial rate of deposition was found. A discordant note, however, can be found in the second paper of Berthiaume and Jachowicz,[13] which describes experiments with unmodified silicone oil: here the rate of deposition from an emulsion with larger drops of silicone oil was found to be higher than that from one with smaller drops. While this result is just the opposite of that predicted, it was interpreted by these authors as being consistent with "the theoretical prediction of increased attractive interactions for larger droplets" according to the Hogg–Healy–Fuerstenau model. Summarizing their work on the deposition of silicone oil from emulsions onto hair fibers, Berthiaume and Jachowicz conclude that, at least in the early stages, the process is generally driven by electrical forces. They also conclude that secondary processes, such as surfactant adsorption, coalescence of deposited oil, and spreading on the fibers, can also play a significant role. The last aspect is discussed in the last section of this chapter.

It should be pointed out that several other techniques, in addition to emulsion depletion analysis and scanning electron microscopy, referred to above, have been used to assess and confirm the deposition of silicone oil onto hair fibers from emulsions. These include atomic absorption,[24] Fourier-transform infrared spectroscopy,[19] electron spectroscopy for chemical analysis (ESCA),[25] and x-ray fluorescence as employed by Gruber and coworkers.[26,27] The results obtained by Gruber et al. are important in the sense that they were obtained under simulated shampooing conditions with realistic formulations containing predispersed (5 to 10 μ) silicone oil droplets: they also demonstrate the utility of the x-ray fluorescence method for obtaining reliable (relative) surface concentrations of deposited silicone oil, if simple precautions are taken, even though x-ray fluorescence is not an intrinsically surface-sensitive technique like ESCA, for example. The authors conclude that silicone oil is deposited onto the shampooed hair under all conditions tested and that the presence of conditioning polycations tends to modulate the deposition, presumably by adsorption on the hair fiber surface. Another finding of interest is that the presence of the higher molecular weight polycations tends to favor deposition. Full explanations of the observed phenomena have yet to be developed.

7.7 VISUALIZING THE DEPOSITION OF OIL: MACROSCOPY

From the successful achievement of conditioning by incorporating oils in shampoo formulations, one can infer that finite amounts of oil can be transferred to hair during washing, rinsing, and drying. These conclusions have been greatly strengthened by the quantitative x-ray fluorescence data of Gruber et al. on hair treated with model shampoos containing silicone oil.

The macrodeposition from silicone emulsions observed by Jachowicz and Berthiaume[18] led these authors to postulate mechanisms involving "spreading and coalescence of silicone oil on the hair fibers." Such macromanifestations suggest the possibility of actual optical observations of these processes, using techniques such as those of Stevenson,[5] who applied them to the opposite phenomenon, viz., of oil removal. One difficulty anticipated in attempting an exact reversal of the technique lies in the manual attachment of an oil droplet to an individual submerged fiber of hair (or even assemblies of hair fibers) so as to permit determination of contact angle, etc. This difficulty can be circumvented by using polished bovine hoof as a model keratin surface.[3,4]

A simplified diagram shows a proposed design for the optical cell (Figure 7.9). Here the oil drop, depending on its density, can be applied to the top or bottom of the polished keratin specimen and viewed through a goniometer optical tube, with or without magnification as required, to establish the contact angle of the applied oil drop. As the oil drops are investigated for attachment and spreading,

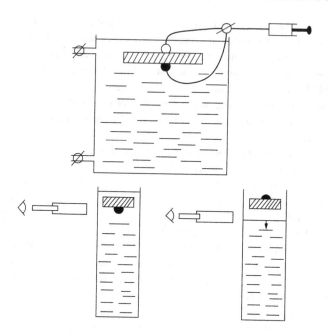

FIGURE 7.9 Schematic of a dilution/optical cell for placement and observation of oil drops on a keratin surface.

they would normally be applied to yield values of the advancing angle. If desired, data on the receding angle could be obtained by withdrawing oil from a preapplied drop. The vessel proposed in Figure 7.9 has the design of a dilution cell. Indeed, the major deposition and spreading of oil, events that represent the opposite of detergency, can be expected to occur at some (perhaps critical) stage of the dilution (rinsing) process.

We have previously drawn attention to the potential complexity of the conditioning processes in hair shampooing.[28] It is believed that the effects of many of the variables involved, e.g., the type and concentration of surfactant and polycation, the conditioning oil itself, the influence of pretreatment of the keratin surface, etc., could be explored conveniently, and in an exploratory way, by use of the proposed dilution cell.

Implicit in the foregoing is the importance of the surface chemistry of hair, referred to earlier: tersely put, keratins display the dual nature of being hydrophobic in air, but hydratable and more hydrophilic in water.[3,4] Although no attachment of a mineral oil drop to a water-immersed keratin surface could be achieved,[4] the superior spreading coefficient of a triglyceride, and especially a silicone oil, is expected to provide enhanced attachment ability. Indeed, the data presented in the previous section of this chapter already point to this. The presence of surfactant in the contacting solution will be inimical to such attachment; it will be more favorable in the rinse — perhaps occurring at some critical dilution level. Spreading will undoubtedly be enhanced as the surface dries.

The effect of the drying process on the spreading of oil could easily be studied for oils heavier than water by withdrawing (diluted) solution to below the level of the keratin surface. Some alteration to the simple procedure or design would be necessary to study the process for oils lighter than water. The drops would need to be captured and transferred onto the (drying) keratin surface, or alternatively, a fresh drop would need to be positioned.

REFERENCES

1. Durham K. *Surface Activity and Detergency.* London: MacMillan, 1961.
2. Evans WP. *Chem Ind* 1969; 893.
3. El Shimi A, Goddard ED. *J Colloid Interface Sci* 1974; 48:242.
4. El Shimi A, Goddard ED. *J Colloid Interface Sci* 1974; 48:249.
5. Stevenson DG. In *Surface Activity and Detergency,* Durham K, Ed. London: MacMillan, 1961, chap. 6.
6. Goddard ED. *Cosmet Toilet* 1987; 102:71.
7. Goddard ED, Faucher JA, Scott RJ, Turney ME. *J Soc Cosmet Chem* 1975; 26:539.
8. Goddard ED, Hannan RB. *J Am Oil Chem Soc* 1977; 54:561.
9. Goddard ED. In *Principles of Polymer Science and Technology in Cosmetics and Personal Care,* Goddard ED, Gruber JV, Eds. New York: Marcel Dekker, 1999, chap. 5.
10. Lochhead RY. *Cosmet Toilet* 1988; 103:23.
11. Pader M, Martin DJ. U.S. Patent 3,533,955, 1970.
12. Pader M. U.S. Patent 4,364,837, 1982.
13. Berthiaume MD, Jachowicz J. *J Colloid Interface Sci* 1991; 141:299.
14. Sukhavinder S, Robbins CR, Cheng WM. WO 94/06409 A1, 1994.
15. Wells RL. U.S. Patent 5,573,709, 1966.
16. Hogg R, Healy TW, Fuerstenau DW. *J Chem Soc Faraday Trans* 1966; 62:1638.
17. Somasundaran P, Shrotri S, Ananthapadmanabhan KP. *Colloids Surfaces A,* 1998; 142:83.
18. Jachowicz J, Berthiaume MD. *J Colloid Interface Sci* 1989; 133:118.
19. Klimisch HM, Kohl GS, Sabourin JM. *J Soc Cosmet Chem* 1987; 38:247.
20. Yahagi K. *J Soc Cosmet Chem* 1992; 43:275.
21. Kitchener JA. *J Soc Cosmet Chem* 1973; 24:709.
22. Van de Ven TGM. *Langmuir* 1996; 12:5254.
23. Spielman LA, Friedlander SK. *J Colloid Interface Sci* 1974; 46:22.
24. Gooch EG, Kohl GS. *J Soc Cosmet Chem* 1988; 39:383.
25. Goddard ED. Unpublished work.
26. Gruber JV, Lamoureux BR, Joshi N, Moral L. *Colloids Surfaces B* 2000; 19:127.
27. Gruber JV, Lamoureux BR, Joshi N, Moral L. *J Cosmet Sci* 2001; 52:131.
28. Goddard ED. *J Cosmet Sci* 2002; 53:283.

8 Emulsions and Their Behavior

P. Somasundaran,[1] Thomas H. Wines,[2] Somil C.
Mehta,[1] Nissim Garti,[3] and Raymond Farinato[4]
[1]NSF Industry/University Cooperative Research Center for
Advanced Studies in Novel Surfactants, Columbia
University
[2]Pall Corporation
[3]Casali Institute of Applied Chemistry, School of Applied
Science and Technology, Hebrew University of Jerusalem
[4]Cytec Industries, Inc.

CONTENTS

8.1 INTRODUCTION

Emulsions are used widely in the cosmetics industry in various products, including conditioners, moisturizers, lotions, creams, sunscreens, and shower gels. An emulsion is essentially a dispersion of droplets of water or oil in a continuous medium of the other. Types of emulsion, depending on the size of the droplets or the nature of their distribution, are macroemulsion or simply emulsion, microemulsion, miniemulsion, and double emulsions:

Macroemulsions — The most common type of emulsions, where the particle sizes of droplets are more than 400 nm. They are visually opaque, but the individual droplets can be easily observed under microscopy. Macroemulsions are thermodynamically unstable, but are kinetically stabilized using surface-active agents.

Miniemulsions — Emulsions with a particle size range in between macro- and microemulsions (about 100 to 400 nm), usually having a blue–white appearance.

Microemulsions — Transparent and most stable form of emulsions, where the particle sizes range from several nanometers to a maximum of about 100 nm. They are a thermodynamically stable form of emulsions and theoretically require an infinite time to break.

Double emulsions — Small droplets of one phase (e.g., oil) dispersed in larger droplets of a second phase (e.g., water) with the latter further dispersed in the former (i.e., oil) as the continuous medium. Problems of phase separation due to differences in geometry of two media are minimized in this case.

The main functions of an emulsion are moisturization and occlusion achieved by their major component, surfactant, on account of its two distinct parts, one hydrophilic and the other lipophilic. In a cosmetic formulation, the hydrophilic part of an emulsion can continuously supply water, and thus is responsible for its moisturizing function, whereas the lipophilic part can prevent water loss from the skin surface, thus performing its occlusive function.[1] The effectiveness of the emulsion results from its rather large oil/water interfacial area, which on account of its positive surface free energy, is also thermodynamically unstable. Emulsions with long-term stability can be obtained, however, by the use of surfactants, which have been called emulsifiers. The emulsifiers accumulate at the oil/water interface and create an energy barrier to flocculation and coalescence of the droplets, and thus impart stability to the emulsion. The emulsifiers can be ionic, nonionic, or zwitterionic surfactants, proteins, or amphiphilic polymers.[2]

8.2 MACROEMULSIONS

Emulsions can be dispersions of either water in oil-continuous medium (W/O) or oil in water-continuous medium (O/W), depending on the amount of the two phases, the nature of the emulsifier, and the way it is prepared. As indicated above, a double emulsion can also be a dispersion of water in oil droplets in water continuum (W/O/W) or oil in water droplets in oil continuum (O/W/O). The behavior of a binary emulsion can be very different for the same amount of oil and water dispersed into each other, depending on whether it is a water-in-oil emulsion or an oil-in-water emulsion or a double emulsion. One of the main factors that decide whether a water-in-oil or an oil-in-water emulsion will be formed is the nature of the surfactant. The nature of emulsifiers is described by a concept known as the hydrophile–lipophile balance (HLB), which is based on the relative fractions of water-compatible and oil-compatible groups in the surface-active agent.

8.2.1 A HYDROPHILE–LIPOPHILE BALANCE (HLB)

The concept of HLB was first introduced by Griffin[3] and later extended by Davies.[4] As per this theory, hydrophobic emulsifiers have a relatively low HLB value and are predicted to be suitable for forming water-in-oil emulsions, whereas hydrophilic emulsifiers have relatively high HLB values and are good for the reverse type of emulsions. Bancroft[5] postulated that upon mixing of the two phases with a surfactant, the emulsifier forms a third phase as a film at the interface between the two phases being mixed. He also predicted that the phase in which the emulsifier is most soluble will become the continuous phase. The continuous phase need not be the predominant quantity of material present. The HLB value can be calculated from the structure of the emulsifier as follows:[6]

$$HLB = 20 * M_H / (M_H + M_L)$$

where M_H and M_L are the molecular weights of hydrophilic and lipophilic moieties, respectively. Davies proposed another method of calculating HLB, which

TABLE 8.1
Classification of Emulsifiers according to the HLB Values

Solubility in Water	HLB Value	Description
Insoluble	4–5	Water-in-oil emulsifier
Poorly dispersible (milky appearance)	6–9	Wetting agent
Translucent to clear	10–12	Detergent
Very soluble	13–18	Oil-in-water emulsifier

is based on a group contribution method, as given below:

$$HLB = \sum hydrophilic - \sum lipophilic + 7$$

A table for contribution by individual functional groups is reported elsewhere.[7] HLB helps to estimate the type of surfactant or combinations of surfactants that are appropriate for a given application. A blend of emulsifiers can also be designed by using a weighted average of the surfactants with individual HLB values. Depending on the HLB value, the following general behavior is observed for an emulsifier (Table 8.1).

In recent years there has been a greater use of silicones as surfactants and oils in the preparation of emulsions. The direct application of the HLB concept to these materials has resulted in very approximate and often misleading values due to the fact that silicones are organic/inorganic hybrids and the thermodynamics of their interactions with the oil and water phases in emulsions scale differently than do the interactions of purely organic amphiphiles. Moreover, the frequent presence of blends of silicone and hydrocarbon surfactants has offered additional challenges for predicting emulsion properties. Also, there have been many new silicone compounds that combine polyoxyethylene (water soluble), silicone (silicone soluble), and hydrocarbon (oil soluble) portions into one molecule. The introduction of these types of molecules and the inability to fit them into the traditional HLB scheme have led to the development of a concept called three-dimensional HLB, first developed by O'Lenick.[8] This system is similar to HLB in terms of the scale used, but it appears in a triangular representation instead of as a linear HLB scale. One side of the triangle represents the HLB system. The three parameters of the three-dimensional HLB system can be calculated as follows:

$$X = 20 * M_H / M \quad Y = 20 * M_L / M \quad Z = 20 - X - Y$$

where X represents the coordinate of the water-compatible portion, Y represents the coordinate of the oil-compatible portion, Z represents the coordinate of the

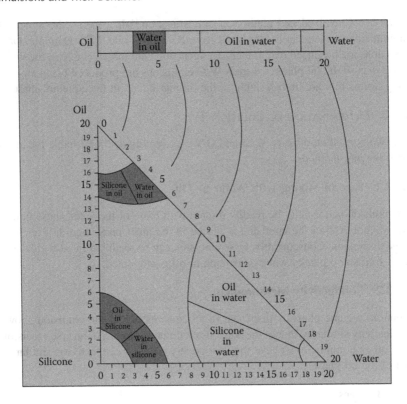

FIGURE 8.1 Hydrophile–lipophile balance (HLB) evolves into three-dimensional HLB. Two-dimensional HLB (A) becomes hypotenuse to the three-dimensional HLB (B). (Reproduced from O'Lenick, A.J., *J. Surfactants Detergents*, 3, 387–393, 2000.)

silicone-compatible portion, and M_H, M_L, and M represent the respective hydrophilic, lipophilic, and total molecular weights.

Pictorially, the three-dimensional HLB system can be represented as shown in Figure 8.1.[9] The triangle used is not equilateral, but a right triangle due to the fact that silicone and hydrocarbon compounds are not equally hydrophobic on a weight basis.

Other methods for surfactant selection based on phase inversion temperature (PIT) and hydrophilic–lipophilic deviation (HLD) are described elsewhere.[11]

8.2.2 TYPE OF MACROEMULSIONS

As mentioned earlier, based on the nature of the dispersed phase, macroemulsions are usually one of two types: oil in water (O/W) or water in oil (W/O). Examples of O/W systems are skin lotions, milk, mayonnaise, and paints. Examples of W/O systems include conditioning agents, butter, and margarine. The type of emulsion formed depends primarily on the nature of the emulsifier and on the ratio of components involved and method of emulsification.[11] In general, the nature of an emulsion formed can be predicted from Bancroft's rule.[12] For example, O/W emulsions are produced by emulsifying agents that are more soluble in the water phase than in the oil phase, whereas W/O emulsions are produced using emulsifying agents that are more soluble in the oil phase than in the aqueous phase.

8.2.3 DETERMINATION OF EMULSION TYPE

The two type of emulsions, W/O and O/W, are readily distinguishable based on the following methods.

8.2.3.1 Ease of Mixing with Water or Oil

An emulsion can usually be readily diluted with more of the outer phase liquid. But when a drop of the emulsion is placed in the inner phase liquid, it tends to resist dispersion. Consequently, O/W emulsion can be readily diluted with water, but it forms two phases when dispersion in oil is attempted.

8.2.3.2 Conductivity Measurement

When an organic phase is dispersed in an aqueous phase, the emulsion shows conductivity similar to that of the aqueous continuous phase. An inverse emulsion with oil as a continuous phase shows a greatly reduced conductivity, similar to that of the oil phase.

8.2.3.3 Dyes

Dyes impart color to a solution when they are dissolved in a solvent. Hence, when an oil-soluble dye is used, it shows color in W/O emulsions, but shows less color in O/W emulsions.

8.2.3.4 Microscopy

The nature of an emulsion can be identified using simple optical microscopy if the two phases of an emulsion have different refractive indices. The phase having the higher refractive index appears brighter under the microscope. Hence, knowing the refractive indices of individual phases, one can determine which phase is continuous.[11] Moreover, if the oil phase has UV or fluorescent groups, then the nature of dispersed and continuous phases can be readily observed using appropriate spectroscopies.

8.2.3.5 Self-Diffusion Constants

Nuclear magnetic resonance (NMR) spectroscopy can be used to measure self-diffusion constants for a molecule in solution. A molecule that is hydrophilic will diffuse much faster in an O/W emulsion than in a W/O emulsion. Conversely, a substrate that is hydrophobic will diffuse much faster in a W/O emulsion than in an O/W emulsion.[13]

8.2.4 Phase Diagrams

Phase diagrams are thermodynamic maps representing the behavior of macroscopic and colloidal systems with respect to the concentrations of individual components and other intensive variables (e.g., temperature and pressure). Emulsions usually involve at least three components: an oil phase, an aqueous phase, and a surface-active agent that stabilizes the interface between the oil phase and water phase. Apart from these three, emulsions often have some co-surfactants or electrolytes or simply other solutes. The other variables that govern a phase diagram are temperature and pressure, the latter often constant at atmospheric pressure in cosmetic applications.

A simple three-component system (oil, water, and surfactant) can be simply represented by a ternary-phase diagram for each temperature. An example of such a simple system is shown in Figure 8.2. The diagram shows five different isotropic regions: the dilute normal micellar solution, L_1, in the left-hand corner; a concentrated micellar solution, L_1', close to the binary water–$C_{12}E_5$ axes; the sponge or bicontinuous phase, L_3, near the left-hand corner; the inverted micellar solution, L_2, which encompasses the pure oil and pure surfactant phases; and the microemulsion, μE, in the center of the diagram. In addition, there is a large lamellar phase region, L_α. The three corners of the fan-shaped microemulsion region connect to three three-phase triangles. At low surfactant concentration, the microemulsion is in equilibrium with L_1 and L_2. For different temperatures, the triangular phase diagram of oil, water, and surfactant varies greatly.[14]

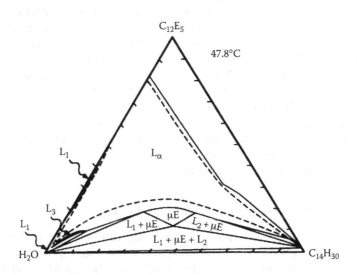

FIGURE 8.2 Phase diagram of the ternary system water–tetradecane–$C_{12}E_5$. (Reproduced from Evans, D.F. and Wennerstrom, H., *The Colloidal Domain Where Physics, Chemistry, Biology and Technology Meet*, VCH Publishers, New York, 1994.)

Many emulsions employ water as the aqueous phase and some hydrocarbon oil as the organic phase. There has been considerable interest in the cosmetics industry over the last few years to use silicone oil as the hydrophobic phase. Silicones are the only class of hybrid organic/inorganic polymers that have been extensively commercialized. Silicones are considered one of the prime delivering agents for skin and hair care products.[15] But since silicones are incompatible with water, as well as most hydrocarbons, a very common mode of their application is in the form of emulsions. Silicone emulsions typically contain water, silicone oil, and a surfactant. Stabilization of silicone oil in water is relatively more difficult than stabilization of hydrocarbon oil in water, and hence the choice of surfactant and the processing equipment are very important. The most common practice of selection of the surfactant is based on the three-dimensional HLB concept described above.[8] The most common processing equipment used for making an emulsion is a homogenizer, which uses mechanical energy to break one of the phases into small droplets.[10]

There has been some work done on the phase diagrams of cyclic silicone oils (D4, D5) and linear silicone chains, water, and a nonionic silicone surfactant called silicone copolyol.[16–18] These phase diagrams show a variety of regions, including simple micellar solutions (L_1 and L_2), microemulsions, and liquid crystalline phases. While some knowledge exists about the behavior of nonionic silicone surfactants, very little is known about ionic silicone surfactants. Although nonionic surfactants are very effective at lowering the interfacial tensions with aqueous systems, they are intolerant to pH variations and hydrolyze to long-chain alcohols. Since long-chain alcohols are irritants, nonionic silicone surfactants are not easily employed under all pH conditions. Moreover, the ionic surfactants are polyelectrolytes, and hence can modify the rheological properties of their formulations, which is a desired outcome in cosmetic products. Our group is evaluating the emulsifying ability of several anionic, cationic, and amphoterically modified silicone polymers. The results indicate that in one case, for example, an anionically modified silicone polymer stabilizes an emulsion of water in oil only at a specific composition of 80% water and 20% silicone oil (D5). The phase diagram is shown in Figure 8.3.

It was observed that 80% water was stabilized as inverse emulsion in a 20% oil phase. Moreover, the droplets are relatively larger, ranging into tens of microns. It is interesting to note that even with just 0.2% surfactant, these concentrated macroemulsions are stable for weeks.

8.2.5 Factors Affecting the Stability of Emulsions

The main reason for phase separation is coalescence of the dispersed droplets, which affects the shelf-life of a cosmetic product. Flocculation leads to sticking together of droplets, which has a similar effect on the emulsion stability as coalescence. The factors that decide the flocculating tendency of dispersed droplets are the same as those that decide the flocculating tendency of solid particles in a dispersion, discussed more in Somasundaran et al.[20]

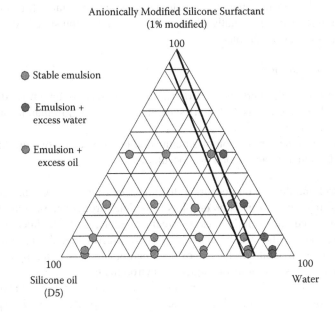

FIGURE 8.3 Three-component triangular phase diagram. The three components are water, cyclic silicone oil (D5), and anionically modified silicone surfactant.

The factors that decide stability of droplets in an emulsion are:[11]

- The physical nature of the interfacial film
- The existence of an electrical or steric barrier
- The viscosity of the interfacial film
- The size distribution of the droplets
- The dispersed phase volume
- Temperature

8.2.6 DESTABILIZATION MECHANISMS

Macroemulsions are thermodynamically unstable, and hence they undergo destabilization after a certain period. Emulsions destabilize due to different mechanisms, some of which follow.

8.2.6.1 Sedimentation/Creaming

During storage, due to the density differences between oils and water, there is a tendency of the oil phase to concentrate at the bottom or top of the emulsion. The rate of separation can be lowered by reducing the droplet size, lowering the density difference between the phases, and increasing the viscosity of the medium.

In addition, the separation/creaming rate depends on the volume fraction of the dispersed phase and is usually slow in concentrated emulsions[21] due to the crowding effect of the droplets.

8.2.6.2 Flocculation

Flocculation is defined as a process by which two or more droplets aggregate. Larger droplets (>2 mm) separate faster, and flocculation promotes creaming and sedimentation.

Flocculation destabilization of an emulsion takes place by two mechanisms: bridging flocculation and depletion flocculation.

- Bridging flocculation occurs in the presence of macromolecular emulsifying agents. Emulsion droplets flocculate through interaction of the adsorbed macromolecules between droplets, and the flocculation depends on the size, type, and amount of macromolecules used in the system. In addition, the rate of flocculation can be affected by the pH and ionic strength of the aqueous environment.
- Depletion flocculation occurs due to exclusion of polymers and the subsequent osmotic flow of the continuous phase from the space between the two dispersed phase droplets. For example the presence of nonabsorbing polymers like polysaccharides (dextran, xanthan, HEC, etc.) induces flocculation of casein-stabilized milk emulsion.[22,23]

Electrical neutralization of charged surfaces of the drop due to addition of a salt of oppositely charged surfactants can also lead to flocculation of drops.

8.2.6.3 Coalescence

Coalescence is the process in which two or more droplets collide and combine with each other, resulting in the formation of one larger droplet. Coalescence involves breaking the interfacial film and is irreversible. Various factors, such as solubility of the emulsifier, pH, salts, emulsifier type and concentration,[24] phase–volume ratio, temperature, and properties of the film, affect the coalescence stability of emulsions.

8.2.6.4 Ostwald Ripening

Ostwald ripening occurs in emulsions with polydispersed droplets. As a result, larger droplets grow at the expense of the small ones.[25] Eventually, the small droplets become very small and solubilize in the continuous medium. This phenomenon is generally observed when the oil is highly soluble in the aqueous phase.

8.2.6.5 Engulfment

In this process, one of the droplets simply engulfs the other droplet, causing a coarsening of the dispersed phase (Figure 8.4).

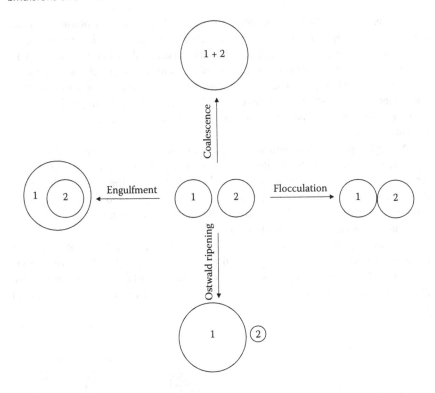

FIGURE 8.4 Schematic diagram illustrating the emulsion destabilization mechanisms

8.3 MINIEMULSIONS

Miniemulsions are very useful for cosmetics from the point of view of polymer latex preparation, where the translucent/transparent appearance of the formulation gives a very attractive product. Moreover, miniemulsions do not cream or settle because the Brownian movement of the sub-micron-sized dispersed droplets mostly offsets the effect of gravity, and hence they result in long-lasting cosmetic products. Miniemulsions are also widely used in the pharmaceutical industry and in drug delivery systems, where certain miniemulsions have been used to kill pathogens and inactivate viral functions.[26,27]

8.4 MICROEMULSIONS

Microemulsions have attracted the attention of many researchers since the pioneering works of Hoar and Schulman in the 1940s.[28] The term *microemulsion* refers to a fluid system that is a transparent single phase on the macroscale, but is heterogeneous on the microscale, with dispersed oil globules in the size range of a few nanometers up to a hundred nanometers; stability is provided by a surfactant layer. In many cases, a co-surfactant, such as a low molecular weight alcohol, is required to form microemulsions, and the aqueous phase can have added salt to change the ionic strength. Reverse microemulsions have water pools dispersed in a continuous nonpolar hydrocarbon phase. Whether a surfactant will tend to form a microemulsion or reverse microemulsion is largely dependent on the critical packing parameters of the surfactant molecule or combination of surfactant and co-surfactant molecule.[29,30] The ratio of the hydrophobe volume to the product of the head group area and molecular length is defined as critical packing parameter.

A third type of microemulsion can also exist, where the characteristics of this microemulsion do not fit into either of the previous classes, and instead is termed a *bicontinuous microemulsion*.[31] The nature of the system fluctuates between water in oil and oil in water and can be pictured as a sponge-like morphology with no real distinct drop structure. The oil-continuous and water-continuous domains exist simultaneously.

Additional structures that are possible with the surfactant/oil/water systems include lamellar phases, vesicles, and liposomes, with the possibility of various geometries for the microemulsions and reverse microemulsions, such as spherical, ellipsoid, and cylindrical shapes. Examples of such structures are presented in Figure 8.5.

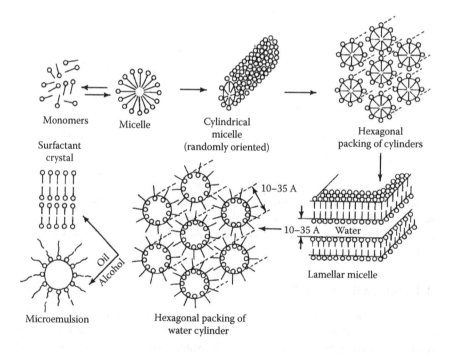

FIGURE 8.5 Possible microstructures formed from surfactant/oil/water systems. (Reproduced from Mittal, K.L. and Mukerjee, P., in *Micellization, Solubilization, and Microemulsions*, Vol. 1, Mittal, K.L., Ed., Platinum Press, New York, 1977.)

In some cases, different organized structures can coexist with each other in two or three phases. These systems have been classified by Winsor[33,34] as type I, oil phase in equilibrium with oil-in-water microemulsion; type II, water phase in equilibrium with water-in-oil microemulsion; and type III, bicontinuous microemulsion in equilibrium with oil and water. These types of systems have been studied for their application to enhanced oil recovery.

Unlike macroemulsions that will phase separate over time, microemulsions are considered to be thermodynamically stable and will retain their composition indefinitely, barring any surfactant decomposition or impurities in the system. The main feature of microemulsions and reverse microemulsions, allowing their stability, is the ultralow interfacial tensions of $<10^{-2}$ dyne/cm. The formation of microemulsions from water, oil, and surfactant can be analyzed from components of the free energies.[35] The water–oil surface area created involves the formation of a surfactant layer, usually spontaneously $(\Delta G)_{\text{surface formation}} < 0$. The self-associated surfactant layer will form readily due to either London–van der Waals attraction in a nonpolar medium or hydrogen bonding and hydrophobic interactions for the nonpolar tails in an aqueous medium. The formation of a surfactant layer will have a penalty for creating surface area when the interface has a small positive energy or interfacial tension, $(\Delta G)_{\text{interfacial tension}} > 0$. Next, the large number of small drops leads to an increase in entropy that is more pronounced as the drop size decreases. This results in a decrease in free energy, $(\Delta G)_{\text{entropy of dispersion}} < 0$. Another significant factor is the interaction energies between the microemulsion drops. Attraction due to London–van der Waals forces arising from charge fluctuations will contribute a negative component to the free energy, $(\Delta G)_{\text{attraction}} < 0$, while repulsion due to double-layer electrostatic or steric factors can lead to an increase in the free energy, $(\Delta G)_{\text{repulsion}} > 0$. The overall free energy from the different free energy contributions will create spontaneous stable microemulsions if their sum is negative:

$$\Delta G_{\text{microemulsion}} = \Delta G_{\text{surface formation}} + \Delta G_{\text{interfacial tension}} + \Delta G_{\text{entropy of dispersion}} + \Delta G_{\text{attraction}} + \Delta G_{\text{repulsion}}$$

The applications of microemulsions include the formation of microgels,[36] polymers,[37] novel drug carriers,[38] and metal colloids.[39] The microemulsions have also been used to model the process in biological membrane systems for studying the transport of materials across cell walls.[40] In cosmetics, microemulsions have found a use for extraction of odorous molecules, such as linalool, citral, and limonene, by solubilization in the micellar core.[41–43] Water-based microemulsions containing Jojoba oil were developed by Shevachman et al., which is uniquely useful in the cosmetics industry as a carrier formulation.[44] Microemulsions containing cyclopentasiloxane (D5)–silicone-based formulations are very effective as cleansing solutions.[45] Such compositions make use of the bicontinuous nature of microemulsions. Other applications of microemulsions in cosmetics include optically clear[46] and temperature-insensitive formulations.[47]

8.4.1 EQUILIBRIUM STUDIES

The goal of equilibrium studies is to determine how composition and temperature can affect the phase behavior and microstructure of a microemulsion system. A phase diagram may be determined by mixing each ratio of a mixture of two components (say oil and surfactant); then a fixed amount of the third phase (water) is added to obtain a mixture of designated composition. These samples are mixed using vortex mixer and allowed to equilibrate at a constant temperature (within 0.1°C). After 24 h of storage, the number of phases and the levels of interfaces are measured. Examination of the phases between crossed polars is done to determine the birefringence of the phases. The sample is again mixed and examined a few days later to check if equilibrium was truly reached in the first observations. Phase equilibrium is said to have been achieved when no further change with time in solution appearance or phase volumes is apparent. The time for equilibrium to be attained varies and is dependent on the composition, viscosity, structure, and vicinity of critical points.[48]

A number of phase conditions are possible in a microemulsion system, including the single-phase states of water-in-oil microemulsion (W/O), oil-in-water microemulsion (O/W), and liquid crystal (LC; lamellar or hexagonal), and various two-phase regions that are composed of the single-phase states in equilibrium with an excess oil or water phase.

The phases in microemulsion have been evaluated using a multitude of analytical techniques,[29] including small-angle neutron scattering (SANS), small-angle x-ray scattering (SAXS), dynamic light scattering (DLS), static light scattering (SLS), nuclear magnetic resonance (NMR),[36] electric birefringence (Kerr effect),[50] time-resolved fluorescence quenching (TRFQ), Fourier-transformed infrared spectroscopy (FTIR),[36] ultraviolet spectroscopy (UV),[39] freeze–fracture electron microscopy (FFEM), vapor pressure osmometry (VPO),[51] viscometry,[50] ultracentrifuge (UC),[52] microwave dielectric determination,[53] electron spin resonance (ESR),[31] ultrasound absorption, and sound velocity[54] and acoustic attenuation spectroscopy for particle size and polydispersity.[55] Thermodynamics has been applied by a number of researchers[35,56,57] to model the equilibrium radius and phase transition conditions for reverse microemulsions.

8.4.2 KINETIC STUDIES

The dynamic or kinetic nature of microemulsion systems can be subdivided into three aspects to facilitate modeling and understanding of the underlying mechanisms:

1. Droplet–droplet collisions (with and without exchange of materials)
2. Equilibrium exchange of surfactant monomers between the microemulsion drops and the bulk continuous phase
3. Fluidity or rigidity of the surfactant layer coating the microemulsion drop

The exchange of surfactant monomers between the droplet and the continuous phase has been associated with rapid fluctuations in the charge of the microemulsion droplet due to momentary imbalances in the charge at the interface.[58] These charge fluctuations can lead to attractive forces between the drops and influence the collision behavior. The fluidity or rigidity of the surfactant layer can affect both the exchange of the monomer surfactant molecules with the continuous phase and the rate of effective collisions between droplets, whereby materials are exchanged between the water pools of reverse microemulsions.

In probing the kinetics of microemulsion systems, various experimental techniques have been employed. Stopped-flow (SF)[59] and continuous-flow integrated output (CFIO)[59] techniques are examples of flow methods where in dynamics induced by mixing, two reactant streams are measured. Other techniques, such as time-resolved fluorescence quenching (TRFQ)[29] and laser photolysis,[60] are employed where dynamics of systems already in a mixed state can be measured. Relaxation or jump techniques offer a way to suddenly disrupt the surfactant monolayer and then monitor how fast a new equilibrium state (surfactant layer repair) is reached. Transport of materials across surfactant layers or solubilization in reverse microemulsion systems, as well as surfactant monolayer rigidity exposed to an external force, can also be evaluated this way.[61] Quasi-elastic neutron scattering[62] has been applied to determine the surfactant monolayer mobility (rigidity); however, in this case the microemulsion system is not perturbed, but instead is monitored under equilibrium conditions.

For reverse microemulsions, electrical percolation[29] is an additional means to obtain information regarding drop–drop interactions, but is less direct and is open to interpretation, depending on the model chosen to explain the sudden increase in electrical conduction (hopping, drop–drop collisions, bicontinuous phase shift).

8.4.3 EFFECT OF ADDITIVES

8.4.3.1 Nonpolymeric Additives

Numerous studies have been conducted on the relatively simple three-component system of water/oil/surfactant, and a baseline has been established of its expected behavior under various experimental conditions (light scattering, electrical percolation, etc.). The addition of a fourth component can produce significant changes in the system behavior, while still maintaining the essential features of the reverse microemulsion, consisting of water droplets coated with surfactant and dispersed in the hydrocarbon solvent. This fourth component can be salts, alcohols, proteins, anionic surfactants, cationic surfactants, nonionic surfactants, or different hydrocarbon solvents. The role of additives in producing changes in the colloidal behavior of reverse microemulsions has been modeled on their effects on the surfactant film rigidity or curvature. The ratio of the volume of the basis of the hydrocarbon tails to the polar head groups has been used to describe these effects and is known as the critical packing parameter, as described earlier:[29,30]

$$R_f = V_H/a_o l$$

where V_H is the hydrocarbon tail volume, a_o is the area of polar head group at interface, and l is the surfactant chain length.

As R_f increases, the film rigidity generally increases. Surfactants with branched or bulky nonpolar tails may lead to poor packing, which leads to R_f ratios that do not support spherical microemulsion geometry. The R_f ratio has been used as a means to predict whether regular microemulsions, reverse microemulsions, or lamellar phases will be formed.

When salts are added, the attractive energy between drops is found to decrease, and this can be explained by a shift in the water pool ionic strength or conductivity. With the salts present, the repulsion between the polar head groups of the charged surfactants decreases due to compression of the electrical double layer. This allows the polar head groups to pack closer together, occupying a smaller area (a_0), leading to a stiffer film that is less penetrable during collisions with other droplets.

The effect of alcohols on the surfactant film rigidity is dependent on the length of the hydrocarbon tail. For short tails (C = 1 to 3), the alcohol is largely water soluble and will not have much penetration into the nonpolar tail region of the microemulsion corona, but will adsorb in the polar head group region. Therefore, the polar head groups will be spread apart, occupying a larger interfacial area, while the hydrocarbon tails will essentially not be affected and will maintain the same volume. The film rigidity is lowered, with a resultant increase in the effectiveness of collisions or attractive interactions. For intermediate alcohols (C = 4 to 7), the alcohol will be located in the surfactant film region, with the nonpolar tails of the alcohol mingling with the nonpolar tails of the surfactant. This will contribute to the total volume of the hydrocarbon tails, with a net effect of increasing the film rigidity. This leads to the droplets being more resistant to collisions or coalescence. For higher-chain alcohols, the solubility increases for the oil phase and the alcohols are no longer located preferentially at the surfactant film interface. The effect of the longer-chain alcohols at low concentration is therefore negligible.

Cationic surfactants such as cetyl trimethyl ammonium chloride and tetramethyl ammonium chloride tend to decrease the rate of effective collisions or attractive drop interactions by partially neutralizing the negatively charged head group of the surfactant forming the microemulsion, allowing for a more compact structure of the mixed surfactant film. Anionic surfactants, as additives, tend to have the opposite effect and are thought to have a disruptive effect on the surfactant packing, thereby allowing an increased penetration by solutes.

When the solvent chain length is changed, the solubility of the nonpolar tails of the surfactant in the hydrocarbon solvent will be influenced. If the solvent has a structure similar to that of the surfactant tails, the highest solubility will be achieved, and this will result in surfactant nonpolar tails swelling preferentially, as compared to the hydrocarbon solvent with different chain lengths. The result is that solvents closely matching the surfactant nonpolar tails will have higher film rigidity and collisions will be less effective than in other solvents. This will also allow for more water to be solubilized before a phase transition.

8.4.3.2 Polymeric Additives

Polymeric additives can have a dramatic effect on microemulsion behavior. Homopolymers will generally be partitioned primarily into one domain, either the aqueous core, the surfactant interface, or the alkane phase. Amphiphilic polymers can be associated with all three regions to some extent, and may preferentially locate at the interface depending on the specific nature of the polymer. A number of parameters can be varied in investigations, including molecular weight, relative size of different portions of the amphiphilic polymers (polar and nonpolar sections), polymer concentration, and relative size of the unperturbed microemulsion droplet to the polymer size.

8.4.3.3 Homopolymer Additives

When a homopolymer is smaller than the microemulsion droplet size, the droplet–droplet attraction decreases. This effect was found to become more pronounced as the molecular weight of the water-soluble polymer increased, as long as the polymer was smaller than the droplet. When the size of the polymer chain approaches the droplet size, then the drop may swell to a larger size under certain conditions. If the chain is larger than the droplet size, the polymer may span multiple reverse microemulsion droplets, creating a structure referred to as a pearl necklace, where the droplets decorate the polymer string.[63] Other structures possibly include less well defined interlinks of the droplets to form polymer-induced clusters or aggregates that have been described as organogels.[64] A schematic is presented in Figure 8.6 showing the cases for a water-soluble polymer being smaller or larger than the microemulsion droplet size and the resultant effect on coalescence of the droplets.

The addition of non-water-soluble polymers to an inverse microemulsion[65] in appreciable concentrations (up to 10%) has the effect of increasing the attraction between the droplets, similar to increasing the solvent chain length.

8.4.3.4 Amphiphilic Polymer Additives

Due to this dual nature of amphiphilic polymers with both hydrophilic and hydrophobic groups, they orient themselves at oil–water interfaces. Wines and Somasundaran's work with the water/heptane/AOT system have shown that hydrophobically modified comb-like polymers reside at the water–heptane interface and occupy a large surface area on the drop.[57] The hydrocarbon graft chains extend into the heptane phase and mingle with the surfactant nonpolar tails, while the hydrophilic groups will be attracted to the water. The overall effect is to disrupt the close packing of the surfactant molecules and allow for a less rigid, more spaced mixed polymer–surfactant film around the water pools. On the other hand, a diblock polymer has the hydrophobic block extending into the heptane, while the hydrophilic block will favor the water pool. The effect on the surfactant film structure will then be to increase the rigidity. Both behaviors are schematically represented in Figure 8.7.

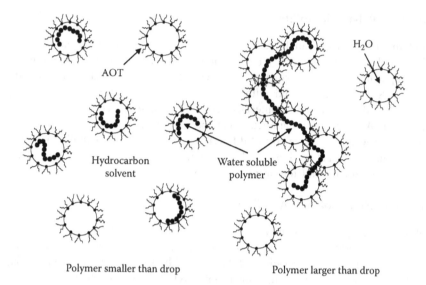

FIGURE 8.6 Possible structures of reverse microemulsion drops with water-soluble polymers. (Reproduced from Wines, T.H., *Effects of Amphiphilic Polymers in Solution on the Behavior of Reverse Microemulsions of Alkane/Water/AOT*, Doctorate thesis, Columbia University, New York, 2002.)

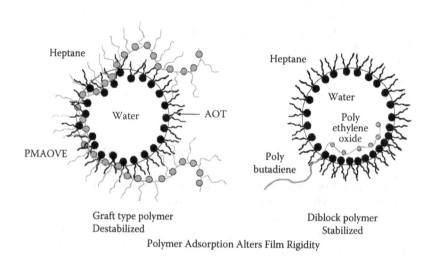

FIGURE 8.7 Adsorption of amphiphilic polymer at reverse microemulsion interface: effect on film rigidity. (Reproduced from Wines, T.H., *Effects of Amphiphilic Polymers in Solution on the Behavior of Reverse Microemulsions of Alkane/Water/AOT*, Doctorate thesis, Columbia University, New York, 2002.)

8.5 MACROEMULSIONS VS. MICROEMULSIONS

The detailed description of macro- vs. microemulsions is given in a review by Wennerstrom et al.,[66] and hence in the present chapter only the main points will be mentioned in brief (Table 8.2).

8.6 DOUBLE EMULSIONS

Double emulsions are complex liquid dispersion systems known also as emulsion of emulsion, in which the droplets of one dispersed liquid are further dispersed in another liquid.[67] The inner dispersed globule/droplet in the double emulsions is separated (compartmentalized) from the outer liquid phase by a layer of another phase.[2,68] A schematic representation of W/O/W double-emulsion droplets is shown in Figure 8.8. The major difference between the inner droplets (W_1/O emulsion) and the globules of the outer emulsion (O/W_2 emulsion) is in the size of the emulsion droplets. The droplet sizes of the inner emulsion (W_1/O) are smaller (1 μm or smaller) than the globule sizes of the outer emulsion (20 to 100 μm).[69]

Double emulsions were considered for close to 60 years as a promising technology. It seems that the numbers of potential applications using these dispersed systems are enormous, yet close examination reveals that the numbers of unsolved obstacles related to the technology are significant, and they retard the possible incorporation of the systems in industrial products.

In 1925, Seifriz[70] was the first to describe, from simple microscopic observations, the existence of emulsion within emulsion, but the uncontrolled droplets' coalescence and film rupture remained unsolved and untreated for over 40 years. An additional 20 years or so passed in which many of the contributions to the

---

TABLE 8.2
Distinction between Macro- and Microemulsion

Macroemulsion	Microemulsion
Droplet size of dispersed phase greater than 400 nm	Droplet size of dispersed phase ranges from 5 nm to about 100 nm
Kinetically stable and hence has a fixed shelf-life	Thermodynamically stable and hence theoretically stable for infinite time unless an external stimulus is used to break it
Visually opaque	Visually transparent
Dispersed phase droplets are polydispersed in size	Dispersed phase droplets are more or less monodispersed
Generally requires intense agitation of the two phases, and the nature of emulsion depends on the technique used for making emulsion	Generally obtained upon mixing the ingredients gently

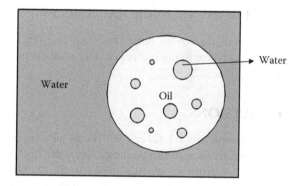

FIGURE 8.8 Schematic presentation of W/O/W double-emulsion droplets.

double emulsions brought mostly descriptive observations and attempts to incorporate drugs and markers within the inner phase.

8.6.1 Method of Preparation

The preparation of double emulsions is both simple and inexpensive. Other advantages of this method are related to the fact that it is considered a soft technique that does not require extreme temperature or pressure conditions and does require only relatively simple equipment.

Preparation of a double emulsion is carried out by three main methods: (1) phase inversion, (2) mechanical agitation, and (3) two-stage emulsification. The two-stage emulsification is the most controlled and frequently used technique. Details on the methods of preparation of double emulsions are given in a review by Garti and Benichou.[71]

8.6.2 Techniques to Evaluate Their Stability

Double emulsions have even less stability than regular emulsions because their droplet sizes have inherent thermodynamic instability. In addition, the release of active material from the inner phase to the outer phase is mostly uncontrolled. The instability and coalescence of double-emulsion droplets can be derived from several possible pathways. It is somewhat difficult to detect if the inner droplets are coalescing first and leading to formation of less compartments in the oil phase, and eventually to the coalescence of the outer droplets, or if the whole droplets are released, as such, to the outer phase without internal coalescence.

The simple and main tool is visual observation by optical microscope. The change in the droplets' size of a double emulsion permits viewing of the final direct consequence of the instability process, but not the ability to distinguish between the individual pathways leading to the size change. Many studies[72] are based on such simple observations, which do not necessarily lead to the correct conclusions regarding the cause of the instability, and as a result, it is difficult to take proper steps to minimize the instability damage caused by the preparation of a double-emulsion sample for microscope observation. To overcome the instability, microslides and coverslips are rinsed with the external continuous aqueous phase of the W/O/W emulsion before use. The W/O/W emulsion samples are placed on a microslide with care to minimize possible destruction of the emulsion structures by shear stress. The samples are then covered with a coverslip and sealed using vacuum grease to prevent water evaporation. Light intensity is kept at a minimum to reduce sample heating. The top and side views using a microscope with a fast digital video camera are also utilized. These novelties, based on simple microscope noninvasive observations, contribute to the understanding of stability and coalescence of the globules in the double emulsion. Confocal scanning light microscopy (CSLM) and the advanced staining techniques of each of the double-emulsion components, including the emulsifiers (if proteins or hydrocolloids), allowed better "peeping" into the internal droplets. Droplet size distribution is given as a function of the volume, and the diameter of globules using the following equation:[73]

$$d_{43} = \frac{\sum_i n_i d_i^4}{\sum_i n_i d_i^3}$$

where n_i is the number of particles with diameter d_i.

Rheological analyses of double emulsion can provide an accurate signature of the structure.[71] The addenda in the inner emulsion alter the rheological property of the double emulsion. As a result, the volume fraction of the inner emulsion W_1/O is changed because of water diffusion. The relationship between the viscosity and the volume fraction is described by the Mooney equation:

$$\ln \eta_r = \frac{K_1 \phi_{primary}}{1 - K_2 \phi_{primary}}$$

where η_r is the relative viscosity of the multiple emulsion (defined as the ratio of the multiple-emulsion viscosity to the external continuous phase viscosity), ϕ primary is the volume fraction of the primary emulsion in the multiple-emulsion system, and K_1 and K_2 are empirical constants dependent on droplet shape and crowdedness. Swelling of the internal aqueous droplets results in a direct increase in $\phi_{primary}$, and hence an increase in viscosity. According to the rheological measurement of double emulsion, we can learn about the stability and internal microstructure of double emulsion.[74] Garti et al. examined the rheology of double emulsion as a function of surfactant concentration and electrolytes. It was observed that Span 83 concentration in the oil phase significantly affected the W/O/W multiple-emulsion stability (Figure 8.9). Both the inner dispersed aqueous droplets and the multiple droplets substantially reduced their sizes as Span 83 concentration in the oil phase increased. The reduced droplet size is believed

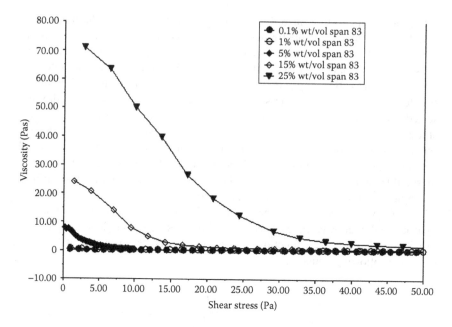

FIGURE 8.9 Viscosity of freshly prepared W/O/W emulsions containing 0.5% w/v sodium salicylate in the inner dispersed aqueous phase, 0.1% w/v Tween 80 in the outer continuous aqueous phase, and varying amounts of Span 83 in the oil phase (25°C).

to provide enhanced kinetic stability to coalescence, in addition to lowered interfacial tension and increased interfacial film strength, as a result of increased surfactant concentration.

Span 83 concentration increases the bulk elasticity of these W/O/W emulsions. The results of storage and loss moduli measurements suggest that the W/O/W emulsions with 20% w/v Span 83 are more elastic (solid like), and thus more stable than those with only 5% w/v Span 83. This is in agreement with the interfacial elasticity data, indicating stronger interfacial film strength, and hence more stable W/O/W emulsions, at higher Span 83 concentrations. However, the concentration of Span 83 in the oil phase appreciably increases the viscosity of the W/O primary emulsion. When the Span 83 concentration reaches 30% w/v, no effective dispersion of the W/O primary emulsion in the external continuous aqueous phase is obtained.

Incorporation of salt in the internal aqueous phase increases the viscosity of W/O/W multiple emulsions because of inner droplet swelling and increased volume fraction ϕ. The swollen droplets may eventually rupture, which destabilizes emulsions. Therefore, a significant increase in viscosity due to salt addition to the internal aqueous phase is an indication of the poor long-term stability of W/O/W emulsions.

The mechanisms of stabilization are discussed in detail elsewhere,[71] and hence will not be discussed here.

8.6.3 Applications

Double emulsions still remain an interesting option for food, pharmaceuticals, and cosmetic addenda entrapment and slow release. Industrial applications of double emulsions include making products such as spreads (margarine replacements) with reduced amounts of fatty ingredients (and in mayonnaise and sauces),[69] improving dissolution rates of certain active matter or solubilization of oil-insoluble materials (the material will dissolve in part in the inner phase and in part at the internal interface, and occasionally at the external interface[2]), slowing and sustaining release of active matter from an internal reservoir into the continuous phase,[75] and protecting sensitive and active molecules from external environmental reactivity, such as oxidation and light.[76] In the flavor industry, encapsulations within double emulsions were used as entrapment reservoirs for masking undesired flavors and odorants.[76] In human pharmaceutical products, double emulsions are used for enhancing the chemotherapeutic effect in cancer, lymphatic absorption of a drug, eternal absorption of a drug, drug immobilization, treatment of drug overdoses, and substitution of red blood cells.[77]

In the cosmetic industry, double emulsions are used in some formulations that will allow a more agreeable aqueous feel than the usual oily texture of a cream. There are also some applications in agriculture and housekeeping products.[75] Calcium thioglycolate, one of the most widely used depilatory agents both in creams and in soaps, was formulated in W/O/W double emulsions using amphiphilic copolymers with controlled release in semisolid form.[68,78] Deposition of water-soluble beneficial agents onto skin from wash-off systems can potentially be achieved by incorporating them in the oil phase of multiple emulsions.[68,79]

ACKNOWLEDGMENT

The authors acknowledge the National Science Foundation (NSF) (Grant EEC-03-28614), and industry/university center for surfactants at Columbia University.

REFERENCES

1. Sakai, Y. et al., Resolving the conflict of a simultaneously highly moisturizing and occlusive emulsion film, *IFSCC Magazine*, 2006; 9(1): 23–28.
2. Sjoblom, J., *Encyclopedic Handbook of Emulsion Technology*, Marcel Dekker, New York, 2001.
3. Griffin, W.C., Classification of surface-active agents by "HLB" *Journal of the Society of Cosmetic Chemists*, 1949; 1: 311–326.
4. Davies, J.T., A Quantitative kinetic theory of emulsion type. I Physical chemistry of the emulsifying agent, *Proceedings of the International Congress on Surface Activity*, 2nd, London 1957, 426–38.
5. Bancroft, W.D., The Theory of Emulsification VI, *Journal of Physical Chemistry*, 1915; 19: 275–309.

6. Stig, E. and Friberg, P.B., *Microemulsion: Structure and Dynamics*, CRC Press, Boca Raton, FL, 2000.

7. Morrison, I.D. and Ross, S., *Colloidal Dispersions: Suspensions, Emulsions, and Foams*, Wiley Interscience, New York, 2002.

8. O'Lenick, A.J., Three-dimensional HLB, *Cosmetics and Toiletries*, 1996; 111(10): 37–38, 41–44.

9. Available from http://www.zenitech.com/documents/hlb_english.pdf.

10. O'Lenick, A.J., Silicone emulsions and surfactants, *Journal of Surfactants and Detergents*, 2000; 3(3): 387–393.

11. Rosen, M.J., *Surfactants and Interfacial Phenomena*, 3rd ed., John Wiley & Sons, Hoboken, NJ, 2004.

12. Bancroft, W.D., The theory of emulsification V, *Journal of Physical Chemistry*, 1913; 17: 501.

13. Berg, T. et al., Insights into the structure and dynamics of complex W/O-emulsions by combining NMR, rheology and electron microscopy, *Colloids and Surfaces A: Physicochem. Eng. Aspects*, 2004; 238: 59–69.

14. Evans, D.F. and Wennerstrom, H., *The Colloidal Domain Where Physics, Chemistry, Biology and Technology Meet*, VCH Publishers, New York, 1994.

15. Newton, J., Stoller, C., and Starch, M., Silicone technologies as delivery systems via physical associations, *Cosmetics and Toiletries*, 2004; 119(5): 69–70, 72–74, 76, 78.

16. Li, X. et al., Phase behavior and microstructure of water/trisiloxane E12 polyoxyethylene surfactant/silicone oil systems, *Langmuir*, 1999; 15(7): 2267–2277.

17. Li, X. et al., Phase behavior and microstructure of water/trisiloxane E12 polyoxyethylene surfactant/silicone oil systems, *Langmuir*, 1999; 15(7): 2278–2289.

18. Hill, R.M., *Silicone Surfactants: Surfactant Science Series*, Marcel Dekker, New York. 1999.

19. Somasundaran, P., Mehta, S.C., and Purohit, P., Silicone emulsions, submitted to *Advances in Colloid and Interface Science*.

20. Somasundaran, P., Runkana, V., and Kapur, P.C., Flocculation and dispersion of colloidal suspensions by polymers and surfactants: experimental and modeling studies, in *Surfactant Science Series*, Vol. 126, *Coagulation and Flocculation*, 2nd ed., CRC Press, Boca Raton, FL, 2005, pp. 767–803.

21. Basu, S., Kandhari, A., and Negi, A.S., Creaming rate of amyl alcohol-in-water emulsions, *Journal of Dispersion Science and Technology*, 2004; 25(6): 823–826.

22. Dickinson, E., Golding, M., and Povey, M.J.W., Creaming and flocculation of oil-in-water emulsions containing sodium caseinate, *Journal of Colloid and Interface Science*, 1997; 185(2): 515–529.

23. Santiago, L.G. et al., The influence of xanthan and λ-carrageenan on the creaming and flocculation of an oil-in-water emulsion containing soy protein, *Brazilian Journal of Chemical Engineering*, 2002; 19(4): 411–417.

24. Ivanov, I.B. et al., The role of surfactants on the coalescence of emulsion droplets, in *Solution Chemistry of Surfactants*, Vol. 2, Mittal, K.L, Ed., Platinum, New York, 1979, pp. 817–839.

25. Meinders, M.B.J., Kloek, W., and Vliet, T.v., Effect of surface elasticity on Ostwald ripening in emulsions, *Langmuir*, 2001; 17: 3923–3929.

26. Solans, C. et al., Nano-emulsions, *Current Opinion in Colloid and Interface Science*, 2005; 10: 102–110.

27. Chepurnov, A.A. et al., Inactivation of Ebola virus with a surfactant nanoemulsion, *Acta Tropica*, 2003; 87: 315–320.

28. Hoar, T.P. and Schulman, J.H., Transparent water-in-oil dispersions: the oleopathic hydro-micelle, *Nature*, 1943; 102: 152.

29. Langevin, D., Structure of reversed micelles, in *Studies in Physical and Theoretical Chemistry: Structure and Reactivity in Reverse Micelles*, Vol. 65, Pelini, M.P., Ed., Elsevier, New York, 1989.

30. Israelachvili, J.N., Mitchell, D.J., and Ninham, B.W., Theory of self-assembly of hydrocarbon amphiphiles into micelles and bilayers, *Journal of the Chemical Society, Faraday Transactions,* 2, 1976; 72: 1525–1568.

31. DeGennes, P.G. and Taupin, C., Microemulsions and the flexibility of oil/water interfaces, *Journal of Physical Chemistry*, 1982; 86: 2294–2304.

32. Mittal, K.L. and Mukerjee, P., The wide world of micelles, in *Micellization, Solubilization, and Microemulsions*, Vol. 1, Mittal, K.L., Ed., Platinum Press, New York, 1977, pp. 1–21.

33. Winsor, P.A., *Solvent Properties of Amphiphilic Compounds*, Butterworth's Scientific Publications, London, 1954.

34. Taber, J.J., *Surface Phenomenon in Enhanced Oil Recovery*, Shah, D.O., Ed., Platinum Press, New York, 1979.

35. Ruckenstein, E., Stability, phase equilibria,and interfacial free energy in microemulsions, in *Micellization, Solubilization, and Microemulsions*, Vol. 2, Mittal, K.L., Ed., Platinum Press, New York, 1977, pp. 755–778.

36. Waguespack, Y.Y. et al., An organogel formed by the addition of selected dihydroxynaphtalenes to the AOT inverse micelles, *Langmuir*, 2000; 16: 3036–3041.

37. Antonietti, M. and Hentze, H.P., Synthesis of sponge-like polymer dispersions via polymerization of bicontinuous microemulsions, *Colloid and Polymer Science*, 1996; 274: 696–702.

38. Attwood, D., *Colloidal Drug Delivery Systems*, Kreuter, J., Ed., Marcel Dekker, New York, 1994.

39. Calandra, P., Goffredi, M., and Liveri, V.T., Study of the growth of ZnS nanoparticles in water/AOT/n-heptane microemulsions by UV-absorption spectroscopy, *Colloids and Surfaces A: Physicochemical and Engineering Aspects*, 1999; 169: 9–13.

40. Chatenay, D. et al., Proteins in membrane mimetic systems: insertion of myelin basic protein into microemulsion droplets, *Biophysics Journal*, 1985; 48: 893–898.

41. Carlotti, M.E. et al., Micellar solutions and microemulsions of odorous molecules, *Journal of Cosmetic Science*, 1999; 50(5): 281–295.

42. Hamdan, S., Dai, Y.Y., and Ahmad, F.B.H., Evaporation from microemulsion with perfume, *Oriental Journal of Chemistry*, 1997; 13(2): 111–116.

43. Nakajima, H., *Microemulsions in Cosmetics*, Surfactant Science Series (Industrial Applications of Microemulsions), Vol. 66, Marcel Dekker, New York, 1997.

44. Shevachman, M., Shani, A., and Garti, N., Formation and investigation of microemulsions based on jojoba oil and nonionic surfactants, *Journal of the American Oil Chemists' Society*, 2004; 81(12): 1143–1152.

45. Watanabe, K. et al., Bicontinuous microemulsion type cleansing containing silicone oil. II. Characterization of the solution and its application to cleansing agent, *Journal of Oleo Science*, 2004; 53(11): 547–555.

46. Wegener, M. et al., Raw Materials and Applications for Microemulsions in Household and Personal Care, paper presented at the World Surfactants Congress, Firenze, Italy, May 29–June 2, 2000.

47. Kluge, K. et al., Temperature-insensitive microemulsions formulated from octyl monoglucoside and alcohols: potential candidates for practical applications, *Tenside, Surfactants, Detergents* 2001; 38(1): 30–34, 37–40.

48. Bellocq, A.-M. and Roux, D., Phase diagram and critical behavior of a quaternary microemulsion system, in *Microemulsions: Structure and Dynamics*, Stig, P.B., Friberg, E., and Bothorel, P., Eds., CRC Press, Boca Raton, FL, 1987, p. 36.

49. Eicke, H.-F., Aqueous nonophases in liquid hydrocarbons stabilized by ionic surfactants, in *Interfacial Phenomenon in Apolar Media*, Eicke, H.-F. and Parfitt, G.D., Eds., Marcel Dekker, New York, 1987, pp. 41–92.

50. Borkovec, M. et al., Two percolation processes in microemulsions, *Journal of Physical Chemistry*, 1988; 92: 206–211.

51. Belocq, A.M., Flexible surfactant films, in *Emulsions and Emulsion Stability*, Vol. 61, Sjoblom, J., Ed., 1985, pp. 204–236.

52. Kabanov, A.V., Reversed micelles as matrix microreactors for chemical processing of macromolecules, *Makromolekulare Chemie, Macromolecular Symposia*, 1991; 44: 253–264.

53. Eicke, H.-F., Surfactants in nonpolar solvents, aggregation and micellization, in *Topics in Current Chemistry: Micelles*, Vol. 87, Boschke, F.L., Ed., Springer-Verlag, Berlin, 1980, pp. 85–145.

54. Letamendia, L. et al., Relaxation phenomenon in critical microemulsion systems, *Colloids and Surfaces A: Physicochemical and Engineering Aspects*, 1998; 140: 289–293.

55. Wines, T.H., Dukhin, A.S., and Somasundaran, P., Acoustic spectroscopy for characterizing heptane/H20/AOT reverse microemulsions, *Journal of Colloid and Interface Science*, 1999; 216: 303–308.

56. Ruckenstein, E. and Karpe, P., Enzymatic super and subactivity in nonionic reverse micelles, *Journal of Physical Chemistry*, 1991; 95(12): 4869–4882.

57. Wines, T.H., *Effects of Amphiphilic Polymers in Solution on the Behavior of Reverse Microemulsions of Alkane/Water/AOT*, Columbia University, New York, 2002.

58. Cametti, C. et al., Electrical conductivity and percolation phenomenon in water-in-oil microemulsions. *Physical Review A*, 1992; 45(8): 5358–5361.

59. Fletcher, P.D.I., Howe, A.M., and Robinson, B.H., The kinetics of solubilisate exchange between water droplets of a water-in-oil microemulsion, *Journal of Chemical Society, Faraday Transactions, 1*, 1987, 83: 985–1006.

60. Atik, S.S. and Thomas, J.K., Transport of ions between water pools in alkanes, *Chemical Physics Letters*, 1981; 79(2): 351–354.

61. Alexandridis, P., *Thermodynamics and Dynamics of Micellization and Micelle-Solute Interactions in Block-Copolymer and Reverse Micellar Systems*, Massachusetts Institute of Technology, Cambridge, MA, 1994.

62. Fletcher, P.D.I., Robinson, B.H., and Tabony, J., A quasi-elastic neutron scattering study of water–in-oil microemulsions stabilized by aerosol AOT, *Journal of Chemical Society Transactions I*, 1986; 82: 2311–2321.

63. Meier, W., Poly(oxyethylene) adsorption in water/oil microemulsions: a conductivity study, *Langmuir*, 1996; 12: 1188–1192.

64. Laia, C.A.T. et al., Light scattering study of water in oil AOT microemulsions with poly(oxy)ethylene, *Langmuir*, 2000; 16: 465–470.

65. Suarez, M.J., Levy, H., and Lang, J., Effect of addition of polymer to water-in-oil microemulsions on droplet size and exchange of material between droplets, *Journal of Physical Chemistry*, 1993; 97: 9808–9816.

66. Wennerstrom, H. et al., Macroemulsions versus microemulsions, *Colloids and Surfaces A. Physicochemical and Engineering Aspects,* 1997; 123/124: 13–26.

67. Garti, N., Double emulsions — scope, limitations and new achievements, *Colloids and Surfaces A: Physicochemical and Engineering Aspects,* 1997; 123/124: 123–124.

68. Garti, N. and Lutz, R., Recent progress in double emulsions, in *Emulsions: Structure, Stability and Interactions,* Pstsev, D.N., Ed., Elsevier Ltd., London, 2004, pp. 557–606.

69. Maa, Y.F. and Hsu, C., Liquid-liquid emulsification by rotor/stator homogenization, *Journal of Controlled Release,* 1996; 38: 219.

70. Seifriz, W., Studies in Emulsions, I: Types of hydrocarbon oil emulsions, *Journal of Physical Chemistry,* 1925; 29: 738.

71. Garti, N. and Benichou, A., Recent developments in double emulsions for food applications, in Friberg, S.E., Larsson, K., and Sjoblom, J. (eds.) *Food Emulsions,* 4th ed., 2004, New York, Marcel Dekker, pp. 281–340.

72. Ficheux, M.-F., Bonakdar, L., Leal-Calderon, F., and Bibetter, J. Some stability criteria for double emulsions, *Langmuir,* 1998; 14: 2702–2706.

73. Tedajo, G.M., Seiller, M., and Prognon, P., pH compartmented W/O/W multiple emulsion: a diffusion study, *Journal of Controlled Release,* 2001; 75(1–2): 45–53.

74. Jiao, J. and Burgess, D.J., Rheology and stability of water-in-oil-in-water multiple emulsions containing Span 83 and Tween 80, *American Association of Pharmaceutical Scientists,* 2003; 5(1): article 7.

75. Pays, K. et al., Coalescence is surfactant–stabilized double emulsions, *Langmuir,* 2001; 17: 7758.

76. Cho, Y.H. and Park, J., Evaluation of process parameters in the O/U/O multiple emulsion method for flavor encapsulation *Journal of Food Science,* 2003; 68: 534.

77. Okochi, H. and Nakano, M., Preparation and evaluation of W/O/W type emulsion containing vancomycin, *Advanced Drug Delivery Reviews,* 2000; 45: 5–26.

78. Gallarate, M. et al., Formulation and characterization of W/O/W multiple emulsion of calcium thioglycolate, *Journal of Dispersion Science and Technology,* 2001; 22: 13.

79. Vasudevan, T.V. and Nase, M.S., Some aspects of stability of multiple emulsions in personal cleansing systems, *Journal of Colloid and Interface Science,* 2002; 256: 208.

9 Role of Surfactant Micelle Charge in Protein Denaturation and Surfactant-Induced Skin Irritation

A. Lips,[1] K.P. Ananthapadmanabhan[1], M. Vethamuthu,[1] X.Y. Hua,[1] L. Yang,[1] C. Vincent,[1] N. Deo,[2] and P. Somasundaran[2]
[1]Unilever Research & Development
[2]Columbia University

CONTENTS

9.1 INTRODUCTION

The skin irritation potential of cleanser surfactants has been investigated extensively in the past using both *in vivo* and *in vitro* techniques.[1,2] Literature results show that, in general, surfactants that interact strongly with stratum corneum proteins, leading to their swelling and denaturation, have a higher potential to cause erythema and itching.[1,2] The tendency of surfactants to interact with model proteins has also been correlated with their harshness toward human skin.

Thus, the higher the tendency of a surfactant to swell stratum corneum[3] or model proteins, such as collagen[4] and keratin,[5] or denature a globular protein such as borine serum albumin (BSA)[6] or dissolve a water-insoluble hydrophobic protein such as zein,[7,8] the higher is its tendency to irritate human skin. The tendency of surfactants to interact with proteins follows the order anionic surfactants > amphoteric surfactants > nonionic surfactants. Prevailing wisdom also suggests that the tendency of anionic surfactants to denature proteins can be reduced by increasing the size and reducing the charge density of the head group. Apart from such empirical guidelines, quantitative structure–function relationships governing surfactant interactions with proteins do not exist at present. In this chapter, a quantitative approach to predicting surfactant interactions with proteins is proposed and its utility is validated using a wide range of surfactants and selected surfactant mixtures. Dissolution of zein, a corn protein, is taken as an example to demonstrate the surfactant interactions with proteins. In principle, such correlations could be established with other examples of surfactant-induced protein damage, such as collagen or corneum swelling, or even *in vivo* irritation test results.

9.1.1 Proposed Model of Surfactant-Induced Protein Swelling and Denaturation

The hypothesis is that surfactant-induced protein damage due to a combination of swelling and, at a local level, the breakup of a secondary protein structure, including denaturation, is the result of formation of micelle-like surfactant aggregates on the protein, leading to an increase in the net charge within the network, which in turn results in an osmotic driven flow of counterions from the bulk solution into the network. Thus, the extent of damage, especially at the local level, should scale strongly with the effective charge density (charge per unit area) of the surfactant aggregate formed on the protein.

Effective charge density, σ, is given by

$$\sigma = e.(\alpha/A) \tag{9.1}$$

where e is the electronic charge, α is the degree of counterion dissociation, and A is the effective area of a surfactant head group in the aggregate. Thus, plots of charge density parameter, σ/e ($= \alpha/A$), vs. protein denaturation or other measures of protein–surfactant interaction should indicate the validity of the above hypothesis.

Since surfactant binding to proteins at high concentrations is primarily associative in nature and governed by the properties of the surfactant,[9] a reasonable estimate of the charge density of the aggregate can be taken to be that of the surfactant micelle under identical solution conditions. In this study, the charge density of the micelles is estimated from measurements of the zeta potential of micelles using a laser Doppler light-scattering technique. An empirical equation proposed by Loeb et al.[12] was used to estimate the charge density from the measured zeta potential values. Such calculations can be refined further with a measure of the size of the micelle and aggregation number of the micelle.

9.2 EXPERIMENT

Surfactants used in this study, and their sources are as follows: sodium dodecyl sulfate (SDS; Sigma Chemicals), sodium laurate (SL; TCI America), potassium laurate (KL; Aldrich Chemicals), dodecyl trimethyl ammonium bromide (DTAB; Sigma Chemicals), cetyl trimethyl ammonium bromide (CTAB; Sigma Chemicals), N-dodecyl-N-N-dimethyl-3-ammonium-1-propanesulfonate (dodecyl sulfobetaine (DSB); SigmaUltra), alkyl polyglucoside (APG; Cognis), Na laureth sulfate (SLES 3 EO, Steol CS 330, Stephan), Na cocoyl isethionate SCI, Unilever synthesized, 92 to 95% pure), monoalkyl phosphate, Na salt (MAP), and cocoamido propyl betaine (CAPB; Goldschmidt).

Surfactant solutions were prepared with distilled and deionized Milli-Q water. The zein solubility measurements were carried out by adding zein powder (4 g) into 40 g of a 5% surfactant solution and equilibrating the mix for 24 h with frequent vigorous shaking. Dissolved zein was separated from the undissolved material by filtering it using a 0.45-μm nylon membrane twice. The dissolved zein concentration was determined using its UV absorption peak at $\lambda \approx 278$ nm. Samples were diluted to the linear absorption range for UV measurements.

The zeta potential of micellar solutions was measured at a concentration of 1% using a laser Doppler light-scattering technique. Specifically, a zeta potential analyzer, ZeatPlus, made by Brookhaven Instruments Corporation, was used to obtain the zeta potential as well as the size of the surfactant micelles. The zeta potential was measured at a pH corresponding to the equilibrium pH of the surfactant solution after zein dissolution. Samples were filtered using a syringe filter with a 0.45-μm nylon membrane prior to the measurement. All experiments were carried out at room temperature (25°C).

9.3 RESULTS

The solubility of zein as a function of surfactant concentration is plotted for two anionic (SDS and SLES), one zwitterionic (CAPB), and a nonionic surfactant in Figure 9.1. The ability of surfactants to dissolve zein follows the order SDS > SLES > CAPB > C12 EO8. This is consistent with the expected skin irritation tendency of these surfactants. Also, while anionic surfactants appear to be more effective, nonionic surfactant is not able to dissolve zein, indicating that charge of the surfactant is a major factor in the dissolution process.

Solubility of zein in 5% surfactant solutions is given in Figure 9.2. Zein solubility in SDS and SL solutions is significantly higher than that in SLES, SCI, and CAPB solutions. APG, a nonionic surfactant, and water show the least amount of protein dissolution. The earlier obtained correlation between skin irritation potential measured in *in vivo* flex wash tests and zein dissolution is given in Figure 9.3a.[10] Also included is the correlation between zein dissolution and *in vivo* patch test results for a number of surfactants.[11] As can be seen, in general, as the zein dissolution increases, the skin irritation potential of surfactants

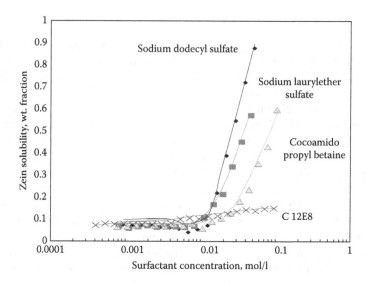

FIGURE 9.1 Solubility of zein in various surfactant solutions. Ability to dissolve zein is in agreement with the expected skin irritation tendency of these surfactants.

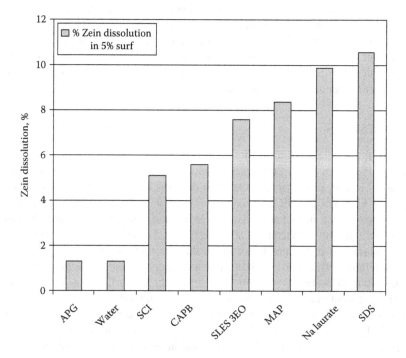

FIGURE 9.2 Solubility of zein in 5% solutions of various surfactants. pH of solutions is 7 except for MAP and Na laurate, which are at 8 and 10 respectively.

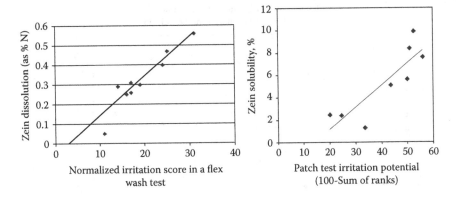

FIGURE 9.3 (a) Correlation between ability of a number of surfactants to dissolve zein and their ability to cause skin irritation in a flex wash test (10). (b) Correlation between zein dissolution and irritation potential as measured in a patch test (11).

measured in a flex wash test[10] and patch test[11] also shows an increase, suggesting that the zein dissolution can be a rough initial predictor of *in vivo* irritation.

The zeta potential of zein particles, as well as zein solubility, as a function of SDS concentration is shown in Figure 9.4. These results show that with an increase in SDS concentration, the zeta potential of zein undergoes a charge reversal, going from positive to negative values. Similarly, the swelling of the protein shows an initial decrease, consistent with the reduction in charge, followed by an increase with an increase in the negative charge. As the values increase to about −50 mV, dissolution of zein is observed. These observations are consistent with the contention that electrostatics play a role in zein dissolution.

The zeta potential of various surfactants measured at the 1 wt% level, along with the data for area per molecule on the micelle surface, as estimated from surface tension measurements, is given in Table 9.1.

9.3.1 CALCULATIONS OF σ (= α/A) (CHARGE DENSITY PARAMETER)

The surface charge density of micelles was estimated from zeta potential measurements based on the assumption of coincidence of the electrokinetic shear plane with the position of the stern layer (Figure 9.5). Another approach, based on measurement of counterion binding using ion-selective electrodes and surfactant area per molecule, calculated from surface tension measurements, yielded a similar trend in results. In this chapter, results obtained using micelle zeta potential measurements are presented.

9.3.2 SURFACE CHARGE DENSITY FROM ZETA POTENTIAL MEASUREMENTS

A semiempirical equation proposed by Loeb et al.[12,13] was used to calculate the surface charge density. The following equation relates zeta potential (ψ_d) to charge

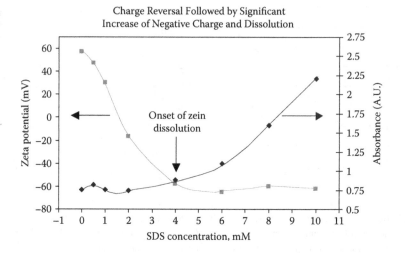

FIGURE 9.4 Zeta potential of zein particles as a function of SDS concentration. Significant increase in solubility of zein is observed only when zein acquires significant negative charge at high SDS levels.

density (σ_d) in the diffused layer, which is equal in magnitude and opposite in sign to the surface charge density:

$$\sigma_d = -\varepsilon \frac{kT}{ze} \kappa \left\{ 2\sinh\left(\frac{ze\psi_d}{2kT}\right) + \frac{4}{\kappa a} \tanh\left(\frac{ze\psi_d}{4kT}\right) \right\} \qquad (9.2)$$

TABLE 9.1
Zeta Potential of Surfactant Micelles Measured at 10% (wt)

Surfactant	Zeta Potential, mV
SDS	−44.3
SDS-C12E07 (7:3)	−40.2
SLES3	−36.0
DTAB	38.0
Na Laurate	−35.8
SLES3-CAPB–2 to 1 wt%	−22.1
SLES3-CAPB–1 to 2 wt%	−19.4
SDS-DSB 1 to 1 wt%	−16.1
CAPB	−10.3
APG	−8.8
DSB	−2.9

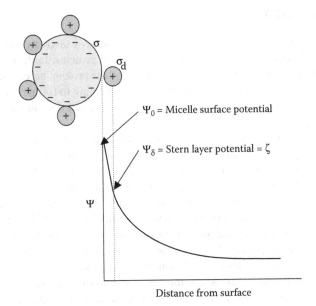

Ψ_0 = Micelle surface potential

Ψ_δ = Stern layer potential = ζ

Ψ

Distance from surface

FIGURE 9.5 Schematic of potential variation from the micelle surface. On the basis of the assumption that measured zeta potential is the same as potential at the shear plane, charge density of the micelle is calculated using the Loeb, Wiersma, & Overbeek approximation.[12]

where k is the Boltzmann constant, T is the temperature, z is the valency of the surfactant ions, e is the charge of proton, and ε is the dielectric constant of the medium. $1/\kappa$ is the Debye length and can be calculated using the equation

$$1/\kappa = (\varepsilon\kappa T/e^2 \ \Sigma \ n_i z_i^2)^{1/2} \qquad (9.3)$$

where n_i is the concentration of ion with z_i as its charge. For univalent–univalent electrolytes, the above equation for the Debye length reduces to[14]

$$1/\kappa = 0.304/\sqrt{[I]} \ \ nm \qquad (9.4)$$

where $[I]$ is the ionic strength ($= \frac{1}{2} \ \Sigma \ n_i \ z_i^2$) and n_i is the ionic concentration in moles per liter. Measurements of counterion binding from ion-selective electrodes were used to correct for the ion concentration in calculating the ionic strength. In cases where the counterion binding data were not available, an iterative procedure was used to obtain a σ_d value that is consistent with changes in the Debye length because of counterion binding to micelles.

9.4 DISCUSSION

It is well recognized that the denaturation of proteins caused by surfactants is due to massive cooperative binding of surfactants to proteins. In the case of zein, the dissolution occurs when the negative charge on the protein increases, resulting in swelling and eventual breakup of the structure, leading to formation of soluble protein–surfactant complexes. A schematic of the protein dissolution process is given in Figure 9.6.

As mentioned earlier, dissolution occurs under conditions of massive cooperative binding of surfactant to the protein. Independent fluorescence experiments using pyrene as the probe further confirmed the formation of hydrophobic aggregates on the protein under conditions of protein dissolution. These observations, as well as the earlier mentioned correlations with zeta potential measurements, led to the hypothesis that protein denaturation should scale with the charge of the surfactant aggregate on the protein. As an initial approximation, micelle charge is thought to be proportional to the charge of the aggregate, and a correlation between micelle charge density and zein dissolution was explored.

The zeta potential of surfactant micelles vs. zein dissolution for a variety of surfactants, including some commercial-grade surfactants, is plotted in Figure 9.7.

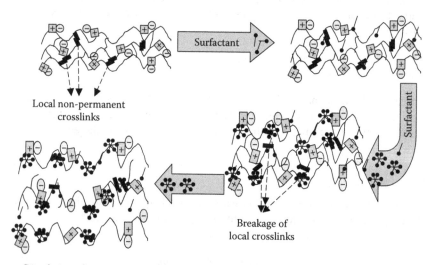

FIGURE 9.6 Schematic of protein swelling and dissolution because of formation of micelle-like aggregates on the protein. Breakage of non-permanent cross links is unlikely to be fully reversible upon removal of surfactants during dilution/rinse. In the case of non-cross-linked proteins such as zein, charge development lead to dissolution where as in the case of cross-linked proteins such as keratin, significant swelling can lead to penetration of more surfactants into deeper layers.

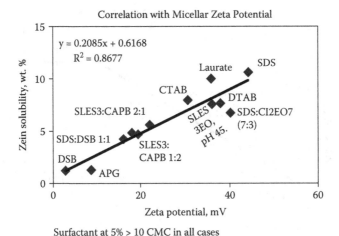

FIGURE 9.7 Correlation between zein solubility in 5% surfactant solutions and the zeta potential of micelles measured at 1% surfactant level.

A plot of zein dissolution vs. our estimates of α/A calculated from the zeta potential data is given in Figure 9.8. Relatively harsh surfactants such as sodium dodecyl sulfate (SDS) and sodium laurate, mild surfactants such as sodium lauryl ether sulfate (SLES) and sodium dodecyl sulfobetaines (DSB), and even nonionic surfactants such as APG are included in this plot. The calculated charge density parameter, α/A, shows strong correlation with the extent of protein dissolution, consistent with our model. It is interesting that the zeta potential also correlates with protein dissolution, albeit less strongly. This is not altogether surprising, since zeta potential is expected to scale linearly with charge density, at least in the low potential range. Even the cationic surfactants cetyl trimethyl ammonium bromide (CTAB) and dodecyl trimethyl ammonium bromide (DTAB) seem to fall on the same correlation line, indicating the generality of the approach to predicting surfactant interactions with proteins.

Figure 9.7 and Figure 9.8 include data for mixtures of sodium lauryl sulfate with sodium dodecyl sulfobetaine (DSB) and sodium lauryl ether sulfates with cocoamido propyl betaines. It is interesting to note that surfactant mixtures also fall on the same line as those for individual surfactants. For surfactant mixtures and commercial surfactants, the composition of the surfactant aggregates may be different from that in the bulk composition and may require a better understanding of the composition of the aggregate for further refinement of the calculations; this will be examined in our future work.

The results presented above support the hypothesis that surfactant interaction with proteins, leading to protein damage involving swelling and breakup of the secondary structure, including denaturation, is essentially controlled by the charge density of the surfactant aggregate formed on the protein. This new insight can be effectively used to assess the relative mildness of surfactants and surfactant

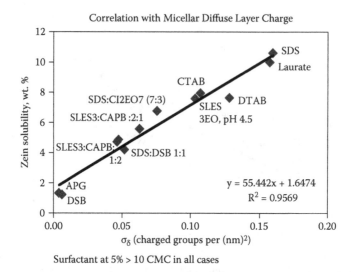

FIGURE 9.8 Correlation between zein solubility in 5% surfactant solutions and the charge density of micelles estimated from micelle zeta potential measured at 1% surfactant level.

mixtures. Since α/A is sensitive to solution parameters such as ionic strength and type and concentration of counterions and additives, this parameter may be a useful predictor of the irritancy potential of even complex surfactant formulations.

9.5 SUMMARY

The results presented here provide a new insight into surfactant interactions with proteins and a novel approach to quantify the relationship between protein interaction and fundamental surfactant properties. The observed correlation between charge density parameter (α/A) of surfactant aggregates (micelles) and protein swelling/denaturation tendency appears to be valid over a wide range of surfactant chemistries, including surfactant mixtures. Note, however, that the relationship between protein swelling/denaturation and clinical irritancy is rather complex. Skin irritation by surfactants is due to penetration of surfactants into living epidermis and the subsequent disruption of epidermal cells, resulting in the release of cytokines and possibly other components, leading to cutaneous inflammation.[2,3] The ability of a surfactant to swell the corneum is an indication of its ability to enhance its own penetration into deeper layers and disrupt the cells in the living layer. This is consistent with the established correlation in the literature between the ability of surfactants to swell the corneum and its irritation potential.

REFERENCES

1. Rhein, L.D., Robbins, C.R., Fernee, K., Cantore, R. J., Surfactant structure effects on swelling of isolated human stratum corneum, *J. Soc. Cosmet. Chem.*, 37, 125, 1986.
2. Rhein, L.D. In *Surfactants in Cosmetics*, Surfactant Science Series, Rieger, M.M., Rhein, L.D., Eds. Marcel Dekker, New York, 1997, p. 397.
3. Imokawa, G. Surfactant mildness. In *Surfactants in Cosmetics*, Surfactant Science Series, Rieger, M.M., Rhein, L.D., Eds. Marcel Dekker, New York, 1997, p. 427.
4. Blake-Haskins, J., Scala, D., Rhein, L.D., Robbins, C.R. *J. Soc. Cosmet. Chem.*, 37, 199, 1986.
5. Robbins, C.R., Fernee, K.M. *J. Soc. Cosmet. Chem.*, 34, 21, 1983.
6. Cooper, E.R., Berner, B. In *Surfactants in Cosmetics*, Surfactant Science Series, Vol. 16, Rieger, M.M., Ed. Marcel Dekker, New York, 1985, p. 195.
7. Gotte, E., Skin compatability of tensides measured by their capacity for dissolving zein, *Tenside*, 15, 313, 1966.
8. Schwuger, M.J., Uber die Wechselwir kung Zwischer Proteinen und an der Modellsubstanz zein, Kolloid, Z. *Polymer*, 233, 898, 1969.
9. Jones, M.N., Surfactant interactions with bio-membranes and proteins, *Chem. Soc. Rev.*, 21, 127, 1992.
10. Lee, R.S. *In-Vitro Screening Methods for Clinical Mildness: Zein Solubilization.* Unilever Research Lab internal report, 1989.
11. Foy, V. and Chang, H. *Multiple Exposure Patch Test to Determine Irritation Potential of Surfactant Solutions.* Unilever internal report, 1997.
12. Loeb, A.L., Wiersma, P.H., and Overbeek, J.Th.G. *The Electrical Double Layer around a Spherical Colloid Particle.* MIT Press, Cambridge, MA, 1961.
13. Hunter, R.J. *Foundations of Colloid Science*, Vol. 1. Clarendon Press, 1993.
14. Rosen, M.J. *Surfactants and Interfacial Phenomena*, 2nd ed. John Wiley & Sons, New York, 1989.

10 Skin Lipid Structure: Insights into Hydrophobic and Hydrophilic Driving Forces for Self-Assembly Using IR Spectroscopy

Mark E. Rerek[1] and David J. Moore[2]
[1]Reheis, Inc.
[2]International Specialty Products

CONTENTS

10.1 INTRODUCTION: SKIN BARRIER FUNCTION AND ORGANIZATION

The stratum corneum (SC) provides the skin's permeability barrier to water, and thus plays a critical role in human physiology; indeed, the development of this barrier function was essential for the evolution of mammalian life in Earth's extremely desiccating terrestrial environment. An effective water barrier is a necessity for viability in the human newborn. In addition to maintaining water homeostasis, the SC provides a barrier to chemical and biological agents entering the body. Furthermore, SC barrier function must remain effective over a wide range of temperature and humidity. Skin must also tolerate a wide range of mechanical stresses, and consequently, the SC must be flexible and have considerable torsional and cohesive strength.

Given these varied requirements, one of the more interesting questions in skin research is, What is the molecular structure and organization of the skin barrier? To properly frame this question, an understanding of the basic composition of the SC is needed. The SC consists of two basic components: anucleated cells, called corneocytes, embedded within an extracellular lamellar lipid matrix. The lamellar bilayer organization of this lipid matrix was first clearly observed using electron microscopy to examine RuO_4 fixed samples.[1] A widely employed analogy for the gross organization of the SC is a brick wall,[2,3] as shown in Figure 10.1. On a macroscopic scale, this is a useful elementary conception of the stratum corneum structure.

In this model, the corneocyte bricks occupy most of the volume of the stratum corneum wall and are surrounded by lipid mortar. The lipid matrix constitutes

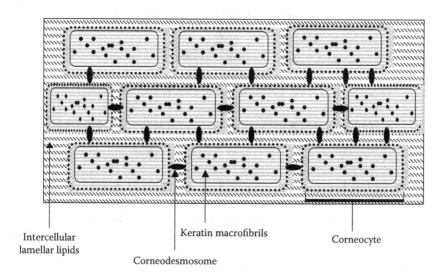

FIGURE 10.1 Bricks-and-mortar model of the stratum corneum.

approximately 20% of the SC volume (about 15% of the dry weight).[4,5] It has been well established, using a variety of tape-stripping and lipid extraction experiments, that the epidermal permeability barrier resides primarily in the lipid bilayers of the SC.

10.2 LIPID ORGANIZATION IN THE STRATUM CORNEUM

The SC lipid bilayers are unique among eukaryotic membranes in terms of composition, organization, and physical properties. The lamellar bilayers of most biological membranes consist of lipids in the liquid crystalline (L_α) state, in which the lipid chains have considerable intramolecular conformational disorder, i.e., *trans/gauche* isomerization, and no specific intermolecular packing organization. Consequently, intermolecular organization in a L_α bilayer is routinely referred to as liquid packing, and the lipid chains in the L_α phase are often described as melted. Aliphatic liquid crystal-forming lipids can undergo reversible transitions between the lamellar gel phase (L_β) and the lamellar L_α phase. In the L_β phase, the hydrocarbon chains are in a fully extended all-*trans* conformation with their chains packed in a hexagonal array. Long-chain lipids can also pack lamellar bilayers with their chains packed in an orthorhombic array. In this phase, the hydrocarbon chains are highly conformationally ordered and packed in a tight crystalline array.[6] These inter- and intramolecular arrangements are illustrated in Figure 10.2.

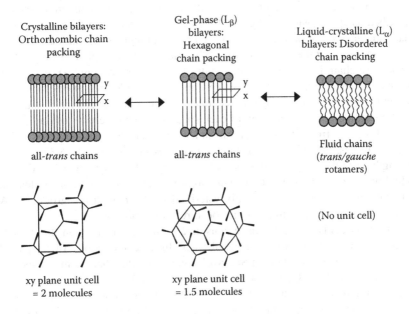

FIGURE 10.2 Chain conformation and packing in lamellar structures.

The majority of lipids in mammalian cell membranes contain mono- and polyunsaturated chains, and consequently, biological membrane bilayers are, on average, in the L_α phase at physiological temperatures. It is important to note that there has been a great deal of recent work on membrane structural heterogeneity and the recognition of the presence of ordered domains (rafts) within biological membranes. There are many excellent reviews of this emerging area of membrane biophysics. However, in contrast to most of the lipids in biological membranes, the hydrocarbon chains of stratum corneum lipids are highly ordered at physiological temperatures. This has been demonstrated in many published reports utilizing a range of techniques, including nuclear magnetic resonance (NMR), x-ray, differential scanning calorimetry (DSC), and Fourier-transformed infrared (FTIR) spectroscopy. A more detailed description of the unique aspects of SC lipid dynamics requires a consideration of the chemical composition of the SC lipids.

10.3 LIPID COMPOSITION IN THE STRATUM CORNEUM

The major lipid species of the SC are ceramides (about 50% by mass), fatty acids (10 to 20% by mass), and cholesterol (25% by mass).[4,5,7] In addition, there are small amounts of cholesterol esters and cholesterol sulfate that, in particular, seem to play a critical role in normal barrier function.[8] There are no phospholipids in the stratum corneum.[5] It is estimated that the skin must synthesize approximately 100 to 150 mg of lipid per day to replace what is lost through normal desquamation. The skin is one of the most active sites of lipid synthesis in the body.[7,9]

Ceramides consist of a long-chain fatty acid and a long-chain amine and are described as sphingosines or phytosphingosines, depending on their amine base chain precursors. For both sphingosine and phytosphingosine ceramides, hydroxylation can occur at the α or ω position of the acid chain, as well as the 6 position of the base chain in sphingosine ceramides (sphinganine ceramides). Esters can also be formed through the ω-hydroxyl group. The major SC ceramides are shown in Figure 10.3 and denoted by their chemical structure nomenclature, along with the reported percent composition of each species. The base chains of human SC ceramides range from 18 to 22 carbons in length.[7,10] For the non-ω-hydroxy fatty acid ceramides, the amide-linked fatty acid chains range from 16 to 32 carbons in length, with the major chain species being either 24 or 26 carbons.[10,11] For the ω-hydroxy ceramides the fatty acid chains are some 30 to 34 carbons in length, with linoleic acid (C18:2) normally esterified to the ω-hydroxy group.[12–14] A review of ceramides and the skin has been recently published.[15]

The fatty acids of the SC have considerably longer chains than those commonly found in other biological membranes. In a detailed study of fatty acid composition in the lower human SC, Norlen et al. reported that the major species of free fatty acid were C22 (11%), C24 (39%), C26 (23%), and C28 (8%).[16] This is in good agreement with other reports of SC fatty acid composition.[4,5,7] There are also some unsaturated fatty acids in the stratum corneum esterified to cholesterol to form cholesterol esters.

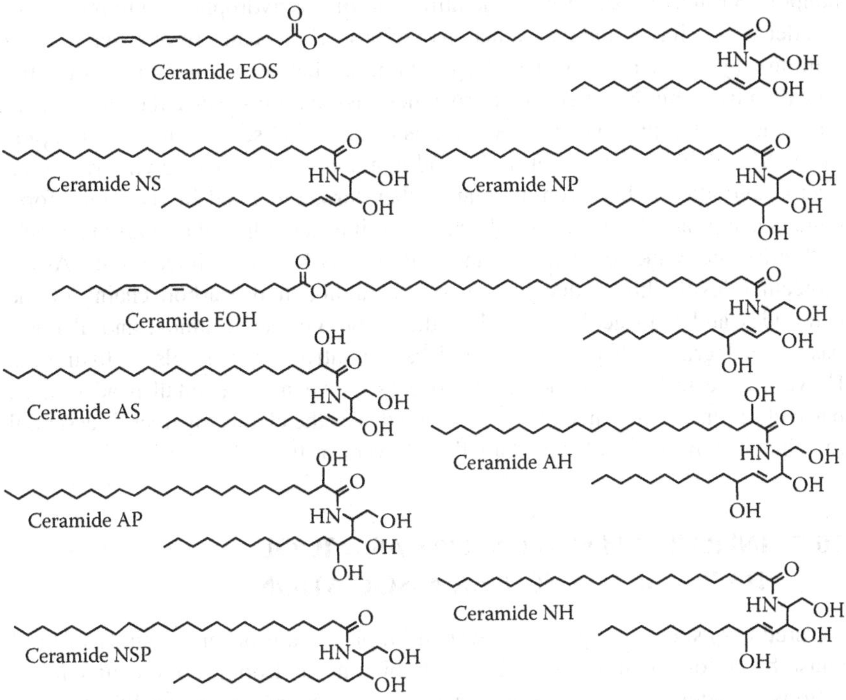

FIGURE 10.3 Ceramides of the stratum corneum.

Most SC lipids are extruded from lamellar bodies present in the keratinocytes of the stratum granulosum, the uppermost layer of the viable epidermis. The SC lipids are synthesized as precursor lipids with more hydrophilic head groups, such as phospholipids, cerebrosides including sphingolipids, and cholesterol esters. At the interface between the stratum granulosum (SG) and SC, the extruded lipids are enzymatically cleaved to generate free fatty acids, cholesterol, and ceramides.[17] These enzymatically modified lipids are generally believed to fuse together exogenously, forming the continuous lamellar bilayers of the SC. At the end of this chapter, we will return to the question of the potential mechanisms by which the barrier cohesion and integrity are achieved.

10.4 LIPIDS AS AMPHIPATHS AND SELF-ASSEMBLY CONSIDERATIONS

The ability of lipids to form membranes and lamellar bilayers in water results from their amphipathic character. Amphipathic molecules have a polar, hydrophilic head group region and a nonpolar, hydrophobic region. In the presence of a polar solvent such as water, the lipid polar groups associate together, while the nonpolar groups associate. It is the attraction of the hydrophobic groups due to van der Waal's forces and the exclusion of hydrocarbon chains from water, thereby minimizing the disruption of hydrogen bonding between water molecules (the so-called hydrophobic effect) that drive these associations. Since these events are spontaneous, the process of association is often called self-assembly. The lipids of the SC are balanced in their polar and nonpolar group areas, giving rise to an overall cylindrical shape (unlike many other surfactants and lipids, which form cone shapes), and hence SC lipids can pack into lamellar bilayer arrangements with efficient cylindrical packing and maximal hydrophobic interactions. At the molecular level, this is due to the long saturated hydrocarbon chains of the ceramides and fatty acids, as well as the carboxylic acid, amide, and alcohol-based head groups that are small and have relatively low levels of hydration. However, the hydrogen bonding that occurs between these small head groups, particularly in the presence of water, which drives the chains together, is essential to achieving the very cohesive lamellar bilayers of the SC.

10.5 INFRARED SPECTROSCOPY AS A TOOL TO PROBE MOLECULAR ASSOCIATIONS

Infrared (IR) spectroscopy is a powerful biophysical tool for the study of lipid phase behavior, including both hydrophobic and hydrophilic molecular inter-actions. Snyder and collaborators have developed an extensive literature of detailed spectra–structure correlations for hydrocarbon chain modes that are directly applicable to biological lipids.[18–20] These modes provide information on both intramolecular and intermolecular interactions. Of particular utility for membrane biophysics is the frequency of methylene stretching modes, which provide information on the conformational order and packing of hydro-carbon chains.[21–23] These modes have been exploited to study the membrane biophysics of biological membranes, both isolated and in intact cells. The methylene scissoring and rocking modes provide information on the chain-packing geometry, while further insights into intramolecular conformation can be obtained from methylene wagging modes.[18,24] In general, the greater the conformational order and the tighter the packing geometry of lipid chains, the stronger and narrower the peaks in the IR spectra. This greatly increases the quality and quantity of information in their IR spectrum. Additionally, IR spectroscopy also provides extensive information on the hydrophilic regions, especially on hydrogen-bonding strength through the hydroxyl stretching, amine stretching, acid carbonyl, and amide I and amide II modes. All protons on these groups are exchangeable by deuterons in the presence of ^2H_2O (D$_2$O). The extent and kinetics of H–D exchange provide further information on band assignment and bond strength.[25] Much of the above will be illustrated by specific examples from both fatty acids and ceramide species. Reviews spe-cifically covering the application of IR spectroscopy to SC lipid biophysics have been published.[26–28]

10.6 OCTADECANOIC ACID: CONFORMATIONAL ORDER, CHAIN PACKING, AND DOMAINS

Although the phase behavior of octadecanoic acid is well documented, it is relevant to revisit this in the context of SC lipids. The fatty acid chains of octadecanoic acid are highly ordered and have orthorhombic packing when both hydrated and nonhydrated. However, as described above, IR is very good at simultaneously presenting both chain order and chain packing, and can do so at varying temperatures. Figure 10.4 shows a plot of the CD_2 stretching (δCD_2) region for hydrated d_{35}-octadecanoic acid as a function of temperature. The initial asymmetric δCD_2 band frequency is very low at 2193.8 cm^{-1}, indicating a high degree of conformational order. As temperature is increased, a very sharp transition is observed with a midpoint (T_m) at 62°C. This transition corresponds to chain disordering/melting. At the same time that the methylene order-to-disorder transition occurs, the acid carbonyl stretch undergoes a sharp transition from 1693 to 1708 cm^{-1} in D_2O. This is consistent with a shift from stronger to weaker hydrogen bonding.

For pure d_{35}-octadecanoic acid, a doublet is observed in the CD_2 scissoring (δCD_2) region that is characteristic of orthorhombic chain packing. The doublet arises through interchain coupling of vibrational frequencies and only occurs between isotopically alike chains. The chains must be very closely packed and have the same unperturbed frequency for this coupling to occur. Octadecanoic acid shows a corresponding doublet in the CH_2 scissoring (δCH_2) region, again characteristic of orthorhombic chain packing. Since the δCD_2 and δCH_2 modes occur at different frequencies, they do not couple. Full splitting is characteristic of domains of 100 chains or greater. When d_{35}-octadecanoic acid and octadecanoic

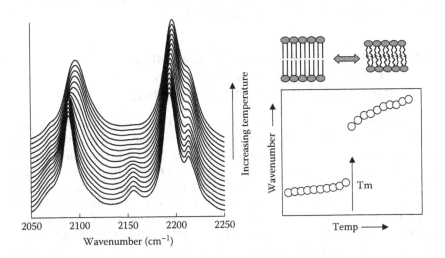

FIGURE 10.4 Thermotropic changes in d_{35}-octadecanoic acid methylene stretching spectra.

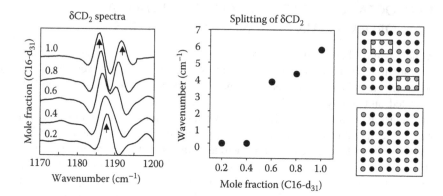

FIGURE 10.5 Detecting and measuring domains of d_{35}-octadecanoic acid from methylene scissoring spectra.

acid are mixed up to a mole fraction of 0.4 d_{35}-octadecanoic acid, no splitting of the δCD_2 band is observed, indicating that on average, a CD_2 chain is not adjacent to other CD_2 chains. Intermediate splitting is observed at mole fractions between 0.4 and 0.8, indicating that the d_{35}-octadecanoic acids are forming domains of an intermediate size. At mole fractions greater than 0.8, full splitting is observed, indicating that the proteated octadecanoic acid molecules are not interrupting most of the large d_{35}-octadecanoic acid domains. Therefore, mixtures of pure deuterated and pure proteated octadecanoic acids can give information on the extent of statistical mixing as a function of mole fraction. This is illustrated in Figure 10.5. This molecular probe of domain size has been exploited to measure domain sizes in binary and ternary lipid mixtures.

10.7 INDIVIDUAL SPHINGOSINE CERAMIDES: CONFORMATIONAL ORDER, CHAIN PACKING, AND HYDROGEN BONDING

The ceramides studied here are ceramide NS, ceramide NP, ceramide AS, and ceramide AP, shown in Figure 10.3. Sphingosine ceramides are characterized by a double bond in the base chain at carbons 4 and 5 and are designated Cer NS (without α-hydroxyl on the acid chain) and Cer AS (with α-hydroxyl on the acid chain). The 4,5 double bond of the sphingosine base permits the two chains to draw into close proximity, allowing very tight packing when hydrated. This is supported by the very low symmetric methylene stretching ($\nu_{sym}CH_2$) frequency of both Cer NS (2847 cm^{-1}) and Cer AS (2846 cm^{-1}).[29] Both Cer NS and Cer AS have higher methylene stretching frequencies in the absence of hydration, indicating that chain packing is less tight. Both Cer NS and Cer AS have orthorhombic chain packing, as evidenced by splitting of their scissoring and rocking methylene modes. This is consistent with previous reports from both NMR and x-ray studies, indicating high conformational order and orthorhombic packing, respectively.[30,31] It is also consistent with monolayer studies, indicating that sphingosine ceramides have lower head group areas than their corresponding saturated phytosphingosine ceramides, allowing close chain packing.[32,33] Further support for high chain order comes from the prominent wagging progression bands observed for both of these ceramides. Second derivative spectra reveal progressions from both acid and base chains.[29] As discussed elsewhere, these modes derive from coupled oscillators and are a characteristic and sensitive measure of fully ordered all-*trans* chains.[18,34]

When Cer NS and Cer AS are packed in their highly ordered orthorhombic phases, they exhibit very sharp bands from their amide and hydroxyl head groups.[25] Cer NS displays two sharp OH/NH stretching bands at 3359 and 3310 cm^{-1}, two amide I bands at 1647 and 1620 cm^{-1} and two amide II bands at 1569 and 1547 cm^{-1}. The most likely explanation for more than one peak for each of these modes is that there are multiple bonding orientations for these groups. The sharpness of the peaks does indicate that there is limited conformational freedom around these bonds, and they are mostly in similar orientation. Most importantly, the frequency of these peaks gives insight into the strengths of their hydrogen bonds; in this case, all of these frequencies indicate strong hydrogen bonding. Similar behavior is observed for Cer AS. Three sharp OH/NH stretching bands at 3443, 3353, and 3266 cm^{-1}, two clear amide I bands at 1645 and 1630 cm^{-1}, and one amide II band at 1523 cm^{-1} are observed. Note that Cer AS has an additional α-hydroxy group on the acid chain and has one more OH/NH stretching band than does Cer NS; it also has one amide II peak and two amide I peaks.

Both Cer NS and Cer AS are thermally stable, such that heating results in only a very small increase in their methylene stretching frequencies until 60°C, where there is a sharp, small increase in Cer NS methylene stretching frequencies (Figure 10.6). At the same temperature, methylene scissoring splitting collapses, signaling a change from orthorhombic to hexagonal chain packing (Figure 10.7). The increase in the methylene stretching frequencies at 60°C reflects greater rotational freedom around the hexagonally packed chains. Coordinated with these packing changes is a large change in the out-of-plane C–H bending mode of the *trans* C=C bond, which is initially split into two peaks at 960 and 980 cm^{-1}. At the orthorhombic-to-hexagonal phase transition, the splitting separation increases, perhaps indicating an increase in ordering near the sphingosine double bond. Since the alkyl chains are increasing in disorder, it appears that the head group area has become more ordered, or more constrained. Further support for a change in the head group hydrogen bonding comes from a reorganization of both the C–O stretch and the C–O–H in-plane bend, as well as loss of one of the two amide II bands at the same temperature. It should be noted that there is no similar change in the amide I band. These processes can all be observed simultaneously, providing an excellent illustration of the power of IR spectroscopy for providing simultaneous information on both intra- and intermolecular lipid dynamics.[29]

Further insight into the molecular dynamics of the Cer NS phase transition at 60°C is obtained by examining the H $\rightarrow$ D exchange of the head groups that

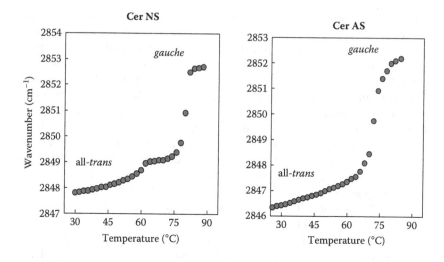

FIGURE 10.6 Thermotropic changes in Cer NS and Cer AS methylene stretching spectra.

occurs when a hydrated film of Cer NS is heated in the presence of D_2O.[25] The change in the peak area of the OH/NH stretch, which decreases with H → D exchange, tracks the changes in the methylene stretching frequency. The change in the normalized amide II band area, which also decreases with H → D exchange, does not track the changes in methylene stretching frequency until the full chain-disordering process is reached at high temperature. These results indicate that as

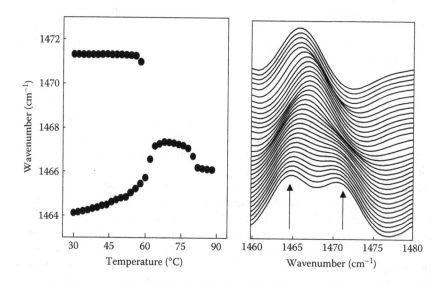

FIGURE 10.7 Thermotropic changes in Cer NS chain packing from methylene scissoring spectra.

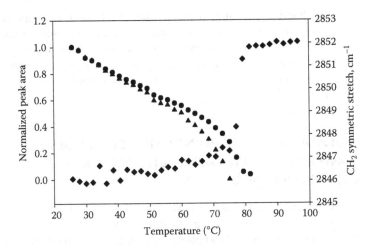

FIGURE 10.8 Thermotropic changes in $v_{sym}CH_2$ (◆), amide II relative integrated area (▲), and vOH/vNH relative integrated area (●) during H → D exchange for orthorhombic phase Cer AS.

the ceramide packing loosens, the hydroxyl protons become accessible (or labile) to D_2O and then undergo H → D exchange. The amide proton, however, is not accessible until complete chain fluidization has occurred. This implies that it is the hydroxyl head groups that are most involved in the solid–solid phase transition.

Cer AS does not exhibit an equivalent solid–solid phase transition, as shown in Figure 10.6. After a gradual increase in methylene stretching frequencies, a sharp chain-disordering transition is observed with a T_m of 78°C precisely as chain orthorhombic packing collapses. Interestingly, the addition of the α-hydroxy group on Cer AS creates tighter chain packing than in Cer NS (lower methylene stretching frequency), yet Cer AS undergoes an order→disorder transition that is 15°C lower than that of Cer NS. Examination of the H → D head group exchange reveals that both the hydroxyl and amide protons undergo a constant rate of exchange, beginning at room temperature and largely completed before chain melting, as shown in Figure 10.8. This implies that the head group region is accessible to D_2O and that the greater efficiency of chain packing in Cer AS is obtained at the expense of tight head group packing.

There is a kinetic barrier to the formation of the optimal orthorhombic chain-packed structures of both Cer NS and Cer AS. Hydrated samples are normally prepared by heating the ceramide above T_m in the presence of water and mixing well to ensure maximum hydration of the head groups. Rapid cooling of these samples results in the formation of a metastable hexagonally packed arrangement that slowly undergoes reorganization to orthorhombic chain packing. These metastable hexagonal phases exhibit looser chain packing and lower conformational order, as reflected by higher methylene stretching frequencies (~2 cm^{-1}) than when orthorhombically packed. The rearrangement of the hexagonal gel phase to form the orthorhombic crystalline phase is faster at intermediate temperatures between room temperature and the orthorhombic-to-hexagonal phase transition temperatures. Once the film achieves orthorhombic chain packing, it forms more readily after heating it through the disordering process again. The somewhat complex kinetics of such processes with SC lipids have been investigated and will be published.

10.8 INDIVIDUAL PHYTOSPHINGOSINE CERAMIDES: CONFORMATIONAL ORDER, CHAIN PACKING, AND HYDROGEN BONDING

The phytosphingosine ceramides do not have a *trans* 4,5 bond on their base chain; however, they have a third hydroxyl group at the 4 position on the base chain (Figure 10.3). This increases the head group area but removes an efficient means of close chain packing by folding back along the *trans* double bond. Monolayer studies by Pascher demonstrated that the head group areas of phytosphingosine ceramides are 3 to 5 Å^2 larger than those of the analogous sphingosine ceramides.[32] Not surprisingly, given this larger head group area, only hexagonal chain packing is observed with the hydrated phytosphingosine ceramides. These ceramides exhibit higher values for their methylene stretching frequencies, consistent with their somewhat looser chain packing. This arises from the greater room between the chains in the hexagonal unit cell of 1.5 molecules, permitting greater rotational movement than with orthorhombic packing, which has a unit cell containing 2 molecules (Figure 10.2). Interestingly, when phytosphingosine and sphingosine ceramides are both hexagonally packed, their methylene stretching frequencies are very similar.

Phytosphingosine ceramides exhibit very different behavior in the head group regions compared to the analogous sphingosine ceramides.[25] Amide I is observed at much lower frequencies, and amide II is observed at higher frequencies; both shifts are indicative of stronger hydrogen bonding. Cer NP has narrow amide I and II peaks; thus, not only is the hydrogen bonding at the amide strong, but this bond is conformationally constrained and limited in orientation. Cer NP also has two sharp peaks in the OH/NH stretching region at frequencies indicative of strong hydrogen bonding. Hydrated Cer NP head group behavior is consistent with the structure elucidated by Dahlén and Pascher for an anhydrous Cer NP analogue with a C24 acid chain.[33] In this structure both the amide and the hydroxyl groups are tightly bound in a regular open V structure. For Cer AP, amide I, amide II, and the OH/NH stretches are broader than Cer NP (or Cer AS), indicating a greater number of hydrogen-bonding orientations or greater conformational freedom of the hydrogen bonds.

Phytosphingosine ceramides have higher chain-disordering temperatures (T_m) than the corresponding sphingosine ceramides, indicating that they are more thermally stable. Cer NP undergoes a chain-disordering process that is 22°C higher than Cer NS, while Cer AP disorders 15°C higher than Cer AS. Given the lower conformational order of the phytosphingosine ceramides at room temperature, it might be expected that the chain-disordering process would occur at lower temperatures due to the already looser chain packing. It appears likely that their increased thermal stability results from the stronger hydrogen bonding of the phytosphingosine ceramides. Indeed, hydration of Cer NP increases the chain-disordering temperature to 115°C from the 110°C of the anhydrous material. However, the addition of the α-hydroxy group on the acid chain lowers thermal stability (even though more hydrogen bonds could be formed), resulting in a 22°C difference in T_m between Cer NP and Cer AP. This compares to the 15°C difference in T_m between Cer NS and Cer AS.

Further insight into the molecular dynamics of phytosphingosine hydrogen bonding has been obtained by examining the H $\rightarrow$ D exchange of the head groups by heating a hydrated film in the presence of D_2O (Figure 10.9). Cer AP begins H $\rightarrow$ D exchange at low temperatures, then stops exchanging between 50 and 85°C, finally undergoing rapid exchange at the chain T_m. This clearly implies that some of the head groups are more accessible than others in Cer AP. This is in contrast to Cer AS, which undergoes gradual continuous exchange (see above).

Cer NP is very resistant to H $\rightarrow$ D exchange. Virtually no exchange is observed below 90°C, indicating exceptional stability for the hydrated Cer NP structure.[25] Between 90 and 98°C (the limit of our experimental technique), rapid exchange of both hydroxyl and amide protons is observed. Exchange occurs before chain disordering. This was also observed in an analogue of Cer NP in which an oleic acid group was substituted for the stearic acid chain. No exchange was observed until about 15°C below the chain-disordering process, and exchange was completed 5°C prior to chain disordering.

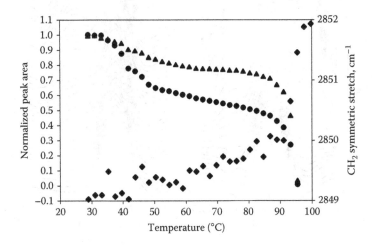

FIGURE 10.9 Thermotropic changes in $\nu_{sym}CH_2$ ($\blacklozenge$), amide II relative integrated area ($\blacktriangle$), and $\nu OH/\nu NH$ relative integrated area ($\bullet$) during H $\rightarrow$ D exchange for orthorhombic phase Cer AP.

10.9 TERNARY SPHINGOSINE CERAMIDE SYSTEMS: CONFORMATIONAL ORDER, CHAIN PACKING, AND HYDROGEN BONDING

Hydrated, ternary equimolar mixtures of Cer NS or Cer AS with cholesterol and d_{35}-stearic acid were prepared by heating the materials to a liquid state and vortexing in the presence of excess water, allowing them to maximally hydrate. Initially, both the ceramides and the stearic acid exhibit hexagonal chain packing with higher methylene stretching frequencies than previously observed in their individual systems. As in the individual systems, the chains undergo an eventual rearrangement to orthorhombic chain packing for both the ceramides and the stearic acid. This can be thermally tracked by following the appearance of splitting in either the ρCH_2 or δCD_2 bands, along with decreases in the methylene stretching frequencies.[36,37] This is shown in Figure 10.10 for Cer AS. Similar changes are observed in the acid carbonyl stretch and amide I bands that go from higher to lower frequencies, indicating stronger hydrogen bonding in the orthorhombic

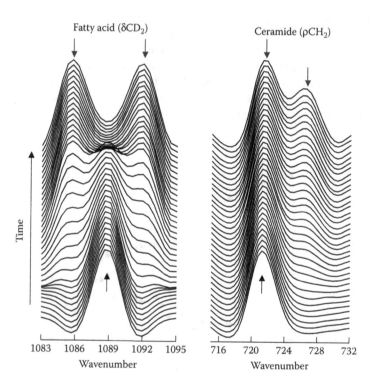

FIGURE 10.10 Time dependence of Cer NS methylene rocking mode and d_{35}-octade-canoic acid methylene scissoring spectra showing chain-packing changes in hydrated, equimolar mixture with cholesterol.

phase/individual domain than in the hexagonal phase (possibly intimately mixed). At the very least, they signal a fundamental change in the hydrogen bonding.

The chain-disordering temperature (T_m) is decreased for both Cer NS and Cer AS by about 20°C when heated in these ternary systems. However, the nature of these transitions is very different. For Cer NS, the chain-disordering process occurs over a very broad temperature range (~20°C). This is indicative of extensive mixing with cholesterol and possibly d_{35}-stearic acid. In contrast, Cer AS undergoes a sharp chain-disordering transition over only several degrees and is very close in temperature to the chain-disordering process for d_{35}-stearic acid, which is also sharp. The lowered and common temperatures indicate a possible eutectic melting between Cer AS and the d_{35}-stearic acid. In the Cer NS system, d_{35}-stearic acid also undergoes chain disordering at a lower temperature than for the pure component, but is some 15°C lower than the Cer NS chain-disordering temperature. Like Cer NS, the disordering process occurs over a broad temperature range, indicating that it also mixes with cholesterol upon disordering.

In both systems, the ceramide and fatty acid orthorhombic chain packing collapse just prior to each component's chain disordering. For Cer AS and d_{35}-stearic acid, the orthorhombic-to-hexagonal chain-packing transition is at similar temperatures, but is at different temperatures for Cer NS and d_{35}-stearic acid.

Upon initial mixing, when the chains of both the ceramides and the d_{35}-stearic acid are in the hexagonal chain-packing configuration, their hydrogen bonding is strongly altered from the individual components. For d_{35}-stearic acid, the acid carbonyl stretch is shifted to a higher frequency by at least 15 cm^{-1}. Amide I of Cer NS in the mixture is a single peak and is shifted to a higher frequency, although compared to pure Cer NS, the peak is broad and difficult to directly compare. This is also true for Cer AS.

Once phase separation/orthorhombic chain packing is observed, the acid carbonyl stretch and the ceramide amide I and amide II bands are similar to the individually hydrated molecules. In the Cer NS system, both amides I and II again split into two bands each. When the d_{35}-stearic acid undergoes the orthorhombic-to-hexagonal phase change, the acid carbonyl stretch undergoes a sharp transition to a higher frequency, indicating weaker hydrogen bonding. A similar effect is observed for Cer NS, where the amide I and II band splitting is lost at the solid phase transition. Interestingly, amide II initially shifts to higher frequency, indicating stronger hydrogen bonding for this mode, before shifting to lower frequency after chain disordering. In the Cer AS system, the amide I and II bands are little changed, as both the solid phase transition and the chain-disordering transition are observed. The d_{35}-stearic acid again undergoes a sharp transition to a higher frequency at the solid phase transition.

From these observations, we can see that at physiological pH and temperatures, there is little interaction between the sphingosine ceramides, fatty acid, and cholesterol when hydrated at equimolar concentrations. Even under fluid conditions when forced to interact, they apparently undergo phase separation to a more stable configuration. These configurations are stable to well above physiological temperatures.

10.10 TERNARY PHYTOSPHINGOSINE CERAMIDE SYSTEMS: CONFORMATIONAL ORDER, CHAIN PACKING, AND HYDROGEN BONDING

The molecular organization and dynamics in the hydrated, equimolar phytosphingosine ceramide, d_{35}-stearic acid, and cholesterol systems are profoundly different from the corresponding sphingosine ceramide ones described above.[38] The most important difference is that ternary phytosphingosine ceramide samples form intimate, homogeneous mixtures in which separate domains are not observed. This interaction is not easy to initiate; it requires heating these systems to above the phytosphingosine ceramide melting temperatures, which is 115°C for Cer NP. Formation of these intimate mixtures appears to be a consequence of the more open phytosphingosine head group, which results in hexagonal chain packing. The more open hexagonal chain array appears to allow much greater mixing with d_{35}-stearic acid, and possibly with cholesterol.

Intimate mixing is demonstrated through several effects. The first is that the d_{35}-stearic acid is hexagonally packed in the ternary phytosphingosine systems. Although hexagonal chain packing can be induced by heating hydrated d_{35}-stearic acid, either alone or in combination with sphingosine ceramides or cholesterol, it always rearranges back to orthorhombic chain packing. We have not been able to observe d_{35}-stearic acid orthorhombic chain packing once hydrated mixtures have been achieved with either Cer AP or Cer NP. From this we conclude that it is the ceramide that dominates the chain-packing orientations in these systems.

The second is that the hydrogen bonding of both the d_{35}-stearic acid and Cer NP and Cer AP is very different from that of the individual hydrated molecules. Both the acid carbonyl stretch and ceramide amide I are shifted to higher frequencies. The weaker hydrogen bonding indicates a very different hydrogen-bonding environment, suggestive of extensive mixing between the ceramide amide and hydroxyl groups with the stearic acid head group.

It is difficult to determine if the head group hydrogen bonding drives the chain packing or if the chain packing drives the hydrogen bonding. However, both the chain conformations and the hydrogen bonding are very stable until very high temperatures. In fact, the third and most surprising observation is the significant increase in chain T_m of d_{35}-stearic acid in these systems (Figure 10.11). In the Cer AP system, the ceramide chain T_m is also increased compared to the individually hydrated molecule. The d_{35}-stearic acid chain-disordering process tracks the phytosphingosine ceramide chain-disordering processes. These disordering processes occur over very wide temperature ranges, indicating that cholesterol is also involved. We have found that hydration is necessary for these interactions; equimolar anhydrous mixtures show separate and sharp chain-disordering processes. Very little change is seen in the acid carbonyl and amide I peaks until chain disordering is almost complete, and this is just a thermal broadening of the peaks.

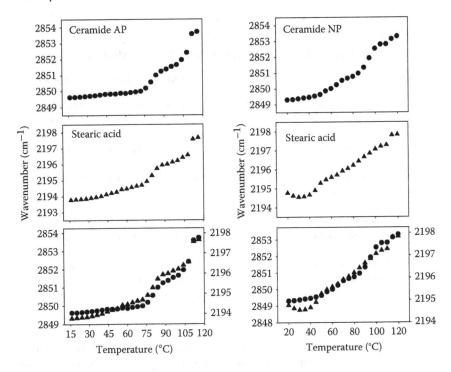

FIGURE 10.11 Thermotropic changes in phytosphingosine ceramide $v_{sym}CH_2$ frequency (●) and d_{35}-stearic acid $v_{asym}CD_2$ frequency (▲) for the hydrated (^2H_2O), equimolar Cer AP, d_{35}-stearic acid, cholesterol skin lipid model system.

10.11 IMPLICATIONS FOR LIPID ORGANIZATION IN STRATUM CORNEUM

We have now examined, in some detail, four of the most common ceramides found in the human stratum corneum.[25,29,35–38] While our work has focused on pure ceramides and three component model systems, we believe the results provide direct relevance toward understanding molecular interactions in the stratum corneum lipid matrix, where ceramides are present with long-chain fatty acids and cholesterol in a roughly equimolar mixture. Table 10.1 summarizes the major findings from our studies, from which several conclusions can be drawn. The first, as has been discussed in detail here, is that there is a fundamental difference between the behavior of sphingosine and phytosphingosine ceramide hydrated, ternary lipid systems. The second conclusion is that it is the ceramide component that drives the behavior of the ternary lipid systems. All four ceramides have the same chain packing in the ternary lipid systems as they do when hydrated individually. When the chains of sphingosines Cer NS and Cer AS pack in orthorhombic subcells and form distinct domains, so do the chains of stearic acid. However, when the chains of the phytosphingosines Cer NP and Cer AP pack in

TABLE 10.1
Ceramide and Fatty Acid Chain Behavior in Ternary Models

Attribute	Cer NS	Cer NP	Cer AP	Cer AS
Stearic acid chain packing	Orthorhombic	Hexagonal	Hexagonal	Orthorhombic
Change in stearic acid chain packing?	No	Yes	Yes	No
Stearic acid chain-disordering T_m	Decreased	Increased	Increased	Decreased
Ceramide chain packing	Orthorhombic	Hexagonal	Hexagonal	Orthorhombic
Change in ceramide chain packing?	No	No	No	No
Ceramide chain-disordering T_m	Decreased	Decreased	Increased	Decreased
Stearic acid/ceramide chain-disordering T_m	Separate	Similar	Similar	Similar
Stearic acid vCO frequency	Similar	Increased	Increased	Increased
Ceramide amide I frequency	Similar	Increased	Increased	Similar

a more open hexagonal structure, the stearic acid chains also pack hexagonally; this is presumably due to incorporation into the more open ceramide matrix along with the cholesterol, as inferred by the broad, synchronous fatty acid and ceramide chain-disordering transitions.

It follows that it is the chain behavior of these ceramides that drives the ultimate organization. For the phytosphingosines, hydrogen bonding is altered in the three-component systems for both the stearic acid and the phytosphingosine ceramides in a way that can be interpreted as lower in bond strength. Yet the stearic acid chain-disordering temperatures are greatly increased, as is the Cer AP chain-disordering temperature. Although little change is seen in both the sphingosine chain packing and hydrogen bonding, the ceramide chain transition is lowered, presumably through solubilization of ceramide in fluid stearic acid. Given the water barrier function of the stratum corneum, it is not surprising that hydrophobic forces drive the functionality.

Finally, these results show that Cer NS, perhaps the most studied skin ceramide in model systems, is the least similar to the other three ceramides in Table 10.1.[11–15,23,24] It is the only ceramide that does not undergo a synchronous disordering transition with stearic acid. It is also the system in which the stearic acid behaves most closely to the hydrated pure molecule, suggesting that Cer NS is the least interactive ceramide of those studied. Conclusions on general ceramide behavior based exclusively on observations from Cer NS model systems should be made with caution.

These results are also consistent with the fundamental ideas in Forslind's domain mosaic model of skin barrier lipid organization.[39] Sphingosine ceramides can form distinct domains, whereas phytosphingosine ceramides can form inti- mate mixtures. The domain mosaic model also highlights the potential role of the more fluid SC lipid precursors at the SG–SC interface. These more fluid precursors are presumably intimately mixed in an L_α-type lamellar organization (typical of most membranes). Enzymatic cleavage of the target head group bonds in these lipids results in an organization that resembles the hydrated melted model mixtures used in our studies. Thus, in the physiological case, mixing is achieved without extremes of temperature or physical force (agitation) by using chemical potential. Presumably, after cleavage, the phytosphingosine ceramides remain intimately mixed with fatty acids and cholesterol, while the sphingosines undergo phase separation to form their individual domains. This sphingosine ceramide phase separation consequently forms fatty acid domains through the ceramide fatty acid separation process.

The combination of both discrete ordered domains and intimate mixtures is necessary to assemble a complex composite material that provides the necessary properties of the SC barrier function. In concert, these properties can produce a structure that is relatively water impermeable, cohesive, and yet mechanically tolerant. Without the appropriate lipid composition and corresponding physical organization, the SC, and hence the skin, would be unable to maintain its key physiological functions, such as maintaining water homeostasis, regulating tem- perature, and communicating sensory signals.

REFERENCES

1. Madison, K.C. et al., Presence of intact intercellular lipid lamellae in the upper layers of the stratum corneum, *Journal of Investigative Dermatology*, 1987; 88, 714–718.
2. Elias, P.M., Epidermal lipids, barrier function, and desquamation, *Journal of Investigative Dermatology*, 1983; 80, 44–49.
3. Williams, M.L. and P.M. Elias, The extracellular matrix of stratum corneum: role of lipids in normal and pathological function, *Critical Reviews in Therapeutic Drug Carrier Systems*, 1987; 3, 95–122.
4. Schaefer, H. and T.E. Redelmeier, *Skin Barrier: Principles of Percutaneous Absorption*, 1st ed., Karger, Basel, 1996, 310 pp.
5. Wertz, P.W. and B. van den Bergh, The physical, chemical and functional prop- erties of lipids in the skin and other biological barriers, *Chemistry and Physics of Lipids*, 1998; 91, 85–96.
6. Small, D.M., The Physical chemistry of lipids: from alkanes to phospholipids, in *Handbook of Lipid Research*, 1st ed., Vol. 4, D.J. Hanahan, Ed., Plenum Press, New York, 1986, 672 pp.
7. Rawlings, A.V., Skin waxes. Their composition, properties, structures and biolog- ical significance, in *Waxes*, R. Hamilton and W. Christie, Eds., The Oily Press, Dundee, 1995, pp. 223–256.
8. Williams, M.L., Lipids in normal and pathological desquamation, in *Skin Lipids*, P.M. Elias, Ed., Academic Press, New York, 1991, pp. 211–262.

9. Elias, P.M., Epidermal barrier function: intercellular lamellar lipid structures, origin, composition and metabolism, *Journal of Controlled Release*, 1991; 15, 199–208.

10. Wertz, P.W. et al., The composition of the ceramides from human stratum corneum and from comedones, *Journal of Investigative Dermatology*, 1985; 84, 410–412.

11. Motta, S. et al., Ceramide composition of the psoriatic scale, *Biochimica et Biophysica Acta*, 1993; 1182, 147–151.

12. Swartzendruber, D.C. et al., Evidence that the corneocyte has a chemically bound lipid envelope, *Journal of Investigative Dermatology*, 1987; 88, 709–712.

13. Robson, K.J. et al., 6-Hydroxy-4-sphingenine in human epidermal ceramides, *Journal of Lipid Research*, 1994; 35, 2060–2068.

14. Wertz, P.W., K.C. Madison, and D.T. Downing, Covalently bound lipids of human stratum corneum, *Journal of Investigative Dermatology*, 1989; 92, 109–111.

15. Harding, C.R., D.J. Moore, and A.V. Rawlings, Ceramides and the skin, in *Textbook of Cosmetic Dermatology*, R. Baran and H.I. Maibach, Eds., Taylor & Francis, London, 2004, pp. 171–187.

16. Norlen, L. et al., A new HPLC-based method for the quantitative analysis of inner stratum corneum lipids with special reference to the free fatty acid fraction. *Archives of Dermatological Research*, 1998; 290, 508–516.

17. Mao-Qiang, M. et al., Extracellular processing of phospholipids is required for permeability barrier homeostasis, *Journal of Lipid Research*, 1995; 36, 1925–1935.

18. Snyder, R.G., Vibrational spectra of crystalline n-paraffins. Part 1. Methylene rocking and wagging modes, *Journal of Molecular Spectroscopy*, 1960; 4, 411–434.

19. Snyder, R.G., Vibrational spectra of crystalline n-paraffins. II. Intermolecular effects, *Journal of Molecular Spectroscopy*, 1961; 7, 116–144.

20. Snyder, R.G., Vibrational study of the chain conformation of the liquid n-paraffins and molten polyethylene, *Journal of Chemical Physics*, 1967; 47, 1316–1360.

21. Snyder, R.G., Hsu, S.L., and Krimm, S., Vibrational spectra in the C-H stretching region and the structure of the polymethylene chain, *Spectrochimica Acta*, 1978; 34A, 395–406.

22. Snyder, R.G., H.L. Strauss, and C.A. Elliger, C-H stretching modes and the structure of n-alkyl chains. 1. Long, disordered chains, *Journal of Physical Chemistry*, 1982; 86, 5145–5150.

23. MacPhail, R.A. et al., C-H stretching modes and the structure of n-alkyl chains. 2. Long, all-trans chains, *Journal of Physical Chemistry*, 1984; 88, 334–341.

24. Snyder, R.G., Vibrational correlation splitting and chain packing for the crystalline n-alkanes, *Journal of Chemical Physics*, 1979; 71, 3229–3235.

25. Rerek, M.E. et al., Phytosphingosine and sphingosine ceramide headgroup hydrogen bonding: structural insights through thermotropic hydrogen/deuterium exchange, *Journal of Physical Chemistry B*, 2001; 105, 9355–9363.

26. Mendelsohn, R. and D.J. Moore, IR determination of conformational order and phase behavior in ceramides and stratum corneum models, in *Sphingolipid Metabolism and Cell Signaling*, Y.A. Hannun and A.H. Merrill, Eds., Academic Press, New York, 2000, pp. 228–247.

27. Mendelsohn, R. and D.J. Moore, Vibrational spectroscopic studies of lipid domains in biomembranes and model systems, *Chemistry and Physics of Lipids*, 1998; 96, 141–157.

28. Moore, D.J., Stratum corneum lipids and barrier function: biophysical studies of molecular organization in sphingomyelin and ceramide [NS] bilayers, *Recent Research Developments in Lipids*, 2002; 6, 55–63.

29. Moore, D.J., M.E. Rerek, and R. Mendelsohn, FTIR spectroscopy studies of the conformational order and phase behavior of ceramides, *Journal of Physical Chemistry B*, 1997; 101, 8933–8940.

30. Kitson, N. et al., A model membrane approach to the epidermal permeability barrier, *Biochemistry*, 1994; 33, 6707–6715.

31. Bouwstra, J.A. et al., A model membrane approach to the epidermal permeability barrier: an x-ray diffraction study, *Biochemistry*, 1997; 36, 7717–7725.

32. Lofgren, H. and I. Pascher, Molecular arrangements of sphingolipids. The monolayer behaviour of ceramides, *Chemistry and Physics of Lipids*, 1977; 20, 273–284.

33. Dahlén, B. and I. Pascher, Molecular arrangements in sphingolipids. Thermotropic phase behaviour of tetracosanoylphytosphingosine, *Chemistry and Physics of Lipids*, 1979; 24, 119–133.

34. Senak, L., D.J. Moore, and R. Mendelsohn, CH_2 wagging progressions as IR probes of slightly disordered phospholipid acyl chain states, *Journal of Physical Chemistry*, 1992; 96, 2749–2754.

35. Flach, C.R. et al., Biophysical studies of model stratum corneum lipid monolayers by infrared reflection-absorption spectroscopy and Brewster angle microscopy, *Journal of Physical Chemistry*, 2000; 104, 2159–2165.

36. Moore, D.J., M.E. Rerek, and R. Mendelsohn, Lipid domains and orthorhombic phases in model stratum corneum: evidence from Fourier transform infrared spectroscopy studies, *Biochemical and Biophysical Research Communications*, 1997; 231, 797–801.

37. Moore, D.J. and M.E. Rerek, Insights into the molecular organization of lipids in the skin barrier from infrared spectroscopy studies of stratum corneum lipid models, *Acta Dermato-Venereologica*, 2000; Suppl. 208: 16–22.

38. Rerek, M.E. et al., FTIR spectroscopic studies of lipid dynamics in phytosphingosine ceramide models of the stratum corneum lipid matrix, *Chemistry and Physics of Lipids*, 2005; 134, 51–58.

39. Forslind, B., A domain mosiac model of the skin barrier, *Acta Dermatol-Venereologica*, 1994; 74, 1–9.

11 Cosmetoceuticals in Modified Microemulsions

Nissim Garti

Casali Institute of Applied Chemistry, Hebrew University of Jerusalem, Jerusalem, Israel

CONTENTS

ABSTRACT

A novel technology to prepare modified reverse microemulsion (denoted NSSL, nanosized self-assembled liquid) vehicles loaded with cosmetoceuticals, based on permitted ingredients that can be progressively diluted with water, was developed recently in our labs. The microemulsion isotropic regions representing water-in-oil (W/O), bicontinuous mesophase, and oil-in-water (O/W) microemulsion structures are presented in a phase diagram so-called U-type. In such compositions in the isotropic regions of the phase diagram, structures can invert from L2 (reverse micelles) to an L1 (direct micelles) phase via W/O, bicontinuous, and O/W regions progressively, without phase separation.

The concentrates (condensed reverse micelles) can be loaded at very high solubilization capacities of guest molecules (lycopene, phytosterols, tocopherols, CoQ10, lutein, antioxidants, aromas, fragrances) that are oil soluble or even mostly insoluble in the water or oil phase. The solubilization exceeds manyfold that of the solubility capacity of each of the phases.

The microemulsion phase transformations were studied by conductivity, viscosity differential scanning calorimetry (DSC), and self-diffusion–nuclear magnetic resonance (SD-NMR) measurements, and the microstructure was determined by small-angle x-ray scattering (SAXS), cryo-transmission electron microscopy (TEM). The loci of the solubilizate at any given water content were determined by following the self-diffusion coefficients of each of the ingredients.

It was concluded that the solubilizates are easily accommodated and tightly packed at the concave, hydrophobic-in-nature, water-in-oil interface and at the bicontinuous interface. Most solubilizates are more loosely packed at the oil-in-water interface and tend to be released from the interface once inversion occurs. Upon inversion to O/W microemulsion droplets, the interface becomes more hydrophilic and convexes toward the water, becoming the continuous phase. The solubilization capacity drops dramatically, and the active matter can be trigger released.

The nutraceuticals are solubilized at higher solubilization capacities if interacting with the surfactant.

Upon entrapping guest molecules, the transition from W/O to bicontinuous, and thereafter to an O/W microemulsion, is occurring, in some cases, at higher levels of water dilution, while in other cases, depending on the nature of the solubilizate, at lower dilutions, indicating that some of the guest compounds add some order to the internal microemulsion organization, while others are destructive to the interface and enhance phase separation or phase transitions.

11.1 INTRODUCTION

Microemulsions have been known to the scientific community as well as to various experts in industry for several decades. Hundreds of studies were carried out by experimentalists, and many theories have been worked out regarding the self-aggregation of surfactants in the aqueous phase (O/W) and oil phase (W/O) to form micellar or reverse micellar structures, respectively, that can be swollen by another liquid phase to form a reservoir of insoluble liquid phase entrapped by a tightly packed surfactant layer.

In spite of the numerous studies and the pronounced potential applications in foods, pharmaceuticals, and cosmetics, only few practical preparations are presently available in the marketplace in which the solubilized molecules are at very low solubilization levels. It is always an open question why these structures did not make their way to final products.

Microemulsion by most common general definition is structured fluid (or solution-like mixture) of two immiscible liquid phases in the presence of surfactant (sometimes with cosurfactant and cosolvent) to form spontaneously and thermodynamically stable isotropic liquid. The surfactants are self-assembled in a continuous phase and can solubilize another phase, other cosolvents, and other guest molecules (solubilizates). Droplet sizes are in the range of a few nanometers to a hundred nanometers.

In theory, in order to form such structures, one must control the interfacial tension between the two phases and reduce it to a value close to zero, and must provide surfactants that will geometrically self-organize in curved structures in proper packing geometrical parameters.

Microemulsions are best studied by composing a proper binary, ternary, or multicomponent phase diagram that will represent the equilibrium situation of the components mixture or the thermodynamic organization of the components. A classical typical phase diagram is shown in Figure 11.1.

Understanding the phase behavior and microstructure of microemulsions is an important fundamental aspect of the efficient utilization of these structured fluids in industrial applications. Today, we have a more profound understanding of the phase behavior and microstructure of microemulsions.[1–6] However, microemulsions in industrial applications are rarely simple ternary systems, but more often complicated multicomponent systems. It is not always clear whether those complex systems have similar droplet sizes and shapes, and what are the roles

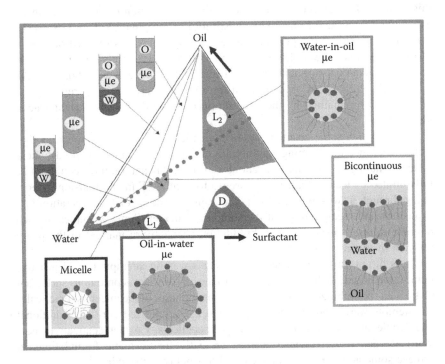

FIGURE 11.1 Typical phase diagram made with water, emulsifiers, and oil phase. Four types of isotropic regions have been identified. Note that the dilution line traverses via a two-phase region and full dilution to the far corner of the water phase is not possible.

of the additional components in stabilizing the interface. Systematic investigations should be useful to understand the microstructure and the effect of the different components on the system.

In recent years, few attempts have been made to formulate and characterize microemulsions that can be used for food, cosmetic, and pharmaceutical purposes.[7,8]

In this effort, normal alkanes have been replaced by oils acceptable in the cosmetics industry, and the majority of preparations are oil continuous (W/O). These papers focused on studying the ability of formulating a microemulsion with triglycerides[9–14] and perfumes[15–17] as the oil component. Some workers[18,19] have studied the phase behavior and microstructure of water-in-triglycerides (W/O) microemulsions based on polyoxyethylene (40) sorbitanhexaoleate. They found that the monophasic area of these systems was strongly dependent on temperature and aqueous phase content. Lawrence and coworkers[11,12] examined the solubilization of a range of triglycerides and ethyl esters in an oil-in-water microemulsion system with nonionic surfactants. They concluded that the solubilization capacity depends not only on the nature of the surfactants, but also on the nature of the oil.

There are few surfactants that can be used in cosmetic formulations. In this respect, Tweens (ethoxylated derivatives of sorbitan esters) are an interesting family of surfactants. The substitution of the hydroxyl groups on the sorbitan ring with bulky polyoxyethylene groups increases the hydrophilicity of the surfactant. The ability of Tweens to form microemulsions in cosmetic and pharmaceutical applications has been studied by a few authors.[20–24] An increased solubility of lipophilic drugs in the microemulsion regime was observed and explained by the penetration of these drugs into the interfacial film.[22–24]

Even though some cosmetic-grade emulsifiers have been mentioned as possible microemulsion-forming amphiphiles, it was almost impossible to use these systems, mainly because the concentrates of oil/surfactant mixtures could not be fully diluted by water or aqueous phases to form an O/W microemulsion without going through a two-phase region and causing a process of fast separation into emulsions and precipitating out the solubilized matter. Some examples of such possible dilution lines stressing the dilution problem are marked in the phase diagram in Figure 11.1.

In addition, in most studies the emphasis was on attempts to add just one immiscible liquid, such as water (or oil) to the oil (or water) continuous surfactant phase, i.e., to solubilize the oil in the core (inner phase) of the micelles. Practically no attempts were made to incorporate into the solubilized core any additional guest molecules, such as drugs or cosmetoceuticals. Cosmetoceuticals (a new term) are active ingredients designed specially for cosmetic formulations to achieve some additional pronounced health benefits to the skin.

The structural and compositional limitations of the presently used cosmetic formulations to make them into formulations loaded with cosmetoceutical ingredients is not an easy task and must be bridged by introducing new

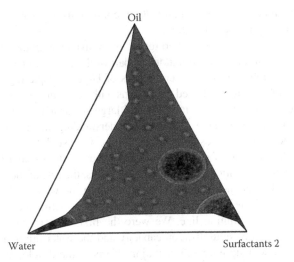

FIGURE 11.2 Typical novel U-type phase diagram composed of selected combinations of cosmetic-grade emulsifiers with progressive full dilution.

concepts in microemulsion preparations. Some of the cardinal points to be solved include:

1. Progressive and continuous dilution by aqueous phase or water without destroying the interface and forming a two-phase region, i.e., formation of a so-called U-type phase diagram that undergoes progressive inversion from W/O to O/W microemulsions (Figure 11.2)
2. Preparation of microemulsions that will be based on the use of permitted cosmetic-grade emulsifiers, oils, cosurfactants, or cosolvents
3. Facilitating the entrapment (cosolubilization capacity) of large loads of insoluble guest molecules within the core of the microemulsion or at its interface
4. Allowing environmental protection to the active addenda (guest molecule) from autooxidation or hydrolysis degradation while stored on the shelf
5. Improving the bioavailability of the entrapped addenda
6. Controlling the release from the vehicle to the water-continuous phase or onto human membranes
7. Use the microemulsions as microreactors to obtain regioselectivity, fast kinetics, and controlled and triggered reactions of active molecules once applied on the skin

A phase diagram with very large isotropic regions is typical of the novel microemulsions that are made from multicomponents. The isotropic regions represent water-in-oil (W/O), bicontinuous mesophase, and oil-in-water (O/W) microemulsion structures. The phase diagrams are known as U-type. In such compositions, within the isotropic regions of the phase diagram, the oil/surfactant-condensed structured mixtures (denoted condensed reverse micelles, L2) can transform to an L1 phase (direct micelles) via an W/O, bicontinuous, or O/W region progressively without any phase separation.

To the best of our knowledge, no reports were available in the literature, prior to the establishment of our formulations as part of the extended new U-type phase diagrams, to comply with these prerequisites of large isotropic regions.[25–38] Most of the early studies were conducted on systems with constant water content (>70%) and with low oil content (ca. 5 to 10%) and large surfactant excess (high surfactant/oil ratios). We enlarged the scope of the understanding of such microemulsions to food applications and cosmetic preparations. Our studies examined various aspects of solubilization of cosmetoceuticals, release patterns, and other thermal and environmental conditions. In some of our studies, the role of the surfactant was examined, but the maximum amounts of the solubilizate were studied and efforts were made to estimate what are the total amounts of active matter that can be entrapped along any dilution line. We were the first to establish the correlation between the maximum solubilization capacity and the water dilution.[25–38]

This review will summarize our major efforts in the development of microemulsions as vehicles for the solubilization of cosmetoceuticals for improved skin penetration and treatment to provide extra health benefits.

11.2 U-TYPE MICROEMULSIONS, SWOLLEN MICELLES, AND PROGRESSIVE AND FULL DILUTION

At first,[25,27] we dealt with water and oil solubilization in the presence of a new set of nonionic ingredients and emulsifiers to form U-type nonionic W/O and O/W cosmetic microemulsion systems. It was recognized that certain molecules destabilize the liquid crystalline phases and extend the isotropic region to higher surfactant concentrations. The additives enable the enlargement of the monophasic region (to be termed the A_T regions) to be as large as possible so that the total amounts of oil and water that can be solubilized are maximized. A pseudoternary phase diagrams for R(+)-limonene-based systems with food- and cosmetic-grade systems, in comparison to those based on no food-grade emulsifiers, such as Brij 96v (C18:1 (EO) 10) is presented in Figure 11.2.[25,27] In these systems, which offer great potential in practical formulations, it is possible to follow the structural evolution of the microemulsion system from an aqueous phase-poor to an aqueous phase-rich region without encountering phase separation.

Figure 11.3 represents a typical cryo-TEM photomicrograph of a microemulsion from a U-type diagram of structures obtained after inversion from an L2 phase into O/W droplets upon dilution with an aqueous phase to 90 wt% water. The droplets' sizes are ca. 8 to 10 nm and are mostly monodisperse. It should be noted that most microemulsions, regardless of the type of oil, surfactant, and cosolvents, consist of droplets of ca. 5 to 20 nm in size and do not grow above these sizes at any water or oil contents.

Various U-type phase diagrams with various types of hydrophilic surfactants, cosolvents, and cosurfactants were constructed, yielding small or large isotropic

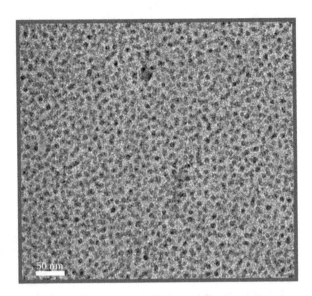

FIGURE 11.3 Photomicrograph of typical O/W droplets derived from a concentrate of W/O after dilution to 90 wt% water content. (From Reference 30. With permission.)

A_T regions. The most successful phase diagram yielded an isotropic region of >75% of the total area of the phase diagram ($A_T > 75\%$). The dilution lines were termed Vm lines. Full-dilution lines are those that can undergo full and progressive dilution to the far water corner (Vm = 100%). An example of such a dilution line is line 64 in Figure 11.2, for which at 60 wt% surfactant phase and 40 wt% oil phase the dilution with aqueous phase is progressive and complete to the far corner (100%) aqueous phase. In dilution line 55 (50 wt% surfactant phase and 50 wt% oil phase) the Wm is only ca. 60% aqueous phase and further dilution will lead to phase separation.

Formation of U-type phase diagrams is essential for formulations that will be based on an oil phase and allowed to mix with water as needed without breaking the structures.

11.3 SOLUBILIZATION OF NONSOLUBLE NUTRACEUTICALS

The growing interest in microemulsions as vehicles for food and cosmetic formulations arises mainly from the advantages of their physicochemical properties. Microemulsions can cosolubilize, together with the inner reservoir, a large amount of lipophilic and hydrophilic nutraceutical and cosmetoceutical additives.

The cosolubilization effect attracted the attention of scientists and technologists for more than three decades. Oil-in-water microemulsions loaded with active molecules opened new possibilities for enhancing the solubility of hydrophobic

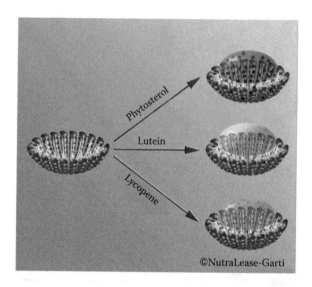

FIGURE 11.4 A schematic illustration of the loading process of various nutraceuticals onto the O/W microemulsion droplets after inversion.

vitamins, antioxidants, and other skin nutrients. This is of particular interest, as it can provide a well-controlled way for incorporating active ingredients and may protect the solubilized components from undesired degradation reactions. [25-30] Figure 11.4 is a schematic illustration of the loading process of various nutraceuticals onto the O/W microemulsion droplets after inversion.

Solubilization of active addenda may therefore be defined as spontaneous codissolving (molecular incorporation) of a liquid-immiscible phase along with an active substance, normally insoluble (or only slightly soluble), in a corresponding solvent in self-assembled surfactants to form thermodynamically stable isotropic structured solution in a nanosized range.

The solubilized active molecules can be certain molecules with nutritional value to the skin or cosmetoceuticals that in most cases are used also in food applications. We will mention a few such examples that were studied in our labs, e.g., lycopene, phytosterols, lutein, tocopherols, CoQ10, and essential oils.

11.3.1 LYCOPENE

In the food and cosmetics industry, supplements have become more prominent in recent years due to the increased public awareness of their health. They play a vital role in today's beneficial effect by improving the nutritional value or nutrients of foods, as well as their texture, consistency, and color. The possibility of enhancing solubility of hydrophobic vitamins, essential oils, deodorants, perfumes, flavors, and other nutrients in oil-in-water microemulsions is of great

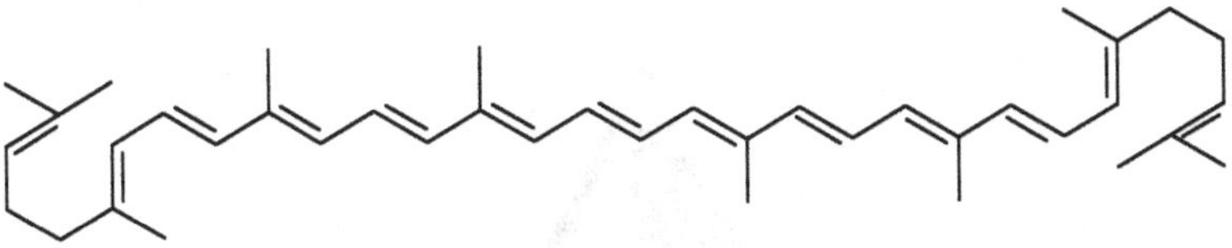

FIGURE 11.5 Molecular structure of lycopene.

interest, as it can provide a well-controlled way for the incorporation of active ingredients and may protect the solubilized components from undesired degradation reactions.[39,40]

The cosmetic industry is adapting these active molecules as nutrients for the skin and as protective antioxidants for fragrances, lotions, and creams.

Lycopene (Figure 11.5) is an essential carotenoid that provides the characteristic red color of tomatoes. It is a lipophilic compound that is insoluble in water and in most food-grade oils. For example, the lycopene solubility in one of the most efficient edible essential oils, R(+)-limonene, is 700 ppm. Several recent studies have indicated the important role of lycopene in reducing risk factors of chronic diseases such as cancer, coronary heart disease, and aging.[39,40] In turn, this has led to the idea of studying the effect of lycopene uptake on human health.

The bioavailability of lycopene is affected by several factors:

1. Food matrix containing the lycopene and, as a result, intracellular location of the lycopene, and the intactness of the cellular matrix. Tomatoes converted into tomato paste enhance the bioavailability of lycopene, as the processing includes both mechanical particle size reduction and heat treatment.
2. Amount and type of dietary fat present in the intestine. The presence of fat affects the formation of the micelles that incorporate the free lycopene.
3. Interactions between carotenoids that may reduce absorption of either one of the carotenoids.[41] The reduced absorption is due to competitive absorption between the carotenoids. On the other hand, simultaneous ingestion of various carotenoids may induce antioxidant activity in the intestinal tract, and thus result in increased absorption of the carotenoids.[42]
4. Molecular configuration (cis/trans) of the lycopene molecules. The bioavailability of the cis-isomer is higher than the bioavailability of the trans-isomer. This may result from the greater solubility of cis-isomers in mixed micelles and yjr lower tendency of cis-isomers to aggregate.[43–47]
5. Decrease in particle size.[48]

Care must be taken in the application of lycopene as a cosmetic additive, since this highly conjugated carotenoid is responsible for the instability of this molecule when exposed to light or oxygen.

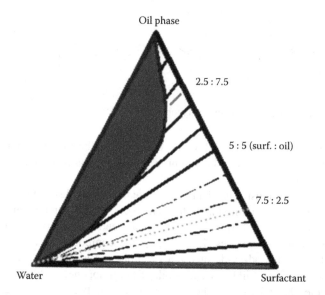

FIGURE 11.6 Pseudoternary phase diagram (25°C) of water/PG/R(+)-limonene/etha-nol/Tween 60 system with constant weight ratios of water/PG (1:1) and R(+)-limonene/eth-anol (1:1). Solubilization of lycopene was studied along dilution line T64.

We explored the ability of U-type microemulsions to solubilize lycopene and have also investigated the influence of solubilized lycopene on the microemulsion microstructure.

Phase diagrams have been constructed, lycopene has been solubilized, and several structural methods have been utilized, including SD-NMR spectroscopy, which was developed to determine the microemulsion microstructure at any dilution point.

The influence of microemulsion composition on the solubilization of lycopene in a five-component system consisting of R(+)-limonene, cosurfactant, water, cosolvent, and polyoxyethylene (20) sorbitan mono fatty esters (Tweens) is shown in Figure 11.6.

Solubilization capacity was defined[44] as the amount of lycopene solubilized in a microemulsion. Figure 11.7 shows the solubilization capacity of lycopene along water dilution line T64, (at this line the constant ratio of R(+)-limonene/eth-anol/Tween 60 is 1/1/3). Four different regions can be identified along this dilution line. At 0 to 20 wt% aqueous phase (region I), the solubilization capacity of lycopene decreases dramatically, from 500 to 190 ppm (reduction of 62%). This dramatic decrease in the solubilization capacity can be associated with the grow-ing interactions between the surfactant and water molecules. The water can also strongly bind to the hydroxyl groups of the surfactant at the interface. When water is introduced to the core, the micelle swells and more surfactant and cosurfactant participate at the interface, replacing the lycopene and therefore decreasing its solubilization. We have concluded that in region I the reverse

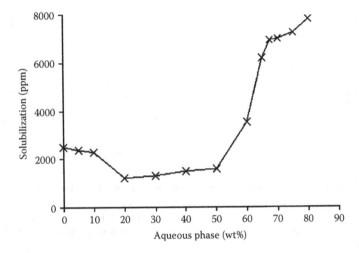

FIGURE 11.7 Solubilization capacity of lycopene along dilution line T64. (From Reference 29. With permission.)

micelles swell gradually and turn more hydrophobic, causing less free volume to be available to the solubilized lipophilic lycopene and a reduction in its solubilization capacity. At 20 to 50 wt% aqueous phase (region II) the solubilization capacity remains almost unchanged (decreased only by an additional 7%). This fairly small decrease in the solubilization capacity could be associated with the fact that the system transforms gradually into a bicontinuous phase, and the interfacial area remains almost unchanged when the aqueous phase concentration increases. Surprisingly, in region III (50 to 67 wt% aqueous phase) the SP increases from 160 to 450 ppm (an increase of 180%). In region IV the solubilization capacity decreases to 312 ppm (a decrease of 30%).

In order to explain the changes in solubilization capacity of lycopene, we characterized the microstructure of microemulsions along dilution line T64, using the SD-NMR technique. Figure 11.8 shows the relative diffusion coefficients of water and R(+)-limonene in empty microemulsions (Figure 11.8a), and microemulsions solubilizing lycopene (Figure 11.8b), as a function of the aqueous phase concentration (w/w). One can clearly see that the general diffusion coefficient behaviors of microemulsion ingredients (R(+)-limonene and water), with or without lycopene, are not very different. The total amount of lycopene does not cause dramatic changes in the diffusion patterns of the ingredients.

It can also be seen that in the two extremes of aqueous phase concentrations (up to 20 wt% and above 70 to 80 wt% aqueous phase), the diffusion coefficients are easily interpreted, while the in-between regions are somewhat more difficult to explain since gradual changes take place. Regions and are difficult to distinguish. However, the structural changes in the presence of lycopene (Figure 11.8b) are more pronounced than those in the absence of lycopene (Figure 11.8a).

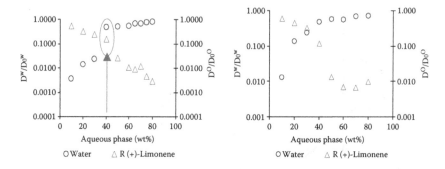

FIGURE 11.8 Relative diffusion coefficient of water () and R(+)-limonene () in micro-emulsions without (a) and with (b) lycopene, as calculated from SD-NMR results at 25°C. was measured in a solution containing water/PG (1:1) and determined to be 55.5*10 to 11 m²sec⁻¹. The diffusion coefficient of R(+)-limonene, was determined to be 38.3*10 to 11 m²sec⁻¹. (From N. Garti. With permission.)

Microemulsions containing up to 20 wt% aqueous phase, and solubilizing lycopene, have a discrete W/O microstructure, since the relative diffusion coefficients of water and R(+)-limonene differ by more than one order of magnitude. Microemulsions solubilizing lycopene and containing 20 to 50 wt% aqueous phase have a bicontinuous microstructure, as the diffusion coefficients of water and R(+)-limonene are of the same order of magnitude. Increasing the aqueous phase concentration to above 50 wt% induces the formation of a discrete O/W microstructure, as the relative diffusion coefficients of water and R(+)-limonene differ by more than one order of magnitude.

From the solubilization capacity and SD-NMR results it is clear that lycopene solubilization is structure dependent.

The four different regions in the solubilization capacity curve are an indication of the microstructure transition along the dilution line. The first region indicates the formation of W/O (L2) microstructure. The second region indicates the transition from L2 microstructure to a bicontinuous microemulsion. In the third region, a transition from a bicontinuous microemulsion to an O/W (L1) microstructure occurs. In the fourth region, a discrete L1 microstructure was found.

While the general behavior of the diffusion coefficients is the same for microemulsions with or without lycopene, the transition point from one microstructure to another is different. Lycopene influences the transition from L2 to bicontinuous microstructure and further to L1 microstructure. In empty microemulsions the formation of a bicontinuous microstructure occurs when the microemulsion contains 40 to 60 wt% aqueous phase, whereas in a microemulsion containing lycopene, a bicontinuous microstructure starts at low aqueous phase content (20 wt%) and continues up to an aqueous phase content of 20 to 50 wt%. It seems that the more water is solubilized in the swollen reverse micelles, the less free interfacial volume there is for the lycopene. It seems that lycopene disturbs both the flexibility of the micelle and the spontaneous curvature. As a result, the interface changes into a flatter curvature (bicontinuous) at an early stage of water concentration, more so in the presence of lycopene than in empty micelles.

The hydrophilic–lypophilic balance (HLB) of the surfactant influences the amount of solubilized lycopene in the aqueous surfactant phase. Tween 60, the hydrophilic surfactant with the lowest HLB value (HLB = 14.9), solubilizes more lycopene than Tween 80 (HLB = 15.2) by 10%. Tween 40 (polyoxyethylene (20) sorbitan monomyristate) decreases the solubilization capacity even further (30%). Replacing Tween 60 with Tween 20 (the most hydrophilic surfactant; HLB = 16.7) will reduce it solubilization capacity lycopene by 88%.

We have also demonstrated that microemulsions stabilized by mixed surfactants enhance the solubilization capacity of lycopene by 32 to 48%, in comparison to microemulsions stabilized by Tween 60 alone.

The use of mixed surfactants increases the solubilization capacity, indicating a synergistic effect. Microemulsions stabilized by a mixture of three surfactants, Tween 60, sucrose ester, and ethoxylated monodiglyceride, have the highest solubilization capacity of lycopene — an increase of 48% — in comparison to microemulsion based on Tween 60 alone.

Synergism phenomena in surfactant mixtures were attributed to Coulombic, ion-dipole, or hydrogen-bonding interactions.[48–50] Therefore, nonionic surfactant mixtures are expected to have a minimum intermolecular interaction and weak synergistic effects. Nevertheless, Huibers and Shah[51] demonstrated a strong synergism in nonionic surfactant mixture, similar to the findings in our study.

Microemulsions that are loaded with lycopene exhibit a stronger synergistic effect than empty microemulsions. Lycopene was solubilized up to 10 times of its dissolution capacity in the microemulsions, in comparison to the lycopene solubility in R(+)-limonene, or any other edible oil. The solubilization capacity and efficiency of lycopene are affected by microstructure transitions from water in oil (W/O) to bicontinuous and from bicontinuous to oil in water (O/W).

11.3.2 PHYTOSTEROLS

An elevated serum cholesterol level is a well-known risk factor for coronary heart disease.[39–48] Most strategies for lowering serum cholesterol require dietary restrictions or the use of drugs. The prospect of lowering cholesterol levels by consuming foods fortified with natural phytonutrients is considered much more attractive.[52]

Phytosterols (plant sterols) are steroid alcohols. Their chemical structure resembles human cholesterol, as can be seen in Figure 11.9. Sterols are made up of a tetracyclic cyclopenta[a]phenanthrene ring system and a long flexible side chain at the C-17 carbon atom. The four rings have trans configurations, forming a flat system.[53–57] Moreover, the sterols create planar surfaces at both the top and bottom of the molecules, since the 20R conformation is preferred in the side chain. This allows for multiple hydrophobic interactions between the rigid sterol nucleus (the polycyclic component) and the membrane matrix.[42–50] Only the side

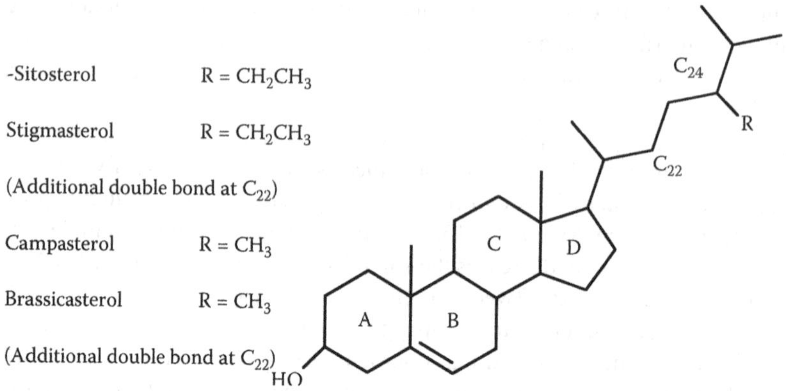

-Sitosterol $R = CH_2CH_3$

Stigmasterol $R = CH_2CH_3$

(Additional double bond at C_{22})

Campasterol $R = CH_3$

Brassicasterol $R = CH_3$

(Additional double bond at C_{22})

FIGURE 11.9 Molecular structure of cholesterol and some abundant phytosterols (R=H–cholesterol; R=CH$_2$CH$_3$–sitosterol; R=CH$_2$CH$_3$ and an additional double bond at C_{22}–stigamsterol; R=CH$_3$–campasterol; R=CH$_3$ and an additional double bond at C_{22}–brassicasterol).

chains of the various sterols are different. These minor differences result in major differences in their biological function.

Peterson et al.[57] reported that the addition of soy sterols to a cholesterol-enriched diet prevented an increase of the plasma cholesterol level. This effect significantly reduced the incidence of atherosclerotic plaque in chick aorta.[58] Since then, numerous clinical investigations have indicated that administration of phytosterols to human subjects reduces the total plasma cholesterol and LDL cholesterol levels.[59,60] Because of their poor solubility and limited bioavailability, high doses (up to 25 g/day) were required to have a noticeable effect.

The exact mechanism by which phytosterols inhibit the uptake of dietary and endogenous cholesterol is not completely understood. One theory suggests that cholesterol in the presence of phytosterols precipitates in a nonabsorbable state. A second theory suggests that cholesterol is displaced by phytosterols in the bile salt and phospholipid-containing mixed micelles, preventing its absorption.[52]

The enhanced phytosterols' solubilization in O/W microemulsions is believed to enhance its effect within the guts. This is due to the fact that the droplet size is in the range of several nanometers.

The activity of phytosterols in cosmetic formulations was not yet fully studied. Our preliminary results indicate that phytosterols are not crossing the skin dermis, but they significantly influence the penetration of cholesterol and other lipids and help to incorporate natural extract of active matter that has been used. The penetration of an extracted bioactive agent was improved in the presence of phytosterols that were solubilized within our NSSL (private communication).

We explored the ability of our unique dilutable microemulsions to solubilize phytosterols and studied the correlation between the solubilization capacity of the phytosterols and the microemulsion microstructure transitions.[38]

The solubilization capacity of phytosterols and cholesterol along dilution line T64 was determined (Figure 11.9).

The solubilization capacity of phytosterols in a reverse micellar solution containing surfactant and oil phase (at 6:4 weight ratio) is 60,000 ppm (6 wt%). As can be seen in Figure 11.3, the solubilization capacity of phytosterols decreases as the aqueous phase concentration increases. In a microemulsion containing 90 wt% aqueous phase, the solubilization capacity is only 2400 ppm, i.e., a decrease of 96% in the solubilization capacity of phytosterols.

A possible explanation for the dramatic decrease in the solubilization capacity could be related to the nature of the molecule and, as a result, the locus of its solubilization at the interface. In the concentrates (without added water) the locus of the phytosterols' solubilization is at the micelle's interface. As dilution takes place and an aqueous phase is added, water-in-oil (W/O) swollen micelles are formed and the hydrophilic OH groups of the phytosterols are oriented toward the aqueous phase, thus causing the molecules to organize between the surfactant hydrophobic chains. This change in the locus of solubilization causes a decrease in solubilization at the interface. Suratkar and Mahapatra[44] observed a similar change in the locus of solubilization of phenolic compounds in sodium dodecyl sulfate (SDS) micelles.

The decrease in solubilization capacity as the aqueous phase concentration increases may be attributed to a microstructure transformation. The structural transformation from W/O via a bicontinuous mesophase to an O/W microstructure forces the phytosterols to solubilize between the hydrophobic amphiphilic chains, being a less preferable location, and thus causing a decrease in the solubilization capacity.

It seems that the phytosterols have a strong effect on the spontaneous curvature of the micelles. As a result, the interface curvature decreases at lower water concentration. This effect is more pronounced in the presence of phytosterols than in empty micelles or lycopene.

The effect of phytosterol on skin penetration is in a process of evaluation. Similarly, the competitive adsorption of cholesterol and phytosterols on the microemulsion's interface and on the skin membrane indicates that reverse microemulsions (W/O) preferentially solubilize cholesterol over phytosterols, but upon dilution and once inversion to O/W microemulsions occurs, the phytosterols are better accommodated at the interface and they displace the cholesterol molecules from the interface (Figure 11.10). It remains to be tested if a similar effect also exists on human skin.

11.3.3 Luteins

There is increasing evidence that the macular pigments, carotenoids lutein and zeaxanthin, play an important role in the prevention of age-related macular degeneration, cataract, and other blinding disorders. The carotenoids are situated in the macula (macula lutea, yellow spot) between the incoming photons and the photoreceptors, and have a maximum absorption at 445 nm for lutein and 451 nm

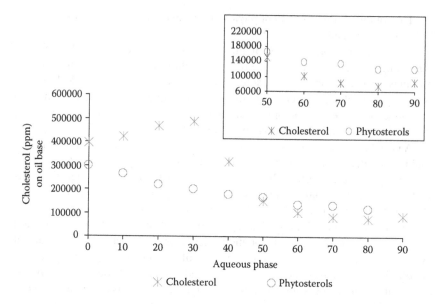

FIGURE 11.10 Competitive solubilization of phytosterols and cholesterol (weight ratio of 1/1) in U-type microemulsions as a function of water dilution.

for zeaxanthin. As a result, lutein and zeaxanthin can function as a blue light filter (400 to 460 nm). The blue light enters the inner retinal layers, thereby causing the carotenoids to attenuate its intensity. In addition to the protection abilities of the macula from blue wavelength damage, these carotenoids can also improve visual acuity and scavenge harmful reactive oxygen species that are formed in the photoreceptors.[62–65]

With aging, some of the eye antioxidant suppliers are diminished and antioxidant enzymes are inactivated. This action appears to be related to the accumulation, aggregation, and eventual precipitation in lens opacities of damaged proteins. The results of this sequence of events are eye disorders.[66,67]

To increase our understanding of the potential benefits of carotenoids in general and lutein in particular, it is important to obtain more insight into their bioavailability and the factors that determine their absorption and bioavailability.

Lutein, a naturally occurring carotenoid (Figure 11.11), is widely distributed in fruits and vegetables and is particularly concentrated in the *Tagetes erecta* flower. Epidemiological studies suggest that high lutein intake (6 mg/day) increases serum levels that are associated with a lower risk of cataract and age-related macular degeneration. Lutein can be extracted as either free form or esterified (miristate, palmitate, or stearate) lutein. Both are practically insoluble in aqueous systems, resulting is low bioavailability.

To improve its solubility and bioavailability, lutein was solubilized in U-type microemulsions based on R(+)-limonene.

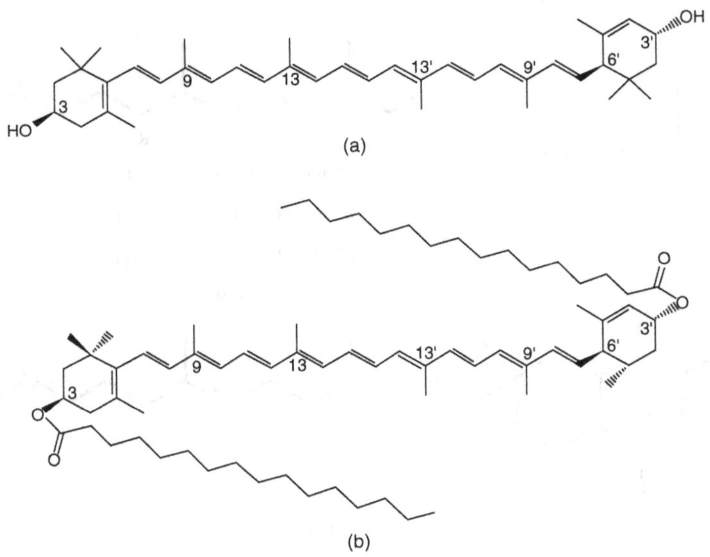

FIGURE 11.11 Chemical structures of (a) free lutein and (b) lutein ester.

Some of the main findings are:[66,67]

1. Reverse micellar and W/O compositions solubilized both luteins better than O/W microemulsion, and maximum solubilization is obtained within the bicontinuous phase.
2. Free lutein is solubilized better than the esterified one in the W/O microemulsions, whereas the esterified lutein is better accommodated within the O/W microemulsion.
3. Vegetable oils decrease the solubilization of free lutein.
4. Glycerol and alcohol enhance the solubilization of both luteins.
5. The solubilization is surfactant dependent in all mesophase structures, but its strongest effect is in the bicontinuous phase.

11.4 VITAMINS

Microemulsions also have potential for enhancing the solubility of hydrophobic vitamins or other nutraceuticals within water-based formulations. The pharmaceutical and medical literature is replete with studies of enhanced micellar delivery of vitamins, in particular vitamin E, vitamin K1, and carotene.

Vitamin E (Figure 11.12), the major lipophilic antioxidant in the human body, has invoked a great deal of interest regarding its disease-preventive and health-promoting effects, as well as its unique chemical structure as a group of amphiphilic homologues exhibiting important interfacial roles in surfactant self-assemblies. Much interest has been devoted to microemulsions as efficient cosmetic

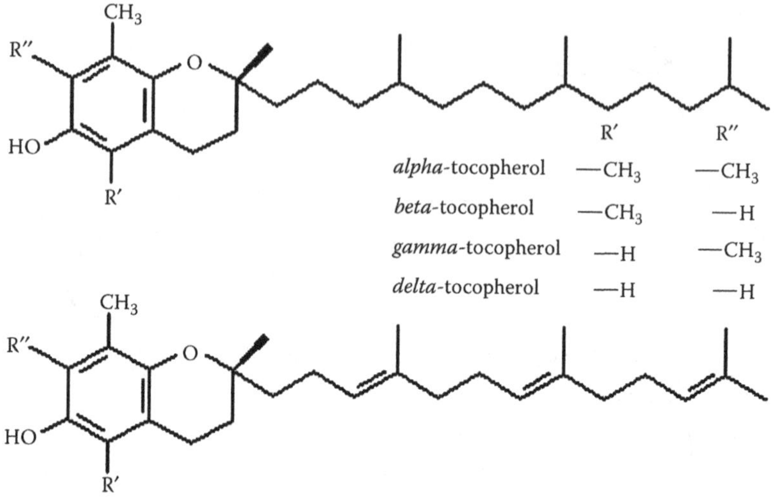

	R′	R″
alpha-tocopherol	—CH$_3$	—CH$_3$
beta-tocopherol	—CH$_3$	—H
gamma-tocopherol	—H	—CH$_3$
delta-tocopherol	—H	—H

Tocotrienols

FIGURE 11.12 Chemical structures of -tocopherols and -tocopherol acebrassicasterol.

and drug delivery systems, enabling the solubilization of hydrophobic active matter in aqueous media and improving their bioavailability.

Therefore, we found it imperative to study the effect of the microemulsion composition on the solubilization capacity of different forms of vitamin E, and to infer the structural transformations from the solubilization data.

The results[38] (Figure 11.13) show that the solubilization capacity of vitamins with free OH head groups in Tween 60-based microemulsions drops abruptly at two dilution levels along a dilution line with a constant surfactant-to-oil ratio, signifying transformations in the microemulsion structure. The number of methyl groups on the vitamin's polar head has an influence on the point at which the solubilization drop occurs, while unsaturation of the hydrophobic tail of the vitamin enhances its solubilization capacity with no observable impact on the solubilization pattern. In contrast to the free OH vitamin forms, the acetate form showed continuous decreases in solubilization capacity along the dilution line. The type of oil used in the microemulsion has a strong influence on the solubilization pattern of the vitamin. Triacetin attained a higher solubilization capacity of vitamin E than R(+)-limonene, with a certain delay in the structural transformations along the dilution line. Medium-chain triglycerides (MCTs), on the other hand, maintained a constant ratio of TocOH to surfactant with increasing level of aqueous phase within a certain range, while the solubilization capacity of D--tocopheryl acetate (TocAc) decreased significantly in the same dilution range. Alcohol cosurfactants and propylene glycol (PG) were found to be vitally important for improving the solubilization capacity of TocAc and TocOH. The latter showed a higher boost of solubilization at

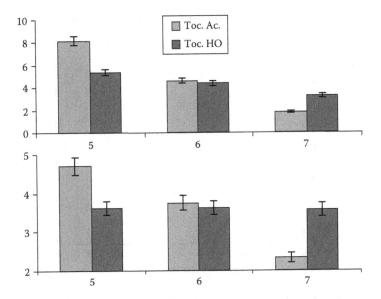

FIGURE 11.13 Solubilization capacities of free tocopherols and tocopherol acetate in U-type microemulsions at several dilutions along dilution line 73 (70% surfactant phase and 30 wt% oil phase). (From Reference 38. With permission.)

high levels of alcohols. TocAc was found to prefer higher concentrations of Tween 60 for better solubilization, while TocOH prefers mild levels. Mixing Tween 60 with diglycerol monooleate (DGM) displayed a pronounced enhancement in the solubilization of TocAc, while causing a significant decrease in that of TocOH.

11.5 WATER BINDING

We examined, by a subzero DSC technique, the nature of the water[30,68] in the confined space of a W/O microemulsion in order to better understand the role of the activity of the entrapped water on the physicochemical properties of the microemulsions and to control enzymatic reactions carried out in the inner phase.[31] We reported (Figure 11.14) that the surfactant/alcohol/PG can strongly bind water in the inner phase so that it freezes below −10°C and acts, in part, as bound water and, in part, as nonfreezable water.[30] Even after complete inversion to O/W microemulsions, the water in the continuous phase strongly interacts with the cosolvent/surfactant and remains partially bound.

We learned that for nonionic microemulsions that also contain polyols and alcohol, the core water is mostly bound to the surfactant head group or to the polyol groups and freezes at subzero temperatures that strongly depend on the nature of the head groups. Such strong binding is important in a reaction that is strongly dependent on water activity (enzymatic hydrolytic reactions).

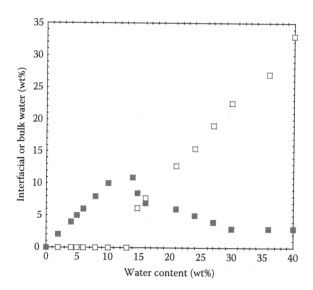

FIGURE 11.14 The amounts (weight percent) of free and bound water in microemulsions based on sugar esters along dilution line 64 (60% surfactant and 40% oil phase). (From Reference 43. With permission.)

11.6 CONCLUSIONS

The present review summarizes ca. 10 years of our research work and more than 20 years of other scientists' work in utilization of microemulsions for the food, cosmetic, and pharmaceutical industries.

We learned that:

1. Microemulsions have high solubilization capacities for oil entrapped in the surfactant micelles and for water in reverse micelles.
2. If the ingredients composing the microemulsions and the cosolvents and cosurfactants are carefully selected, one can form a variety of cosmetic microemulsions.
3. U-type microemulsions with progressive full dilution with the aqueous phase or water can be formulated.
4. Microemulsions of W/O and bicontinuous structures, as well as O/W microemulsions, can solubilize guest molecules at their interface at high solubilization capacities, in some cases up to 100-fold of the solubility of the nutraceuticals in the corresponding solvent.
5. Molecules such as lycopene, vitamin E, tocopherols, tocopherol acetate, beta carotene, lutein, phytosterols, and CoQ10 can be quantitatively solubilized.
6. Microemulsion provides some oxidative protection to the nutraceuticals.

7. Various other molecules, such as aromas, flavors, and antioxidants, can be solubilized in microemulsions.

8. The water that is entrapped at the core of a W/O microemulsion can be strongly bound to the surfactant head group and will restrict the water activity. Thus, upon adding more water, the reaction by the enzyme or regents can be triggered.

REFERENCES

1. Shinoda, K., Lindman, B. Organized surfactant systems: microemulsions. *Langmuir* 1987, 3, 135–149.

2. Solans, C., Pons, R., Kunieda, H. Overview of basic aspects of microemulsions. In *Industrial Applications of Microemulsions*, Solans, C., Kunieda, H., Eds., Marcel Dekker, New York, 1997, Vol. 66, pp. 1–17.

3. Ezrahi, S., Aserin, A., Garti, N. Aggregation behavior in one-phase (Winsor IV) microemulsion systems. In *Handbook of Microemulsion Science and Technology*, Kumar, P., Mittal, K.L., Eds., Marcel Dekker, New York, 1999, pp. 185–246.

4. Regev, O., Ezrahi, S., Aserin, A., Garti, N., Wachtel, E., Kaler, E.W., Khan, A., Talmon, Y. A study of the microstructure of a four-component nonionic microemulsion by cryo-TEM, NMR, SAXS, and SANS. *Langmuir* 1996, 12, 668–674.

5. Kahlweit, M., Busse, G., Faulhaber, B., Jen, J. Shape changes of globules in nonionic microemulsions. *J. Phys. Chem.* 1996, 100, 14991–14994.

6. Billman, J.F., Kaler, E.W. Structure and phase-behavior in 4 component nonionic microemulsions. *Langmuir* 1991, 7, 1609–1617.

7. Dungan, S.R. Microemulsions in foods: properties and applications. In *Industrial Applications of Microemulsions*, Solans, C., Kunieda, H., Eds., Marcel Dekker, New York, 1997, Vol. 66, pp. 148–170.

8. Gasco, M.R. Microemulsions in the pharmaceutical field: perspectives and applications. In *Industrial Applications of Microemulsions*, Solans, C., Kunieda, H., Eds., Marcel Dekker, New York, 1997, Vol. 66, pp. 97–122.

9. Alander, J., Warnheim, T. Model microemulsions containing vegetable-oils. 1. Nonionic surfactant systems. *J. Am. Oil Chem. Soc.* 1989a, 66, 1656–1660.

10. Alander, J., Warnheim, T. Model microemulsions containing vegetable-oils. 2. Ionic surfactant systems. *J. Am. Oil Chem. Soc.* 1989b, 66, 1661–1665.

11. Malcolmson, C., Lawrence, M.J. Three-component non-ionic oil-in-water microemulsions using polyoxyethylene ether surfactants. *Colloids Surf. B Biointerfaces* 1995, 4, 97–109.

12. Warisnoicharoen, W., Lansley A.B., Lawrence M.J. Nonionic oil-in-water microemulsions: the effect of oil type on phase behavior. *Int. J. Pharm.* 2000, 198, 7–27.

13. von Corswant, C., Engström, S., Söderman, O. Microemulsions based on soybean phophatidylcholine and triglyceride phase behavior and microstructure. *Langmuir* 1997, 13, 5061–5070.

14. von Corswant, C., Söderman, O. Effect of adding isopropyl myristate to microemulsions based on soybean phosphatidylcholine and triglyceride. *Langmuir* 1998, 14, 3506–3511.

15. Hamdan, S., Lizana, R., Laili, C.R. Aqueous and nonaqueous microemulsion systems with a palm oil-base emollient. *J. Am. Oil Chem. Soc.* 1995, 72, 151–155.

16. Kanei, N., Tamura, Y., Kunieda, H. Effect of types of perfume compounds on the hydrophile-lipophile balance temperature. *J. Colloid Interface Sci.* 1999, 218, 13–22.

17. Tokuoka, Y., Uchiyama, H., Abe, M., Christian, S.D. Solubilization of some synthetic perfumes by anionic-nonionic mixed surfactant systems 1. *Langmuir* 1995,11, 725–729.

18. Joubran, R.F., Cornell, D.G., Parris, N. Microemulsions of triglyceride and non-ionic surfactant: effect of temperature and aqueous phase composition. *Colloids Surf. A* 1993, 80, 153–160.

19. Trevino, S.F., Joubran, R., Parris, N., Berk, N.F. Structure of a triglyceride micro-emulsion: a small-angle neutron scattering study. *J. Phys. Chem. B* 1998, 102, 953–960.

20. Constantinides, P.P., Scalart, J.P. Formation and physical characterization of water-in-oil microemulsions containing long- versus medium-chain glycerides. *Int. J. Pharm.* 1997,158, 57–68.

21. Prichanont, S., Leak, D.J., Stuckey D.C. The solubilization of mycobacterium in a water-in-oil microemulsion for biotransformations: system selection and char-acterisation. *Colloids Surf. A Physicochem. Eng. Aspects* 2000, 166, 177–186.

22. Park, K.M., Kim C.K. Preparation and evaluation of flurbiprofen-loaded micro-emulsion for parenteral delivery. *Int. J. Pharm.* 1999, 181, 173–179.

23. Radomska, A., Dobrucki, R. The use of some ingredients for microemulsion preparation containing retinol and its esters. *Int. J. Pharm.* 2000, 196, 131–134.

24. Trotta, M., Morel, S., Gasco, M.R. Effect of oil phase composition on the skin permeation of felodipine from O/W microemulsions. *Pharmazie* 1997, 52, 50–53.

25. Garti, N., Yaghmur, A., Leser, M.E., Clement, V., Watzke, H.J. Improved oil solubilization in O/W food-grade microemulsions in the presence of polyols and ethanol. *J. Agric. Food Chem.* 2001, 49, 2552–2562.

26. Yaghmur, A., Aserin, A., Garti, N. Furfural-cysteine model reaction in food-grade nonionic O/W microemulsions for selective flavor formation. *J. Agric. Food Chem.* 2002, 50, 2878–2883.

27. Yaghmur, A., Aserin, A., Garti, N. Phase behavior of microemulsions based on food-grade nonionic surfactants: effect of polyols and short-chain alcohols. *Colloids Surf. A* 2002, 209, 71–81.

28. Yaghmur, A., Aserin, A., Tiunova, I., Garti, N. Structural behavior of nonionic surfactants in the presence of propylene glycol in nonionic microemulsions studied by DSC. *J. Thermal Anal. Cal.*, 2002, 69, 163–177.

29. Spernath, A., Yaghmur, A., Aserin, A., Hoffman, R.E., Garti, N. Food grade microemulsions based on nonionic emulsifiers: media to enhance lycopene solu-bilization. *J. Agric. Food Chem.* 2002, 50, 6917–6922.

30. Spernath, A., Yaghmur, A., Aserin, A., Hoffman, R.E., Garti, N. Phytosterols solubilization capacity and microstructure transitions in Winsor IV food-grade microemulsions studied by self-diffusion NMR. *J. Agric. Food Chem.* 2003, 51, 2359–2364.

31. Yaghmur, A., Aserin, A., Antalek, B., Garti, N. Microstructure of five-component food grade oil-in-water microemulsions by PGSE-NMR, conductivity, and viscosity. *Langmuir* 2003, 19, 1063.

32. Garti, N., Amar, I., Yaghmur, A., Spernath, A. Interfacial modification and struc-tural transitions induced by guest molecules solubilized in U-type nonionic food-grade microemulsions. *J. Disper. Sci. Technol.* 2003, 24, 397–410.

33. Garti, N., Yaghmur, A., Aserin, A., Spernath, A., Elfakess, R., Ezrahi, S. Solubilization of active molecules in microemulsions for improved solubilization, and environmental protection. *Colloids Surf. A* 2004, 230, 183–190.

34. de Campo, L., Yaghmur, A., Garti, N., Leser, M.E., Glatter, O. Food-grade microemulsions: structural characterization. *J. Colloid Interface Sci.* 2004, 274, 251–267.

35. Yaghmur, A., de Campo, L., Glatter, O., Leser, M.E., Garti, N. Structural characterization of five-component food grade oil-in-water nonionic microemulsions. *Phys. Chem. Chem. Phys.* 2004, 6, 1524–1533.

36. Yaghmur, A., Fanun, M., Aserin, A., Garti, N. Food grade microemulsions based on nonionic emulsifiers as microreactors for selective flavor formation by Maillard reaction. In *Self-Assembly*, Robinson, B.H., Eds., 2003, pp. 144–151.

37. Yaghmur, A., Aserin, A., Abbas, A., Garti, N. Reactivity of furfural-cysteine model reaction in food grade five-component nonionic microemulsions. *Colloids Surf. A* 2005, 253, 223–234.

38. Garti, N., Zakharia, I., Spernath, A., Yaghmur, A., Aserin, A., Hoffman, R.E., Jacobs, L. Solubilization of water-insoluble nutraceuticals in nonionic microemulsions for water-based use. *Prog. Colloid Poly. Sci.* 2004, 126, 184–189.

39. Dungan, S.R. Microemulsions in foods: properties and applications. In *Industrial Applications of Microemulsions*, Solans, C., Kunieda, H., Eds., Marcel Dekker, New York, 1997, Vol. 66, pp. 148–170.

40. Holmberg, K. Quarter century progress and new horizons in microemulsions. In *Micelles, Microemulsions, and Monolayers*, Shah, O., Eds., Marcel Dekker, New York, 1998, pp. 161–192.

41. Dungan, S.R. Microemulsions in foods: properties and applications. In *Industrial Applications of Microemulsions*, Solans, C., Kunieda, H., Eds., Marcel Dekker, New York, 1997, Vol. 66, pp.

42. Garti, N., Clement, V., Fanun, M., Leser, M.E. Some characteristics of sugar ester nonionic microemulsions in view of possible food applications. *J. Agric. Food Chem.* 2000, 48, 3945–3956.

43. Garti, N., Aserin, A., Fanun, M. Non-ionic sucrose esters microemulsions for food applications. Part 1. Water solubilization. *Colloids Surf. A Physicochem. Eng. Asp.* 2000, 164, 27–38.

44. Suratkar, V., Mahapatra, S. Solubilization site of organic perfume molecules in sodium dodecyl sulfate micelles: new insights from proton NMR studies. *J. Colloid Interface Sci.* 2000, 225, 32–38.

45. Bramley, P.M. Is lycopene beneficial to human health? *Phytochemistry* 2000, 54, 233–236.

46. Rao, A.V., Agarwal, S. Role of lycopene as antioxidant carotenoid in the prevention of chronic diseases: a review. *Nutr. Res.* 1999, 19, 305–323.

47. Cooke, J.P. Nutraceuticals for cardiovascular health. *Am. J. Cardiol.* 1998, 82, 43S–46S.

48. Van het Hof, K.H., West, C.E., Weststrate, J.A., Hautvast, J.G.A.J. Dietary factors that affect the bioavailability of carotenoids. *J. Nutr.* 2000, 130, 503–506.

49. Lindman, B., Olsson, U., Söderman, O. Characterization of microemulsions by NMR. In *Handbook of Microemulsion Science and Technology*, Kumar, P., Mittal, K.L., Eds., Marcel Dekker, New York, 1999, pp. 309–356.

50. Hou, M.J., Shah, D.O. Effects of the molecular structure of the interface and continuous phase on solubilization of water in water/oil microemulsions. *Langmuir* 1987, 3, 1086–1096.

51. Huibers, P.D.T., Shah, D.O. Evidence for synergism in nonionic surfactant mixtures: enhancement of solubilization in water-in-oil microemulsions. *Langmuir* 1997, 13, 5762–5765.
52. Hicks, K.B., Moreau, R.A. Phytosterols and phytostanols: functional food cholesterol busters. *Food Technol.* 2001, 55, 63–67.
53. Pietronen, V., Lindsay, D.G., Miettinen, T.A., Toivo, J., Lampi, A.M. Review — plant sterols: biosynthesis, biological function and their importance to human nutrition. *J. Sci. Food Agric.* 2000, 80, 939–966.
54. IUPAC. *The Nomenclature of Steroids* (Recommendations 1989), International Union of Pure and Applied Chemistry and International Union of Biochemistry and Molecular Biology. Available at http://www.chem.qmw.ac.uk/iupac/steroid/.
55. Nes, W.R. Multiple roles for plant sterols. In *The Metabolism, Structure and Function of Plant Lipids*, Stumpf, P.K., Mudd, B.J., Nes, W.R. Eds., Plenum Press, New York, 1987, pp. 3–9.
56. Bloch, K. Sterol structure and function. *J. Am. Oil Chem. Soc.* 1988, 65, 1763–1766.
57. Peterson, D.W., Nichols, C.W., Schneour E.W. Some relationships among dietary sterols, plasma and liver cholesterol levels and atherosclerosis in chicks. *Proc. Soc. Exp. Biol. Med.* 1951, 78, 1143–1147.
58. Pelletier, X., Belbraouet, S., Mirabel, D., Mordret, F., Perrin, J.L., Pages, X., Debry, G. A diet moderately enriched in phytosterols lowers plasma cholesterol concentrations in normocholesterolemic humans. *Ann. Nutr. Metab.* 1995, 39, 291–295.
59. Jones, P.J.H., MacDougall, D.E., Ntanios, F., Vanstone C.A. Dietary phytosterols as cholesterol-lowering agents in humans. *Can. J. Physiol. Pharmacol.* 1997, 75, 217–227.
60. Miettinen, T.A., Puska, P., Gylling, H., Vanhanen H., Vartiainen, E. Reduction of serum cholesterol with sitostanol-ester margerine in a mildly hypercholesterolemic population. *N. Engl. J. Med.* 1995, 333, 1308–1312.
61. Ostlund, R.E., Spilburg, C.A., Stenson, W.F. Sitostanol administered in lecithin micelles potently reduces cholesterol absorption in humans. *Am. J. Clin. Nutr.* 1999, 70, 826–831.
62. Handelman, C.R. *Nutrition* 2001, 17, 818.
63. Vandamme, Th.F. *Prog. Retinal Eye Res.* 2002, 21, 15.
64. Hou, M.J., Kim, M., Shah, D.O. *J. Colloid Interface Sci.* 1988, 123, 398.
65. Hadden, W.L., Watkins, R.H., Levy, L.W., Regalado, E., Rivadeneira, D.M., Van Breemen, R.B., Schwartz, S.J. *J. Agr. Food Chem.* 1999, 47, 4189.
66. Amar-Yuli, I., Aserin, A., Garti, N. Microstructure transitions derived from solubilization of lutein and lutein esters in food microemulsions. *Colloids Surf. B* 2004, 33, 143–150.
67. Amar-Yuli, I. and Garti, N. *Progress in Structural Transformation in Lyotropic Liquid Crystals Colloids and Surfaces* (in print).
68. Regev, O., Ezrahi, S., Aserin, A., Garti, N., Wachtel, E., Kaler, E.W., Khan, A., Talmon, Y. A study of the microstructure of a four-component nonionic microemulsion by cryo-TEM, NMR, SAXS, and SANS. *Langmuir*, 1996, 12, 668–674.

Part III

SURFACTANTS IN FINISHED
PRODUCTS

12 Surfactants in Lip Products

Robert W. Sandewicz
Revlon Research Center

Lip products are unique among all color cosmetics formulations. They represent a significant portion of the total value of the cosmetics industry. There are many good reasons for this. These products typically are worn daily, and usually are reapplied several times throughout the course of a day. They are easy to use and are offered in an incredible selection of shades. Women often start using lip cosmetics in their preteen years, and may continue to use them well into their golden years. Certain lip products (i.e., lip treatment balms) are not gender specific, and therefore can be used by men, women, and children.

Unlike other pigmented cosmetics products, lip formulations are applied directly to a mucous membrane. Therefore, they must be toxicologically innocuous. They are tasted continuously and, due to close proximity of the upper lip and the nose, are smelled readily as well. Because the lips and surrounding tissues are highly innervated, it is particularly important for lip cosmetics to exhibit smooth application and emollient textures. In addition to embellishing the surfaces of the lips, lip products also provide moisturization and can act as a barrier against chapping. Many lip products also incorporate sunscreen actives, to protect lip tissue from UV attack.

Because of their widespread appeal, lip products are offered in a wide variety of forms. In the minds of most observers, the familiar 0.500-inch diameter molded bullet (sometimes referred to as a pomade) probably represents the archetypal lip product. However, there are many other types of lip products sold commercially, including liquid lip color, glosses, balms, liners, etc. They are characterized by a wide range of physical forms, from liquid to gel to solid. Products may either be largely nonvolatile or incorporate one or more volatile carriers, such as cyclomethicone, low molecular weight dimethicone, or isododecane.

The vast majority of lip products are anhydrous formulations. By definition, anhydrous technology is oriented toward the chemistry of lipophilic ingredients, such as waxes, oils, fats, and hydrophobic polymers. Simply stated, the artful blending of oleochemicals with various colorants represents the very heart of lip product formulation technology. Skillful formulation techniques are needed to

achieve an oftentimes contradictory series of aesthetic and performance requirements: smooth application, great comfort, high gloss, intense color impact, long
wear, and ease of removal. Fortunately, modern raw ingredient technology gives
lip product development chemists the power they need to create high-performance
formulations. The industry today is blessed with a mind-boggling selection of
fatty ingredients, plus a huge array of silicones and related materials. These
ingredients give lip product chemists a formidable toolbox with which to work.
Somewhat ironically, perhaps the most common cosmetic tool is often conspic-
uously absent from this toolbox: water.

Lipsticks containing water have been sold occasionally. Such products use
one or more surfactants (typically low hydrophile–lipophile balance (HLB) nonionics) to emulsify a relatively modest quantity of water (i.e., <20% w/w) into
an oily vehicle. Emulsified lipsticks usually have elegant textures and can provide
lip treatment benefits. Emulsion lip products historically have not had long lives
in the marketplace. One of the main reasons for this may involve difficulties
related to color stability. In contrast to most cosmetic emulsion products, virtually
all lipsticks contain significant levels of organic colorants. Most of these colorants
are "lakes" derived from water-soluble organic dyes. Residual dyes will dissolve
readily in water, promoting shade drift and staining of users' lips. While this
situation might be perceived as somewhat beneficial in the case of red dyes, the
stain resulting from yellow or blue dyes very likely would be regarded as unat-
tractive. Water-in-oil (W/O) emulsion lipsticks present special preservation challenges and must be tested carefully to ensure microbiological safety. As is the
case for all emulsified formulations, emulsion lipsticks require a higher degree
of manufacturing precision than is normally required for anhydrous lipsticks.
Special precautions are needed to blend, heat, charge, and disperse the internal
water phase during bulk manufacture. Additionally, shade drift problems can
frustrate shade-matching efforts. Because modern anhydrous raw ingredients offer
lipstick formulators great latitude to develop a wide array of appealing textures,
elegant, highly functional lip products can be produced without the use of water
and classical emulsion chemistry.

Given that lip products rely so overwhelmingly on anhydrous chemistry, it
should not be surprising that conventional surfactants have been used very sparingly
in lip product formulations. Nevertheless, emulsion technology may still be required
for lip product development, albeit in a somewhat counterintuitive sense.

Many cosmetic chemists would automatically assume that emulsions must
contain water. This is understandable, since a great many eye, face, hair, and skin
product formulations contain emulsified water. However, if one considers the
broader definition of an emulsion as a mixture of two immiscible liquids, it
becomes apparent that lipstick formulators routinely need to combine two or more
incompatible ingredients (even though both may be oils), and thus might need
to think more like "true" emulsion chemists.

In order to underscore this point, one may take a brief look at certain older
lipstick formulations. Until fairly recently, mineral oil had been a fairly common
ingredient in lip products. It was used to produce high gloss and a lubricious

texture. It does not disperse pigments very well, however, so lipstick chemists often used another time-honored ingredient — castor oil — to provide adequate pigment dispersion. Compatibility problems arose between these two ingredients, even though both are correctly described as lipophilic. Formulators needed to devise a means of coaxing these immiscible oily materials into a homogeneous, stable product. The classical answer was to use a third ingredient to act as a cosolvent or coupling agent to improve miscibility, much as a surfactant would be used to promote miscibility between oil and water. Oleyl alcohol was often used successfully in such a role. While not regarded as a surfactant in a traditional sense, the architecture of oleyl alcohol can be regarded as roughly amphiphilic (it has a terminal hydroxyl head attached to a C-18 monounsaturated tail). It is reasonable to think that the polar hydroxyl group would preferentially affiliate with castor oil (a hydroxylated, unsaturated triglyceride), while the 18-carbon chain would align more closely with mineral oil (mostly linear hydrocarbons). Lanolin and its many derivatives exhibit varying degrees of surface activity and historically have been used successfully in many lip products, both as couplers and as emollients.

Contemporary lip product formulations generally eschew mineral oil (and sometimes lanolin products), but they still may contain numerous lipophilic ingredients having varying degrees of mutual miscibility. For example, dimethicone may be incorporated to provide a high degree of emolliency; this is particularly true of lip products that assert antichapping claims. Cyclomethicones or low molecular weight dimethicones may be used as volatile carriers in transfer-resistant formulations. Modern formulators may use phenyl silicone fluids or various fatty esters as coupling agents, to ensure that dimethicone blends properly with other base ingredients. Volatile hydrocarbons, such as isododecane, are often used as carriers in long-wearing lipstick formulations. Care must be exercised to ensure compatibility of such materials within the overall formulation.

One can make an additional case for the use of surfactants in anhydrous lip products. These products often carry sizable quantities of colorants: a typical lipstick may incorporate 5 to 15% of pigments and pearls, while the color payload of a lip liner might exceed 20%. Colorants invariably are particulate materials that must be wetted thoroughly by the lip product base, to prevent agglomeration and streaking.

Certain inorganic pigments (notably titanium dioxide and iron oxides) may exhibit floatation (manifested as discontinuities and streaks at the surfaces of stick products) if not dispersed properly. Organic pigments must be dispersed carefully in oils to promote a smooth, nongritty texture, as well as to achieve maximum development of colorant strength. Incompletely dispersed organic pigments (especially red lakes) can produce a speckled appearance and may cause streakiness or grittiness on application. Some formulators might take a process-intensive approach to solve these problems, opting for use of high-energy dispersion equipment to achieve smooth pigment incorporation. Such equipment may be expensive, however, and often requires some degree of expertise on the part of the operator to prevent degradation of colorants due to excessive heat and shear. Other formulators might consider a surface-active approach, by experimenting with one or more wetting agents at various levels, to facilitate smooth and complete pigment dispersion. The combination of a judiciously selected dispersion vehicle (i.e., a grinding oil) and a wetting agent may provide smoother dispersions with less reliance on brute force. As is the case with coupling agents, some degree of experimentation is needed to match the right oil with the right wetting agent.

Pigment dispersions typically are evaluated for fineness of grind by using a Hegman gauge to measure particle size. Most lip product formulators seek a Hegman score of 7.0 NS when testing dispersions. As a possible experiment to rank the efficacy of several wetting agents, one might compare percent wetting agent vs. number of mill passes required to achieve a Hegman score of 7.0 NS.

One also might consider using surfactants to influence a very important part of lip product performance: application. Users of lip products (especially stick-type formulations) are very conscious of the degree of effort needed to deposit a product film across their lips. Excessive dragginess or slipperiness typically are regarded negatively, while just the right amount of "cushion" is highly prized. The judicious use of appropriate surfactants might improve wetting of lip surfaces, and thus facilitate smooth, even film deposition. As with all other surfactant usage, experimentation is needed. Excessive amounts or improperly chosen surfactants might compromise wear, by making the resultant product film somewhat vulnerable to attack by water and aqueous foods and beverages.

Overall, it is reasonable to conclude that surfactants rightfully belong in the toolbox of the modern lip product chemist. When used properly, they likely will bring important benefits to lip product formulations. Nevertheless, some general considerations should be made when contemplating the use of surfactants in lip product formulations:

1. *Taste, odor, and irritation potential*: The lips are very sensitive. Lip products may be applied to lips that are cracked and chapped. Irritation must always be considered. Raw ingredient taste and odor are critical to lip product acceptability, even if flavors or fragrances are used. Surfactant taste and odor must be evaluated carefully; this can be problematic for ingredients that are highly propoxylated. Make certain that the surfactant does not interact negatively with fragrances, flavors, sunscreen actives, or antimicrobial agents.

2. *Product integrity*: The classic indication of anhydrous ingredient compatibility is clarity when mixed and melted. This same rule of thumb holds true for coupling agents and surfactants used in anhydrous systems. Clarity is a welcome sign of mutual miscibility, while haziness (however slight) is often an indicator of incipient phase separation and incompatibility. Achievement of clarity can be a good guide to surfactant type and amount, especially when trying to blend incompatible materials. It is reasonable to believe that low-HLB surfactants will be more suitable in anhydrous systems than their high-HLB counterparts.

It is also important to make certain that surfactants do not affect product–package compatibility.

3. *Aesthetics and performance*: An exquisite application must be balanced with gloss, comfort, color aesthetics, and wear properties. Colorants must be compatible with a surfactant; observe test samples to see if unusual color changes occur over time, especially under accelerated temperature conditions. Make certain that use of a surfactant does not compromise any important attribute, especially wear. Lip products are constantly exposed to moisture when in use, so it is important to ascertain that surfactant use, even at low levels, does not render the lip product vulnerable to attack by water, beverages, or aqueous foods.

4. *Thermal and structural properties*: Lip product structure can be assessed by a variety of thermal and physical test methods (e.g., accelerated temperature studies, differential scanning calorimetry (DSC), crush-and-break tests, penetration, viscosity, etc.). Surfactant use conceivably could have a significant impact on the outcomes of some or all of these tests.

5. *Manufacturing processes and filling operations*: Lip products routinely are manufactured and filled while melted. They are often exposed to high heat (80 to 85°C) for prolonged periods. Lip product formulators and process engineers must collaborate to study the behavior of any new lip product formulation as it is scaled up. Will malodor, bad taste, or color changes develop over the course of 16 h at elevated temperatures? Will a surfactant cause any other problems in the manufacturing environment? Will use of a surfactant inhibit the release of bullets from molds or interfere with stick flaming?

Albert Einstein once said, "More important than knowledge is imagination." This expression could well be the mission statement of all cosmetic chemists, but it is particularly relevant to the use of surfactants in lip product formulations. Surfactants have not enjoyed historical widespread use in lip cosmetics. Nevertheless, they may offer formulators some significant benefits as new, high-performance lip products are created to satisfy future market needs.

13 Surfactants in Liquid Foundation

Jane Hollenberg
JCH Consulting

CONTENTS

13.1 INTRODUCTION

Foundation refers to skin tone color cosmetics intended to be applied to the face, and usually the neck, to enhance the wearer's appearance. A successful product evens out skin tones, obscures imperfections, and augments skin color without appearing artificial. Types of foundation formulations include pressed and loose powders, anhydrous wax/oil or wax/volatile solvent systems, and emulsions. In the U.S., emulsified foundations, first introduced in the mid-1950s, continue to be the most popular form, especially the fluid formulations, referred to as liquid makeup.

Foundation emulsions are oil-in-water or water-in-oil systems containing a combination of pigments and fillers to match the range of skin tones. Composition of foundation makeup varies widely, depending on the degree of coverage desired, whether the product is positioned for oily, normal, or dry skin, and the intended type of finish, ranging from matte to dewy. The formulations consist of an oil phase, a water phase, and a pigment phase, which must be combined to form a homogenous product that remains physically stable, preferably without phase separation, for a shelf-life of 2 years. To permit these immiscible phases to be blended with one another and to stabilize the resulting dispersion, surface-active agents are required.

13.2 CRITERIA FOR SURFACTANT CHOICE

Because foundations are leave-on products that are usually in contact with the skin for an entire day, the surfactant combinations used must be nonirritating and nonsensitizing. The total level of emulsifier is kept as low as possible, often by utilizing combinations of surfactant types. For example, anionic/nonionic blends are common in oil-in-water systems.

Low foaming potential is an additional requirement for the emulsifiers and wetting agents used in foundation to minimize entrapment of air during manufacture. Foundation emulsions are especially prone to foam development. The step of dry pigment addition, followed by the high-shear agitation required for adequate dispersion, can generate a significant amount of foam, which should not be stabilized by the surfactant system. Once air is entrained in a foundation emulsion, dissipation is difficult due to the relatively high viscosity of the external phases needed to suspend the pigments. Additionally, the common viscosity control agents, such as magnesium aluminum silicate, xanthan gum, or cellulose gum, tend to stabilize foam in water-based emulsions.

Liquid makeup is usually finger applied, causing contamination of the bulk during each use, requiring a robust preservation system. To minimize the level of preservatives required, the surfactant system should not inactivate the formula preservatives. Adequacy of preservation must be carefully checked when combining ethoxylated compounds and parabens, because of their known interaction.

Finally, the surfactants must be compatible with the pigments and fillers commonly used in foundations. Titanium dioxide is the white pigment most often used to provide coverage and tint the shades of foundations. Zinc oxide sometimes replaces titanium dioxide in shades for darker skin to provide coverage without an ashy effect. By blending the three shades of iron oxide, red, yellow, and black, with or without white pigment, all skin tones can be matched. The surface electrical charge of the pigments and fillers affects emulsifier choice. At the near-neutral pH of most foundations, most titanium dioxides, iron oxides, talcs, and micas are negatively charged, causing coalescence with cationic surfactants, whereas anionic surfactants repel these pigments, creating stable dispersions.

Two functions are performed by the surfactants incorporated into liquid foundation formulations: emulsification and pigment wetting. While some surfactants perform both functions, in other cases, particularly in oil-in-water formulations, a wetting agent is combined with the emulsification system.

13.3 WETTING AGENTS

Surfactants used to wet dry materials into liquids, whether aqueous or nonaqueous, are referred to as wetting agents. The function of a wetting agent is to reduce the interfacial tension between the solid material and the dispersing medium, allowing the medium to spread over the surface, displacing air. To be effective in a given system, a wetting agent should have affinity for both the pigment and the vehicle, improving compatibility between the liquid and the solid phase, as does a coupling agent between two immiscible liquids. In aqueous media, only a small amount of wetting agent, as little as 0.05%, is needed to achieve a marked improvement in wetting. When dispersing solids in oils or silicones, higher amounts, from 0.5 to 1%, are often required. In water or oil, the objective of good wetting is to achieve full color development, lack of striation or flotation, and a close relation between the mass tone and skin tone of the product.

Either anionic or nonionic wetting agents are generally used in oil-in-water foundations when the pigments and fillers are incorporated in the water phase. Sarcosines and phosphate esters are examples of anionic wetting agents that are effective in water-based formulations. Lecithin or a derivative, a natural ingredient composed primarily of the amphoteric phosphatidyl choline, wets oxides very well but has the disadvantage of being a nutrient for bacteria. Among the nonionic surfactants, those of intermediate hydrophile–lipophile balance (HLB), such as Polysorbate 61 or Polysorbate 81, are the most useful in coupling the somewhat hydrophobic pigments and fillers into water phases. Water soluble silicone glycol copolymers also wet pigments well, as do some fluorocarbon surfactants. If the pigments are to be incorporated into the oil phase, whether in oil-in-water or water-in-oil formulations, low-HLB surfactants, such as polyglyceryl esters or sorbitan esters, are employed, often performing the dual function of wetting and emulsification.

13.4 EMULSIFYING AGENTS

13.4.1 OIL-IN-WATER FOUNDATIONS

Anionic surfactants have been most frequently used as the primary emulsifiers for oil-in-water foundations because of their compatibility with the pigments and fillers, the slip they exhibit during rub-out on skin, and the relative ease of achieving stable emulsions. The original liquid makeups, first formulated in the 1950s, were emulsified with fatty acid soaps, particularly triethanolamine-stearate. Co-emulsifiers included glyceryl monostearate, fatty alcohols, or lanolin alcohols. As the use of nonionic emulsifiers became common, the use of nonionic pairs such as polysorbate 80 (20 mol ethoxylated sorbitan monooleate)/sorbitan oleate in combination with an anionic soap became the most common emulsifying system for oil-in-water foundations. Table 13.1 is an example of an oil-in-water anionic/nonionic emulsion foundation. Lecithin is the wetting agent used to wet the pigments into the water phase. The primary emulsifier, the triethanolamine-stearate soap, is formed *in situ* during the emulsification step as the stearic acid of the oil phase and the triethanolamine of the water phase combine.

Triethanolamine soaps have been preferred over sodium or potassium soaps due to greater water solubility and emulsifying capability. Because of recent concerns of possible carcinogenicity of triethanolamine, some formulators choose other alkalis, such as aminomethyl propanol or tromethamine. When formulating fluid makeups, a combination of liquid (isostearic) and solid (stearic) fatty acids is often used to maintain pourability.

TABLE 13.1
Oil-in-Water Foundation[a]

Phase	Ingredient	Percentage
	Water Phase	
1	Deionized water	54.43
1	Lecithin	0.05
1	Triethanolamine	1.00
2	80% Titanium dioxide and talc	8.00
2	80% Yellow iron oxide and talc	1.90
2	80% Red iron oxide and talc	1.20
2	80% Black iron oxide and talc	0.15
2	Talc	2.75
3	Magnesium aluminum silicate	1.00
3	Propylene glycol	4.00
4	Cellulose gum	0.12
4	Propylene glycol	2.00
5	Polysorbate 80	0.80
5	Methyl paraben	0.20
	Oil Phase	
6	Propylene glycol dicaprate/dicaprylate	10.00
6	Octyl dodecyl stearoyl stearate	5.00
6	Glyceryl stearate SE	1.50
6	Sorbitan monooleate	1.50
6	Stearic acid	2.00
6	Propyl paraben	0.10
7	Imidazolidinyl urea	0.30
7	Deionized water	2.00
		100.00

[a] *Manufacturing procedure:* The oil phase (6) is combined and heated to 75 to 80°C with stirring. The phase (2) 80% extender pigments are prepared in advance by hammer milling the pigment/talc combinations to deagglomerate the pigments. Phase (1) is combined and heated to 75 to 80°C. Phase (2) is added while homogenizing slowly. Phase (3) is blended and added to combined Phases (1), (2), then combined phases (1) to (3) are heated to 85 to 90°C for 15 min with homogenization. Phases (1) to (3) are cooled to 75 to 80°C, and phase (4) is blended and added. The remaining water phase ingredients of phase (5) are added.

Emulsification: The oil phase (6) is added to the water phase (1 to 5) while homogenizing. Temperature and agitation are maintained for 15 min. The batch is cooled to 45°C. Phase (7) is combined and added. The batch is cooled to 30°C with paddle mixer agitation.

Phosphate emulsifiers offer an alternative to soap systems that require no amine. The pH of soap emulsions is 7.5 to 8.5; the potassium salt of cetyl phosphate, however, is an excellent primary emulsifier that is effective at pH 6 to 7, permitting claims of "pH balanced" or "pH of the skin."

Glyceryl monostearate, either pure or the partially saponified or partially ethoxylated self-emulsifying grades, and the fatty alcohols, cetyl, cetostearyl blends, and stearyl, continue to be very much in use as co-emulsifiers and viscosity control agents. Even 0.1% incremental adjustments in fatty alcohol content can change viscosity by 1000 centipoises.

There are hundreds of nonionic emulsifiers available to the formulator, including the sorbitan esters, ethoxylated ethers, sucrose esters, polyglyceryl esters, etc. Just as liquid fatty acids are helpful when formulating fluid soap systems, so are liquid nonionic emulsifiers useful in avoiding gelation. The liquid emulsifiers, often oleates or isostearates, are less efficient emulsifiers than their straight-chain counterparts, so blends are often employed. Isostearates may be preferred over oleates for their lower potential for malodor formation. Table 13.2 is an example of a liquid foundation containing a phosphate emulsifier as the primary anionic emulsifier and a sucrose cocoate/sorbitan monolaurate nonionic emulsifier pair.

Although purely nonionic foundation oil-in-water emulsions are possible, difficulties in achieving a stable emulsion, a nontacky feel, adequate preservation, and uniform pigment wetting are reasons to utilize anionic systems whenever possible. Similarly, careful pH adjustment of the aqueous pigment dispersion to the acid range can make cationic foundations feasible, but a strong benefit in performance would have to be achieved to justify the effort.

13.4.2 Water-in-Oil Foundations

Polymeric emulsifiers have made possible the formulation of cosmetically elegant water-in-oil or water-in-silicone emulsion foundations. The water-in-oil emulsions produced using low-HLB conventional emulsifiers or lanolin derivatives were too heavy and greasy to be suitable for foundations.

With the introduction of the dimethicone copolyol emulsifiers in the early 1980s, lightweight water-in-silicone foundations with exceptional spreading and blending characteristics were achieved. Subsequently, alkyl-modified dimethicone copolyols became available, specifically designed to form water-in-oil emulsions. PEG-30 dipolyhydroxystearate is another polymeric water-in-oil emulsifier that can be used alone or in combination with the silicone glycol copolymers.

The dimethicone copolyol emulsifiers that are primary emulsifiers for water-in-cyclic silicone foundations include PEG/PPG 18/18 dimethicone, PEG-10 dimethicone, bis-PEG/PPG 14/14 dimethicone, and PEG/PPG 20/15 dimethicone. The emulsifier is incorporated at a level of 2 to 5% in the silicone phase. About 0.2 to 1.0% of a low-HLB conventional co-emulsifier, such as a polyglyceryl ester, sorbitan ester, or low mole percent ethoxylated ether, is generally added to

TABLE 13.2
Oil-in-Water Foundation[a]

Phase	Ingredient	Percentage
	Water Phase	
1	Deionized water	48.81
1	PEG-12 dimethicone	0.05
1	10% Potassium hydroxide	1.30
2	80% Titanium dioxide and talc	10.00
2	80% Yellow iron oxide and talc	2.25
2	80% Red iron oxide and talc	1.10
2	80% Black iron oxide and talc	0.25
2	Talc	0.40
3	Magnesium aluminum silicate	1.00
3	Butylene glycol	4.00
4	Cellulose gum	0.12
4	Butylene glycol	2.00
5	Methyl paraben	0.20
	Oil Phase	
6	Di-PPG-3 myristyl ether adipate	14.00
6	Diethyl hexyl maleate	5.00
6	Cetyl alcohol	0.62
6	Steareth-10	2.00
6	Steareth-2	0.50
6	Dicetyl phosphate, ceteth-20 phosphate, cetearyl alcohol	4.00
6	Propyl paraben	0.10
7	Imidazolidinyl urea	0.30
7	Deionized water	2.00
		100.00

[a] Manufacturing procedure is similar to that of the Table 13.1 formulation.

improve emulsion stability. Very low levels (0.01 to 0.1%) of a hydrophilic emulsifier can be added to the water phase to lower the surface tension, facilitating the dispersion of the phase into droplets. In addition to serving as emulsifiers, both the dimethicone copolyols and the low-HLB conventional emulsifiers act as wetting agents for the pigment and fillers. Table 13.3 is a water–in-silicone foundation disclosed in U.S. Patent 5,143,722, assigned to Revlon. It should be noted that INCI names are changed to correspond to nomenclature current as of June 2005. The primary emulsifier is PEG/PPG 18/18 dimethicone, supplied at a level of 10% in cyclomethicone. The low-HLB co-emulsifier also incorporated in the oil phase is laureth-9.

The polymeric emulsifiers are specific to the type of oils the emulsion can contain. A material incompatible with the emulsifier will cause the polymer to curl up and become less functional. Only small amounts of oil other than cyclic

TABLE 13.3
Water-in-Silicone Foundation[a]

Ingredient	Percentage
Silicone Phase	
Cyclomethicone	12.00
Dimethicone/10 cs	5.00
Cyclomethicone (and) PEG/PPG 18/18 dimethicone	20.00
Laureth-9	0.50
Propyl paraben	0.10
Pigments (coated with methicone):	
Red iron oxide	0.70
Yellow iron oxide	1.50
Black iron oxide	0.20
Talc	3.30
Titanium dioxide	8.50
Water Phase	
Deionized water	38.00
Sodium chloride	2.00
Propylene glycol	8.00
Methyl paraben	0.20
	100.00

[a] *Manufacturing procedure*: Stir together the ingredients of the oil phase. Disperse the pigments in the oil phase using a high-speed disperser or high-shear mill. Combine the ingredients of the water phase. Stir in the water phase using a high-speed stirrer or homogenizer.

siloxanes can be utilized in formulations in which the primary emulsifier is a dimethicone copolyol. The alkyl dimethicone copolyols, lauryl PEG/PPG 18/18 methicone and cetyl PEG/PPG 10/1 dimethicone, are intended for use with hydrocarbons. Experimentation is required to determine the level of other ingredients, such as the more nonpolar esters and silicones, that can be incorporated without weakening the emulsion. In both types of water-in-oil emulsions, a salt is added to the water phase to favor the migration of the polymer to the oil–water interface to optimize stability. Table 13.4 is a water-in-oil foundation in which cetyl PEG/PPG 10/1 is the primary emulsifier, with polyglyceryl-4 isostearate as the co-emulsifier.

Further developments in water-in-silicone emulsion technology that will expand makeup formulators' capabilities include polymeric emulsifiers compatible with a broader range of oil phase ingredients and compounds combining silicone elastomers with silicone emulsifiers to simultaneously provide emulsification and viscosity control.

TABLE 13.4
Water-in-Oil Foundation[a]

Ingredient	Percentage
Oil Phase	
Cetyl PEG/PPG 10/1 dimethicone	0.45
Polyglyceryl-4 isostearate, cetyl 10/1 dimethicone, hexyl laurate	1.75
Cetyl dimethicone	1.80
Propyl paraben	0.10
Pigment Grind (all pigments and fillers are treated with triethoxycaprylyl silane)	
Ethyl hexyl palmitate	7.00
Phenyl trimethicone	2.20
Titanium dioxide	7.50
Yellow iron oxide	0.70
Red iron oxide	0.35
Black iron oxide	0.03
Talc	3.82
Dimethicone/10 cs	1.30
Cyclomethicone (and) dimethicone cross-polymer	15.00
Water Phase	
Deionized water	51.85
Diazolidinyl urea	0.20
Sodium chloride	0.50
Butylene glycol	5.30
Methyl paraben	<u>0.15</u>
	100.00

[a] *Manufacturing procedure*: Pigments are milled in the oils of the pigment grind using a high-shear disperser, then combined with the remaining ingredients of the oil phase. The ingredients of the water phase are combined and heated to 50°C with stirring until homogenous, then cooled to 30°C. The water phase is slowly added to the oil phase with stirring or low-speed homogenization. When emulsification is complete, homogenize for 5 min. Cool to 30°C with paddle mixer agitation.

PEG-9 polydimethyl siloxyethyl dimethicone is an example of an emulsifier that can be utilized with cyclic and low molecular weight linear silicones, hydrocarbons, and many esters. The addition of high molecular weight esters is still not recommended. PEG-12 dimethicone cross-polymer is an elastomeric emulsifier capable of forming the emulsion and maintaining viscosity in water-in-silicone and water-in-silicone-in-water emulsions to satisfy the need for improved stability and easier manufacture.

14 Surfactants for Nail Care

Steven W. Amato, M.S., M.B.A.
Nail Care Research & Development, Coty, Inc.

CONTENTS

14.1 THE MARKETPLACE

The global hand and body care market reached $8.12 billion in 2003, with an average 5-year growth rate of 2.6%. It is expected to reach $9.04 billion in 2008. Globally, hand care was 26.4% of the hand and body care market. The Asia-Pacific region was the largest segment of the market at 35.8%, followed by Europe at 25.6%, the U.S. at 24.0%, and the rest of the world at 14.6%.[1] The hand and body care segment is 27.8% of the global skin care market.[2]

The global makeup market value reached $23.65 billion in 2003, with a 5-year average growth rate of 4.3%. It is expected to grow to $28.8 billion by 2008. Globally, nail makeup was 9.2% of that total market in 2003. The U.S. was the leader at 32.2% of the value share, followed by Europe at 28.3%, the Asia-Pacific region at 23.7%, and the rest of the world at 15.8%.[3] The professional salon business is strongest in the U.S., and a significant number of people derive their income from nail care and related services. For 2002, there were an estimated 51,571 nail salons and 368,818 licensed nail technicians nationwide. Ninety-nine percent of the salons offered manicures, 96% offered pedicures, and over 50% offered skin care and massage services. Skin care and massage were the third and fourth fastest growing salon services, after nail powder and glue and other spa services.[4]

14.2 NAIL CARE BASICS

Proper nail care begins with excellent care of the hands and feet. This is because the growth and condition of the nail relies on the health of the skin of the fingers and toes. First, let us define some of the key parts of the nail structure. The main parts of the nail are the *nail plate*, the term for the nail itself, which rests on the *nail bed*, or the fleshy tip of the finger. The nail plate grows out of the *nail root*, which is embedded underneath the skin at the base of the nail. Beneath the nail root is the *nail matrix*, which contains nerves together with lymph and blood vessels that produce nail cells and control the rate of nail growth. The *lunula*, or half moon area, at the base of the fingertip is where the matrix connects to the nail bed. The skin of the finger is attached to the top of the nail by the cuticle that functions to protect and seal the area between the nail and nail bed. The nail is made primarily of keratin and, like hair and skin, needs moisture to remain smooth and flexible. The condition of the nail is often a reflection of one's general health and is often used as a diagnostic tool for heart and lung health.[5,6*]

Common problems that people experience with their nails, including chipping, splitting, peeling, and brittleness, are a result of overexposure to harsh

---

* Definitions were adapted from *Milady's Art and Science of Nail Technology*, 2nd ed., MILADY, 1997. Reprinted with permission of Delmar Learning, a division of Thomson Learning: www.thom-msonrights.com; fax, 800-730-2215.

chemicals found in removers, cleansers, and nail treatment items. A number of treatment products are available that can help to mitigate these effects. Some of these are nail moisturizers, strengtheners, and hardeners. Additional products that are used to treat conditions that may affect the nail include antibacterial fluids, antifungal creams and fluids, and corn and callus softeners and removers.

14.2.1 CLEANSING

Good nail health begins with proper cleansing and moisturizing. Some studies indicate that frequent and proper hand cleansing can significantly reduce transmission of diseases; however, care must be taken against overwashing. Two major groups of microorganisms are found on skin: resident flora, which normally reside there, and transient flora, contaminants that are the primary cause of hospital infections from cross-contamination in a hospital environment. Plain soap and water can physically remove one level of microbes and, in fact, may aid in the dispersal of bacteria on the skin of the hands.[7] In order to kill microorganisms, an antiseptic agent is necessary. Such cleansers typically contain alcohol and additional antimicrobial agent.[8] Alcohol cleansers may be too defatting and cause irritant contact dermatitis, especially when followed by soap and water cleansing. In addition to alcohol solutions, several other antibacterial agents are used. These include chlorhexidine gluconate, iodine and iodophors, quaternary ammonium compounds, triclosan, and others. Chlorhexidine gluconate is cationic, and formulations containing anionic and nonionic emulsifying agents may reduce its activity. Iodine and iodophors are often stabilized with a polymer and an ethoxylated nonionic surfactant to reduce irritation from the iodine. Among the most frequently used quaternary ammonium compounds are the alkyl benzalkonium chlorides. They are not compatible with anionic surfactants. Triclosan is nonionic and can be formulated with a variety of surfactants. The activity level of triclosan can be affected by the micelles formed by the surfactant; however, it seems to be formulation dependent and needs to be investigated for each case.[9]

Work site cleansers many be caustic and abrasive, they may contain sensitizers such as lanolin or limonene, or perfumes, and they may contain irritants such as alcohol. Antibacterial cleanser formulations containing alcohol are very typical of those that are used in medical facilities. Anionic and cationic surfactants are more harmful than nonionic surfactants, and increased concentrations of surfactant cause severe damage to the skin. The normal pH of the skin is in the range of 4.5 to 5.5, and hand and foot cleansers and treatment products can help maintain the health of the skin when they are formulated to be pH neutral to mildly acidic. A publication on the website for the Electronic Library of Construction Occupational Safety provides a list of acceptable hand soaps and cleansers.[10]

Skin irritation is a major concern when formulating surfactant systems that are intended to have skin contact. Protein denaturation by the adsorption of the surfactant onto charged sites on the skin is a major factor in deciding which surfactant to use. The ability of the surfactant to adsorb onto the skin and penetrate cell membranes seems to determine degree of skin irritation. In general, the order of denaturation is anionics > cationics > amphoterics > amine oxides > ethoxylated nonionics. For anionic surfactants of the series $C_{12}H_{25}(OC_2H_4)_{XSO4Na}$, no denaturation occurs when X = 6 or 8. The addition of cationic surfactants to anionic surfactants tends to reduce their degree of irritation.[11] The medical community for the control of disease transmission recommends the use of cleansers for home use. Specific recommendations are:

1. Use soap and running water.
2. Rub your hands together, creating friction.
3. Wash all surfaces of your hands, including the backs of hands, wrists, between fingers, and under fingernails.
4. Wash hands for at least 60 sec.
5. Rinse well.
6. Dry the hands with a paper towel.
7. Turn the faucet off with a paper towel instead of bare hands.[12]

An interesting innovation in the hand cleanser segment is HandClens®[13] from Woodward Laboratories, Aliso Viejo, CA. Clinical studies sponsored by the company show that with a strict regimen of antibacterial cleanser use, the illness and class absenteeism rates were reduced by approximately one third.[14–16] The product form is a liquid with a broad-spectrum bactericide; it is supplied for refillable wall-mount dispensers or over the counter as a clear liquid in a pump dispenser. The pumping action combined with the surfactants present converts the liquid to foam for ease of use. The ingredient listing is as follows:

Active Ingredient: benzalkonium chloride. Inactive ingredients: water, cocamidopropyl betaine, propylene glycol, allantoin, cetrimonium chloride, quaternium 12, cocamidopropylamine oxide, diazolidinyl urea, quaternium 15, methyl paraben, propyl paraben, Ext. D&C Violet No. 2, D&C Green 5, fragrance, TEA, citric acid.

The commercial formula contains the nonionic cocamidopropylamine oxide, the cationic cetrimonium chloride, and the amphoteric surfactant cocamidopropylbetaine. The specific blend of surfactants improves the permeation of the active ingredients, and the presence of a keratolytic agent such as allantoin further enhances the activity of the benzalkonium chloride.[17,18]

14.2.2 HAND, FOOT, AND NAIL TREATMENTS

Following is a discussion of several products for maintaining the health and appearance of the hands, feet, and nails. These include hand and nail cream, hand lotion, cuticle conditioner, cuticle remover, specialty medical products, and exfoliating cuticle scrub.

14.2.2.1 Hand and Nail Cream

A good starting formula for a moisturizing hand cream is illustrated in Table 14.1 (from International Specialty Products[19]):

TABLE 14.1
Refreshing Hand Cream with Vital™ ET and Prolipid® 141, Formula 10890-123-2

Ingredients	Weight %	Supplier
Phase A		
Deionized water	65.70	
Carbomer (Carbopol 980)	0.30	Noveon
Disodium EDTA	0.10	Dow Chemical
Glycerin	2.00	
Phase B		
Petrolatum	6.00	Penreco
Ethylhexyl palmitate (Ceraphyl® 368)	9.50	ISP
Glyceryl dilaurate (Emulsynt™ GDL)	2.00	ISP
Isodecyl oleate (Ceraphyl® 140A)	1.50	ISP
Glyceryl stearate (and) behenyl alcohol (and) palmitic acid (and) stearic acid (and) lecithin (and) lauryl alcohol (and) myristyl alcohol (and) cetyl alcohol (Prolipid® 141)	4.00	ISP
Phase C		
Triethanolamine (99%)	0.40	
Deionized water	5.00	
Phase D		
Disodium lauraminodipropionate Tocopheryl phosphates (Vital™ ET)	3.00	ISP
Diazolidinyl urea (and) iodopropynyl Butyl carbamate (Germall® Plus)	0.50	ISP

Procedure:

1. Combine ingredients in Phase A; heat to 75°C and mix until uniform.

2. Combine ingredients in phase B; heat to 75°C and mix until uniform.

3. Add Phase B to Phase A with homogenization.

4. Add Phase C to Phases A and B with homogenization.

5. Cool batch to 45°C and add Phase D.

6. Q.S. for water loss.

This formula has passed a 28-day double-challenge efficacy test. However, the preservative system has not been optimized to its lowest effective level. The pH should be approximately 6.19 and is helpful for maintaining the acidity of the skin. The Prolipid 141 complex is formulated with a balance of surfactant ingredients that offer a wide range of pH compatibility and skin protection through lamellar gel formation. The Vital ET is an effective antiswelling and antiredness agent.

The information contained in this chapter and the various products described are intended for use only by persons having technical skill and at their own discretion and risk after they have performed necessary technical investigations, tests, and evaluations of the products and their uses. While the information herein is believed to be reliable, we do not guarantee its accuracy, and a purchaser must make its own determination of a product's suitability for the purchaser's use, protection of the environment, and the health and safety of its employees and consumers of its products. Neither ISP nor its affiliates shall be responsible for the use of this information, or of any product, method, or apparatus described in this chapter. Nothing herein waives any of ISP's or its affiliates' conditions of sale, and *we make no warranty, express or implied, of merchantability or fitness of any product for a particular use or purpose*. We also make no warranty against infringement of any patents by reason of purchaser's use of any product described in this chapter.

14.2.2.2 Hand Lotion

Table 14.2* details a good starting formula for a Conditioning Hand and Body Lotion[20]; it is nongreasy and has a long-lasting silky afterfeel.

---

* Although the information and recommendations in this publication are believed to be accurate and are given in good faith, Uniqema makes no representation or warranty as to the completeness or accuracy of any information given. Suggestions made concerning uses or applications are only the opinion of Uniqema, and users should undertake their own tests and analyses to determine the suitability of these products for their own particular purposes. However, because of numerous factors affecting results, Uniqema *makes no representation or warranty, express or implied, including without limitation the warranties of merchantability and fitness for a particular purpose, with respect to information or the product to which the information refers.*

Nothing contained herein is to be construed as a recommendation to use any product, process, equipment, or formulation in conflict with any patent or other intellectual property right, and Uniqema makes no representation or warranty, express or implied, that the use thereof will not infringe any patent or other intellectual property right, including without limitation copyright, trademark, and designs of any third party.

Any trademarks herein identified, including without limitation Uniqema and the ICI Roundel, are trademarks of the ICI Group of Companies. The ICI Group of Companies shall mean Imperial Chemical Industries PLC, and all companies or other legal entities owned directly or indirectly by Imperial Chemical Industries PLC. Uniqema is the trading name of Unichema Chemie BV, which is registered in the Netherlands: No. HR29009483, Registered Office Buurtje 1, 2802 BE, Gouda, The Netherlands. Uniqema is an international business of Imperial Chemical Industries PLC. Uniqema operates through ICI-affiliated companies in relevant countries, for example, ICI Americas, Inc., Unichema, a division of Indopco, Inc., and Mona Industrie, Inc., in the U.S.© 2002 Uniqema

TABLE 14.2
Conditioning Hand and Body Lotion

Ingredients	Weight %	Supplier
Part A		
Arlasilk™ phospholipid SV (stearamidopropyl PG-dimonium chloride phosphate (and) cetyl alcohol)	3.00	Uniqema
Propylene glycol	2.00	
Germaben II (propylene glycol (and) diazolidinyl urea (and) methyl paraben (and) propyl paraben	0.40	ISP
Titanium dioxide	0.40	
Triethanolamine (99%)		
Water	84.60	
Part B		
Cetyl alcohol	2.00	
Arlatone™ MAP 160 (cetyl phosphate)	1.00	Uniqema
Hexyl laurate	4.00	
Monasil™ PCA (PCA dimethicone)	2.00	Uniqema
Total	100.00	

Procedure:

Heat Parts A and B separately to 65°C. Slowly add B to A with homogenization and continue blending for an appropriate time. Stir cool to 40 to 45°C, add fragrance, and package.

Typical properties: viscosity = 100,000 cP, pH = 6.4.

The Arlasilk Phospholipid SV is compatible with skin mantle pH and helps with skin feel. The Arlatone MAP 160 helps with Silicone deposition.

14.2.2.3 Cuticle Conditioners and Moisturizers

These products are helpful to maintain the suppleness of the cuticle. This is important because the cuticle is a barrier against infection. Dried and cracked cuticles not only make the manicure difficult, but also can provide sites for entry of bacteria and fungus. These products typically contain good moisturizers or humectants such as urea, hyaluronic acid and its derivatives, phospholipids, sodium PCA, glycerin, and others. The role of surfactants will be to assist penetration into the cuticle and make the cream or lotion more effective for its intended purpose.

Table 14.3 gives an example formula of a cuticle conditioner with a neutral pH[21]:

14.2.2.4 Cuticle Removers

Cuticle removers are used when the cuticle is too large and intruding onto the nail plate. They can be in the form of a fluid, lotion, or cream and are applied to

TABLE 14.3
Cuticle Conditioner with Neutral pH

Material	Weight %
Polyoxyethylene lanolin wax	7.5
Stearyl alcohol	6.0
Dewaxed lanolin	2.0
Mineral oil (65/75 Saybolt)	15.0
Decyl oleate	4.0
Isopropyl palmitate	2.0
Propyl paraben	0.10
Deionized water (Q.S.)	100.0
Methyl paraben	0.10
Glycerin	5.00
Special oat flour (The Quaker Oats Co.)	2.00
Quaternium 15	0.10

Procedure:

Weigh oil phase ingredients 1 through 7; begin heating and stirring. Heat to 70 to 73°C. Weigh water phase ingredients 8 through 11 and begin heating and stirring. Heat to 70 to 73°C and add the water phase to the oil phase. Both should be 70 to 73°C. Cool to 40°C and add ingredient 12. Fill at 25 to 30°C.

the cuticle area followed by gentle massage to the area. Cuticle removers generally contain either sodium hydroxide or potassium hydroxide and are extremely alkaline. A pH of 10 or higher is not unheard of. The cuticle will become soft and washes off with gentle rubbing. The use of surfactants can assist in the penetration of the ingredients and speed up the softening of the cuticle. Table 14.4 provides an example formula[22].

TABLE 14.4
Cuticle Remover

Material	Weight %
Water	86.8
Sodium hydroxide	3.0
Sodium lauryl sulfate	1.0
Cetyl alcohol	9.0
Perfume	0.2
Total	100.0

14.2.2.5 Specialty Medical Products

There are several products on the market that make use of surfactants not only because of their emulsifying ability or stabilizing ability, but also due to their property of permeation enhancement of pharmaceutically active ingredients. These include corn and callus treatments, ingrown toenail treatments, topical antifungals, topical skin protectants, and topical antimicrobials (including antibiotics) and are covered by monographs in the U.S. Code of Federal Regulations (CFR) 21. Unless specific protectant claims are made, many of the ingredients listed in the monograph are used in skin creams and lotions without the allowed claims. Typically, antifungal products disclaim their use directly on the nail, due to the fact that the Food and Drug Administration (FDA) monograph does not recognize the efficacy of topical treatments for nail fungus. An ingredient list for a currently popular antifungal cream, Lotrimin Ultra,[23] Schering Plough Healthcare Products, Inc., Memphis, TN, is as follows:

Active ingredient: Butenafine hydrochloride, 1%
Other ingredients: Benzyl alcohol, cetyl alcohol, diethanolamine, glycerin, glyceryl monostearate SE, polyoxyethylene (23) cetyl ether, propylene glycol dicaprylate, purified water, sodium benzoate, stearic acid, white petrolatum

The nonionic emulsifiers glyceryl monostearate SE, polyoxyethylene (23) cetyl ether, and propylene glycol dicaprylate contribute to a nonirritating cream base.

An interesting antimicrobial treatment product is Mycocide NS®[24] nail solution from Woodward Laboratories, Aliso Viejo, CA. The product claims to help kill germs and other microbes that attack the skin surrounding and under the nail, thereby helping to prevent nail diseases. It is covered by at least two U.S. patents[17,18] and teaches the use of optimized surfactant blends to enhance the efficacy of the active antimicrobial agent, benzalkonium chloride, which is present in the commercial product at 0.1% by weight. The other ingredients are water, hydroxypropyl methylcellulose, cocamidopropyl betaine, cocamidopropylamine oxide, propylene glycol, allantoin, cetrimonium chloride, quaternium 12, quaternium 15, diazolidinyl urea, methyl paraben, propyl paraben, triethanolamine, and citric acid.

The key teaching is the optimization of a blend of nonionic, cationic, and amphoteric surfactants. The nonionic surfactant content is optimal between 1.5 to 5.0 wt%, the cationic surfactant content is optimal between 0.75 to 1.5 wt%, and the amphoteric surfactant is optimal between 3.0 and 5.0 wt%. The commercial formula contains the nonionic cocamidopropylamine oxide, the cationic cetrimonium chloride, and the amphoteric surfactant cocamidopropyl betaine. The presence of a keratolytic agent such as allantoin further enhances the activity of the benzalkonium chloride. This is additionally supported by a research paper presented by Wadhams et al.[25] that demonstrates the efficacy of Mycocide NS as

TABLE 14.5
Exfoliating Cuticle Scrub

Material	Weight %	Supplier
Phase A		
Deionized water	Q.S to 100.0	
Benzophenone-4	0.05–0.50	
Disodium EDTA	0.01–1.0	
Butylene glycol	1.0–4.0	
Glycerin, USP (99.5%)	1.0–4.0	
Multifruit acid complex	0.1–1.0	Barnet
Methyl paraben	0.1–0.50	
Phase B		
Aloe Vera Gel 10X	0.1–0.50	
Phase C		
Ultragel 300	0.5–2.0	Cosmetic Rheologies Ltd.
Phase D		
Polyethylene powder	1.0–5.0	
Phase E		
Propyl paraben	0.05–0.50	

Note: Fragrance as desired.

Procedure:

1. Combine ingredients in Phase A at ambient temperature in a vessel equipped for homogenization and side sweep-type mixing; mix until uniform with side sweep, then homogenize.

2. Add Phase B to Phase A with homogenization.

3. Add Phase C to Phases A and B with side sweep mixing.

4. Add Phase D gradually with side sweep mixing: homogenize on slow speed until uniform. Excessive speed will break down the exfoliant.

5. Mix the ingredients for Phase E in a side vessel until uniform.

6. When Phases D and E are uniform, add Phase E into Phase D and mix until uniform.

7. Q.S. for water loss.

Approximate pH = 3; viscosity range = 600 to 900 centipoise, Brookfield LVT viscometer, Spindle 4, 12 RPM.

This basic cuticle scrub starting formula is courtesy of Coty, Inc.[26]

an effective cure for nail plate disease, specifically the treatment of pedal onychomycosis (fungus-infected toenails). The authors believe that due to the fluidity of this formula and the unique surfactant delivery system, the product penetrates the nail plate more effectively than a cream-type formulation.

14.2.2.6 Exfoliating Cuticle Scrub

Regular use of an exfoliant helps to remove the outer layer of dead skin on the hands, feet, and cuticle. The massaging action upon application of the product stimulates blood flow and assists in the generation of new skin cells. The physical result is that the skin feels softer and appears fresher. Exfoliants need to be pH balanced in the same manner as skin cleansers and soaps.

Table 14.5* gives an example of a starting formula for a cuticle scrub.

14.3 PROFESSIONAL SALON PRODUCTS

The professional salon environment is one that requires more stringent adherence to sanitizing, disinfecting, and cleansing than one typically does at home. This is due in part to the fact that nail technicians are licensed and there are strict guidelines that are set by each state in the U.S. Examples of basic guidelines for nail technicians, which is a code of conduct, and an example of a footbath preparation procedure can be found on the *Nail Magazine* website.[27,28] The salon must be careful to do preservice sanitization on all nonliving surfaces in the salon. The most often used disinfectants are quaternary ammonium compounds, phenolics that are usually formulated to pH 11 or higher, alcohol, and bleach. A step-by-step procedure for preservice sanitization will include:

1. Wash implements thoroughly with warm water and soap.
2. Rinse implements in plain water.
3. Completely immerse implements in an Environmental Protection Agency (EPA)-registered, hospital-level disinfectant.
4. Wash hands with an antibacterial soap.
5. Rinse implements and dry with a clean towel.
6. Follow a state regulation-approved storage procedure.
7. Sanitize the manicure table with disinfecting or sanitizing solution.
8. Disinfect the table surface with an EPA-registered disinfectant.
9. Wrap the client's cushion in a clean towel.
10. Refill disposable materials.
11. Use a sanitizing hand wash on your own hands in front of the client.

The manicuring and pedicuring procedures are designed so that cross-contamination from one extremity to another extremity is unlikely. Examination of the procedures gives insight to the types of commercial products that are useful to the salon industry.

---

* The information contained in this chaper and the various products described are intended for use only by persons having technical skill, and at their own discretion and risk after they have performed necessary technical investigations, tests, and evaluations of the products and their uses. While the information herein is believed to be reliable, there is no guarantee of its accuracy and a user must make its own determination of a product's suitability. Coty, Inc., shall not be responsible for the use of this information, or of any product, method, or apparatus described in this chapter.

A basic manicure procedure is as follows:

1. The clients wash their own hands with an antibacterial soap.
2. Remove the nail polish, starting with the hand that is other than the one they favor. If right-handed, begin with the left hand.
3. Shape the nails: rectangular, round, oval, or pointed.
4. Place fingers in a soaking solution while working on the other hand.
5. Remove the fingers from the soak solution and clean the nails with a nailbrush.
6. Dry the hand and gently push back the cuticle.
7. Apply a cuticle remover to the nails of the recently brushed hand. Place the other hand in the soak solution while continuing to work on the first hand.
8. Loosen the cuticles using an orangewood stick or the spoon end of a steel pusher.
9. Clip excess cuticles or hangnails if permitted by state regulations.
10. Clean under the free edge of the nail with a cotton-tipped orangewood stick. Remove the hand that is in the soak bath and brush the first hand over the bath to remove any last bits of polish and cuticle.
11. Repeat steps 5 to 10 on the other hand.
12. Bleach the nails (optional) with a 6% hydrogen peroxide solution if the nails are yellow, avoiding the cuticles and skin of the client to avoid irritation.
13. Buff with a chamois buffer (optional).
14. Apply cuticle oil.
15. Bevel the nails to remove any rough edges or cuticle particles.
16. Apply a hand lotion to the hand and arm with a sanitary spatula and perform a hand and arm massage.
17. Remove traces of cuticle oil so that the nail polish will adhere better to the nail.
18. Apply the polish. This usually includes a base coat, colored nail polish, a topcoat, and, optionally, an instant dry to prevent smudging.

A basic pedicure procedure is as follows:

1. Remove shoes, socks, and hose, and roll pant legs to the knee.
2. Spray or wipe feet with an antiseptic.
3. Soak feet in a sanitizing bath.
4. Rinse the feet.
5. Dry the feet.
6. Remove polish, if any.
7. Clip the nails.
8. Insert toe separators.
9. File the nails.
10. Use a foot file to remove dry skin and callus growths.

11. Remove toe separators and rinse the foot.
12. Repeat steps 7 to 11 on the other foot.
13. Brush the nails with a nailbrush. Rinse, dry, and insert toe separators.
14. Apply a cuticle remover to soften the cuticles.
15. Push back the cuticle with an orangewood stick. Clip hangnails only if permitted by state regulators.
16. Remove toe separators; dip the foot into the sanitizing bath and brush with a nailbrush to remove any bits of nail polish and cuticle.
17. Apply a lotion and massage the foot.
18. Place foot on a clean towel and repeat steps 13 to 18 on the other foot.
19. Remove traces of lotion from the toenails of both feet with cotton balls soaked with nail polish remover.
20. Apply polish and dry thoroughly.
21. Powder the feet.
22. Replace hose and shoes.

The previous procedures are from *Milady's Art and Science of Nail Technology.*[29]*

14.3.1 HAND SOAKS AND FOOT SOAKS

These are used prior to the start of the manicure to cleanse and sanitize the client's hands and feet and to soften skin, calluses, and cuticles. They are typically alkaline, with a pH in the range of 8 to 10, and contain detergents, foam boosters, and antimicrobial agents. An example of an ingredient listing of Pedi Redi Plus™, a currently available powder for salon foot soak use, follows: sodium chloride, sodium sesquicarbonate, chloramine-T, sodium tripolyphosphate, fragrance, maltodextrin, isopropyl palmitate, oleamide DEA, dimethicone. May contain: FD&C Blue No. 1, FD&C Yellow No. 5, FD&C Red No. 33, FD&C Red No. 40.[30]

14.4 SURFACTANTS IN NAIL POLISH

Nail polish is a complex combination of ingredients brought together to make a fluid that, upon drying, creates a decorative film on the nails. In the fluid state it needs to be stable to the environment and resistant to variations in temperature, exposure to light, and mechanical shocks. Once applied to the nail, it is required to dry evenly in such a manner that it does not form a skin that traps solvent. Trapped solvent can lead to solvent popping, which leaves circular surface defects.

The drying film must allow for recoating of itself with good flow and intercoat adhesion. Polymeric coatings tend to shrink as they dry due to chemical or physical changes. One reason is due to solvent evaporation. The area of the coating is constrained to remain in the original wet film size by its initial adhesion to a relatively rigid substrate. Early on, the changes in volume are accommodated by changes in thickness due to fluid flow. Once the coating has dried sufficiently so

---

* Reprinted with permission of Delmar Learning, a division of Thomson Learning: www.thommsonrights. com; fax, 800-730-2215.

that it can no longer flow, additional chemical changes or additional solvent loss produces an internal strain in the plane of the coating that increases as it reaches its ultimate dry state. There will be some viscoelastic relaxation processes occurring; however, this internal strain is never completely compensated, and the cohesive and adhesive properties of the film may be compromised. The extreme case is when the coating spontaneously detaches upon final drying due to the internal stresses and strains.[31] The film must remain somewhat porous on the microscopic level and allow the dried film to breathe, i.e., allow moisture from perspiration to pass through. The dried film must last on the nail for several days and retain its gloss, resistance to chipping, abrasion, and peeling.

The coating will adhere best to the nail if the surface is free of foreign matter such as dirt, oil, moisture, and weak boundary layer materials. This is a very difficult task to achieve because the nail, although not living tissue, is attached to the living body and is subject to constant contact with one's own body oils and moisture. Surfactants can help the nail polish to overcome these interfering materials to some degree. First let us look at the basic theories of adhesion and see how surfactants can assist the adhesion and rheology of nail coatings.

14.4.1 THEORIES OF ADHESION

The mechanism of adhesion may be one or a combination of various factors. Some major theories are mechanical, adsorption, electrostatic, and diffusion.

The mechanical adhesion theory requires that the adhesive material must penetrate cavities on the surface of the substrate and displace trapped air at the interface. Mechanical anchoring of the coating is essential to this theory.

The adsorption theory postulates that adhesion results from molecular contact between two materials and the surface forces that occur. The process of establishing this intimate contact is called wetting. For a coating to wet a solid surface, the coating should have a lower surface tension than the critical surface tension of the solid substrate. After the substrate becomes wetted, it is proposed that permanent adhesion arises from molecular attraction through electrostatic bonds, covalent bonds, metallic bonds, and van der Waal's forces.

The electrostatic theory states that a double layer of electrical charge forms between the coating–substrate interface and these charges resist separation. Empirical evidence of the presence of electrostatic forces is that electrostatic discharges occur when many adhered materials are forcibly separated.

The diffusion theory states that there is an intermingling of molecules of coating and substrate. This is believed to occur in solvent systems on polymeric substrates.[32]

14.4.2 WETTING, PENETRATION, SPREADING, AND COHESION

Wetting is generally taken as the processes that encompass adhesion, penetration, spreading, and cohesion. Adhesion is the process of face-to-face contact, and for coatings, it typically involves the contact of a smooth liquid surface with that of a rough substrate surface. Spontaneous adhesion occurs for contact angles less than 90°. If the contact angle is greater than 90° and the surface is rough, adhesion may not occur. Penetration is usually taken to be the permeation of a liquid into the porous surface of a substrate. Penetration can be considered analogous to the surface energy conditions of capillary action. Penetration occurs when the contact angle is less than 90° and may not occur when the contact angle is greater than 90°. Spreading refers to a liquid flowing over a surface as a duplex film. This means that the film is not a monolayer, but sufficiently thick to have distinct properties at the liquid–substrate interface and the liquid–air interface. Retraction will occur for contact angles over 90°. Cohesive forces occur when two faces of the same liquid are brought together, they adhere, and the surface energies are neutralized by each other and the surface molecules merge to become bulk molecules.[33]

14.4.3 Practical Applications

Surfactants can be found in nail polish in two main components: the monochromatic colorant grinds and the nail polish base. Most prevalent in the monochromatic colorant grinds are surfactants appropriate for the deagglomeration and dispersing of the pigment; they will vary by the nature of the formulation and colorant itself. Silicones and silicates are often used for flow and leveling properties and antifoaming properties. Foam is produced when a gas is introduced into a solution whose surface film has viscoelastic properties. The foam can be reduced or eliminated by addition of a surfactant that reduces or eliminates those viscoelastic properties of the gas–liquid interfacial film.[34]

These can be added at any stage of the formulation; however, silicones are often added to the uncolored nail polish base. The most prevalent silicone used in nail polish is dimethicone, which can be in the range of 10 to 1000 centistokes, depending upon the nature of the formulation. Most typically used are those grades between 500 and 1000 centistokes, as they contribute to improved flow and leveling properties. Typical usage levels are between 0.01 and 0.5 wt% of the total formula, depending upon the desired property enhancement.

14.4.4 Rheology

The nail polish needs to have a rheological profile that helps to maintain product stability in the container, have good flow-off of the applicator onto the nail surface, level well on that nail surface to have as near a defect-free appearance as possible, and allow for good adhesion from that application to the nail. Choice of rheological additive is contingent upon whether the nail polish is solvent-borne or waterborne. The rheological profile has an influence over flow, leveling, gloss, brush resistance, film thickness, hiding power, sedimentation tendency, and pigment stabilization. When the rheological profile is inadequate, syneresis processes can occur.[35] Rheological additives can help to reduce flocculation of the particulates that are dispersed in the wet nail polish. A surfactant film at the interface between those two phases stabilizes the dispersion of solid particles in liquids. The surfactant produces steric or electrical barriers to the aggregation of the dispersed solid particles. Elimination of those barriers allows flocculation.[36] Care must be taken to balance the stabilizing properties against the commercially desired attributes of stability that contribute to appearance in the package, flow-off of the applicator, and appearance of the dried film. Formulating to a relatively high viscosity at high shear can contribute to surface defects of the nail polish film, including streaking, poor wetting, adhesion, and leveling. The coating will not last as long as one with a viscosity profile that is optimized for the specific type of applicator used. Most often this is a brush. The typical shear rate range for brushing is between 5000 and 20,000 reciprocal seconds. It is helpful to understand the shear rates that a coating will be subjected to during manufacture, packaging, storage (pigment-settling processes), and application to aid in formulating a stable product that will also be acceptable to the consumer.[37]

Nail polish formulations typically are pseudoplastic and thixotropic in character. Pseudoplasticity describes a condition where the viscosity decreases with increasing shear rate. It is also known as shear thinning. The viscosity instantaneously returns to the original low-shear value when the shear stress is removed. Thixotropy describes a condition that occurs where viscosity decreases when a constant shear rate is applied over a period. When the shear force is removed, the viscosity returns to approximately the original value, with a time delay. Nail polish benefits from the shear-thinning property for spreading and flow on application, and the thixotropic property plays a role in storage stability. Many coatings scientists will speak of determining a thixotropic index, which refers to measuring the instantaneous viscosity at two different shear rates and determining a value based upon dividing the lower-shear-rate viscosity result by the higher-shear-rate viscosity result. This is in fact a determination of a shear-thinning index. This index gives insight toward the storage stability and application properties of the coating. The exact higher shear rate to use as a reference will vary based upon a company's experience of relating consumer acceptance with the measured properties of that coating. Typical ranges for the high-shear viscosity are 350 to 1000 centipoise, as measured with a Brookfield LVT rotational viscometer equipped with spindle 4 and set at 60 rpm. The reading is taken after 60 sec of elapsed rotational time at 25°C. The lower shear rate is typically 6 rpm, and the index range most often found useful is 1.5 to 3.0. The use of rheological additives can assist the formulator in optimizing these processes to obtain the desired storage and application properties of the nail polish.

14.4.5 MONOCHROMATIC PIGMENT GRINDS

The desired effects of surfactants in the pigment grind are to improve pigment wetting, aid in deagglomeration and dispersion, develop the color strength as fully as possible, improve gloss, and improve storage stability. The initial immersion and subsequent wetting of the pigment, followed by the ultimate distribution and colloidal stabilization of the pigment, occur simultaneously. During the immersion and wetting phase there are three considerations: (1) the surface energy of the pigment particle, (2) the energy of the particle in vapor plus the work done to create a space in the liquid that is equal to the volume of the pigment, and (3) the work done to

TABLE 14.6
Paste Concentrate

Material	Weight %
Calcium octoate (5% calcium metal in mineral spirits)	12.5
Octoic acid (2-ethylhexoic acid)	12.5
A carrier resin (a cellulosic, a polyester, toluenesulfonamide/formaldehyde resin, others)	50.0
Toluene	50.0
Total	100.0

fill the space in the liquid with the pigment particle. The spaces between pigment powder particles can be treated as capillaries, and it is necessary to consider the pressure required to force a liquid into the capillary. The selection of a surfactant is based upon its ability to enhance the liquid penetration of agglomerates. To improve wetting, it is desired to maximize the surface energy ($\lambda_{LV} \cos \theta$, where θ is the contact angle) at the liquid–vapor interface and decrease the contact angle; however, the addition of a surfactant that adsorbs onto the particle at the vapor (air) interface will tend to decrease both the surface energy at the liquid–vapor interface and the contact angle and lead to better wetting. The dominant effect needs to be determined by experimentation. Additionally, pigment geometry, chemistry, and particle size will have a measurable effect on the surface wetting by the vehicle on the pigment, and therefore the resultant rheology of the finished coating formula.[38]

An interesting surface-active agent treatment for inorganic pigments in a mill base is presented in U.S. Patent 5,133,966.[39] It described therein an organometallic salt plus an organic acid buffering solution for pretreating the inorganic pigment. First, an additive paste is prepared as in Table 14.6. Next, the paste is let down with a thinning solution as in Table 14.7.

This mixture is then milled thoroughly to at least 8+ on the Hegman scale. The duration of milling will be dependent upon various factors, including rheology of the mill base, the type of milling equipment, and the milling media (if present).

Next, a monochromatic pigment suspension is formulated. Typically, such a pigment suspension formula is used for the rapid color matching of finished coating shades. Thus Table 14.8.

It is reported that this pretreatment and letdown process provides a finished nail polish whose shades are more stable against pigment agglomeration, settling, or floatation, and improve the hiding power and gloss.

14.4.5.1 Rheological Additives for Solvent-Borne Nail Polish

The major additives for solvent-borne nail coatings are organoclays, castor waxes, and polyamide waxes. The two major classes are bentonites and hectorites. They most often require the presence of a polar solvent to activate the clay during the dispersion phase. Bentonites develop edge-to-edge hydrogen bonds between

TABLE 14.7
Let Down Phase

Material	Weight %
Toluene	4.07
Butyl acetate	35.26
Additive (from above)	1.63
This is followed by the addition of inorganic pigment and other mill base ingredients with agitation:	
Titanium dioxide	41.19
Butyl acetate	0.56
Toluene	2.25
Stearalkonium hectorite	0.43
RS π second nitrocellulose	7.86
Camphor	1.86
Toluenesulfonamide/formaldehyde resin (80% in butyl acetate is typical)	2.64
Total	100.00

hydroxyl groups found on the clay's platelet edges. In most cases, an additional polar activator is used in combination with the polar solvent. Hectorites are similar to bentonites; however, there are more negative charges on the surface. They have an ability to thicken water, and the organically modified versions find use in solvent-borne nail polish. Complete dispersion is required to develop optimum gel development.

Stearalkonium bentonite and stearalkonium hectorite are the major organoclays found in solvent-borne nail polish today. Typical usage levels are between

TABLE 14.8
White Monochromate Pigment Solution

Material	Weight %
Toluene	25.78
Titanium dioxide paste from Stage 2	22.00
Butyl acetate	13.38
Nitrocellulose (RS π second is typical)	9.53
Ethyl acetate	8.92
Toluenesulfonamide/formaldehyde resin (80% in butyl acetate is typical)	8.40
Dibutyl phthalate	6.00
Isopropyl alcohol	4.26
Camphor	1.38
Stearalkonium hectorite	0.25
Benzophenone-1	0.10
Total	100.0

0.8 and 1.5 wt% of the total formulation. They can be used either alone or in combination. U.S. Patent 6,740,314[40] teaches the use of a polymeric urea in combination with stearalkonium bentonite or stearalkonium hectorite to enhance the suspension and gloss properties of metallic pigments in a nail polish.

Castor oil-derived waxes require heat and shear to become activated and are synergistic with organoclays. Polyamide waxes help to form chain entanglements over time, subject to sufficient shear force and time elapsed.

14.4.5.2 Rheological Additives for Waterborne Systems

Rheological additives for waterborne systems include various materials with either chemical, electronic, or space-filling properties. These include nonassociative thickeners, associative thickeners, cellulosic, organoclays, organowaxes, metal organic gellants, and natural gum derivatives.

Associative thickeners form network structures with the pigments and the latex particles and include aqueous swellable emulsions, called HASE, for hydrophobically modified anionic soluble emulsion; polyurethane thickeners, called HUER, for hydrophobically modified ethylene oxide urethane rheology modifier; and hydrophobically modified polyether. HASE thickeners are anionic and provide psuedoplasticity. HUER types are nonionic and do not rely on alkali for activation. The polyethers are relatively new and offer a trade-off of properties between HASE and HUER types of thickeners.

Nonassociative thickeners are primarily from the ASE (alkali swellable emulsion).

14.4.5.2.1 Class
Nonassociative thickeners are typically high molecular weight acrylic polymers that contribute pseudoplasticity to waterborne formulations. They rely on alkali for property development and are pH dependent.

14.4.5.3 Cellulosics

These include carboxymethyl cellulose (CMC), hydroxyethyl cellulose (HEC), hydrophobically modified HEC (HMHEC), methyl cellulose (MC), methyl hydroxyethyl cellulose (MHEC), methyl hydroxypropyl cellulose (MHPC), ethyl hydroxyethyl cellulose (EHEC), and hydrophobically modified EHEC (HM_EHEC).

Cellulose thickeners are the dominant class of thickeners for waterborne coatings despite competition from synthetics. They are generally classified as ionic or nonionic. The former includes CMC; the latter includes all others (HEC, EHEC, MHEC, MHPC, and HPC). Some are soluble in cold or hot water (CMC and HEC), some are soluble in cold water (MHEC, MHPC, and HEC), and some are soluble in water with solvents (HPC).

The MHEC and MHPC types are associative cellulosics and are hydrophobically modified. They function primarily by chain entanglements and hydrophobic association with the latex and pigment.

The cellulosics fulfill many functions in a waterborne coating, including thickener, surfactant, dispersing agent, emulsion stabilizer, rheology modifier, protective colloid, and more. Cellulosics help adjust formulas for brushability, pigment stabilization, and syneresis control.

14.4.6 SURFACTANTS AS PROTECTIVE COLLOIDS: SURFACE-ACTIVE OLIGOMERS AND POLYMERS USED IN WATERBORNE SYSTEMS

Although they do not have the typical hydrophilic head and hydrophobic tail, they can be used to stabilize and disperse. They are most often referred to as protective colloids.

14.4.6.1 Anionics

Sodium polyacrylate is used in dispersing inorganic powders, especially titanium dioxide, iron oxides, calcium carbonate, and aluminum hydroxide.

A copolymer of olefin and sodium maleate is a good dispersant for organic and inorganic powders, but has a high foaming property. Polyphosphates work well on inorganics. Sodium tripolyphosphate had been used until the 1970s, but it was discontinued due to eutrafication of lakes.

Carboxymethyl cellulose is used in pigment dispersion and as an antisoil redeposition agent.

14.4.6.2 Cationics

Initially water soluble, *cationic cellulose* complexes with anionics to form a nonsoluble material unless an excess of anionic surfactant is present.

Cationic starch is used as a dispersing agent for emulsion polymerization.

14.4.6.3 Nonionics

Polyvinyl alcohol is used as a stabilizer for emulsion polymerization.

The preceding synopsis of rheological additives is abstracted from the SpecialChem4Coatings website with the permission of the editors.[41]

14.4.7 EFFECT OF POLYMER CONCENTRATION ON VISCOSITY OF WATER-SOLUBLE SYSTEMS

Solutions of polymers in organic solvents are mostly Newtonian in behavior; however, that is not the case for polymers in water-soluble systems. Water-soluble systems tend to be non-Newtonian, and the polymer concentration to viscosity relationships is not well understood. Many of these water-soluble systems are based upon carboxyl terminated polymer chains that are neutralized by amine salts to achieve solubility in water alone or, more commonly, in water and cosolvent blends. At a certain point, the polymer solution converts to a dispersion of micelles that may or may not have a hazy appearance.

Typically, these water-soluble systems are further reduced with additional water to achieve the final coating concentration. Because these polymers are typically hydrophobic and the hydrophilic salts are low in concentration, the addition of water causes the diluted solution to entrain less water, and as a result, the final viscosity tends to be lower than would be predicted from a simple dilution alone. Dilution of water-soluble cosolvent systems tends to initially drop in viscosity, similar to solvent-soluble systems; however, they differ in that somewhere in the range of 30 to 50% polymer concentration there is a plateau where relatively small changes in viscosity occur. Thereafter, a drastic reduction of viscosity typically occurs. Because the water-to-cosolvent ratio is important for controlling micelle formation, it can be used indirectly to control viscosity behavior. The use of two cosolvents can be advantageous because one, which is more volatile, can be used to reduce sagging of the coating, while the lower-volatility cosolvent can help to control leveling and film formation with sufficient open time to prevent solvent "popping," which leads to surface defects of the dried coating.[42]

Another important contributing factor to the rheology of coatings is pigment geometry and pigment-packing factors. One scheme for assessing the dispersibility of pigments is based upon calculating structure ratings for the pigment. It is based upon determining a packing factor that is derived from knowledge of the critical pigment volume concentration (CPVC) in the binder (typically determined by oil absorption values), specific surface area of the pigment, and the pigment density. Pigments can be classified into soft textured (easy to disperse) and hard textured (difficult to disperse). Simplified, finer-particle-size pigments are typically more difficult to disperse than coarser and less densely packed ones. In practice, combinations of coarse and fine pigments are used, and it is expected that the fine pigments can fill in some of the voids between the coarser ones.[43]

14.4.8 SOME EFFECTS OF CRITICAL PIGMENT VOLUME CONCENTRATION

Typical nail coatings are formulated so that the commercial product is well below the CPVC. When the pigment volume concentration (PVC) is lower than the CPVC, air voids are minimized and the pigment particles are separated. Above the CPVC, air voids are present. Knowledge of the CPVC allows the formulator to determine what properties of the coating will be affected and in what direction based upon the actual PVC of the formula. Glossy enamels are typically binder rich and below the CPVC. The use of surfactants can allow for reduction of entrapped air at the surface of and within the structure of pigment particles, thereby increasing the amount of PVC for a given product viscosity. This can afford an increased hiding power at a given coating viscosity.

Waterborne coatings exhibit a latex critical pigment volume concentration because the dispersion of pigment particles in latex exhibits different behavior than the dispersion in solvent systems. One difficulty arises because the latex particles may be at or very near the particle size of the pigment that they are expected to disperse. When a latex coating is drying, the latex particles dry around the pigment particles as the water evaporates or permeates the substrate. The resultant concentration of pigment in the dried coating is the latex pigment volume concentration (LPVC). The latex particle size determines the achievable PVC. The smaller the latex particle size, the more they are able to move around in a latex coating as drying occurs, and therefore can enhance the coating's ability to penetrate interstices of the substrate. The latex particle size is controlled during the polymer synthesis by the nature of the surfactant used to stabilize that polymerization reaction.[44]

The emulsion polymerization process typically consists of monomers, a surfactant, a water-soluble polymerization initiator, and water. The surfactant is initially in the form of micelles that form when the concentration of said surfactant exceeds the critical micelle concentration (CMC). As monomer is added and free radicals are generated, most of them are captured by the micelles and polymerization begins. Generally, the higher the surfactant concentration, the more rapid the emulsion polymerization will be, and the percentage of monomer converted will be greater than at lower surfactant concentrations. This is so because increasing the surfactant increases the number of particles per unit volume of emulsion. The resultant latex may already be in the form used for the coating. Most often the surfactant, coagulants, and initiator fragments remain in the final product.[45]

14.4.9 Examples of Waterborne Nail Polish

One of the most commercially successful waterborne nail polishes to date is Aube from Kao Corporation. A recent ingredient list is as follows: water, (alkyl acrylate/ethylhexyl acrylate/hema/styrene) copolymer, PEG-2 diethyl, ethanol, Dimethicone, sorbitan laurate, glyceryl stearate, sorbitan sesquioleate, fragrance, sodium lauryl sulfate, BHT, (Na/Mg) silicate, oxybenzone-3, betaine, methyl paraben, ethyl paraben, octyldodeceth-25, sodium trilaureth-4 phosphate, iron oxides, titanium dioxide, mica, silica, (Ca/Al) borosilicate, Red 226, Blue 404.[46]

This formula offers a proprietary copolymer and a complex surfactant system, including anionics and nonionics, which is designed to help penetrate the nail plate, emulsify the natural fats and oils on the nail, and aid in pigment suspension and stabilization. It is currently considered the most long lasting of its class.

One major market for waterborne nail polish is the children's segment. A recent commercial product has the following ingredient listing: acrylates copolymer, water, laureth-23, mica, titanium dioxide, imidazolidinyl urea, and ammonium hydroxide. May contain: D&C Red No. 7 Calcium Lake, D&C Red No. 27 Aluminum Lake, FD&C Blue No. 1 Aluminum Lake, and FD&C Yellow No. 5 Aluminum Lake.[47]

The children's nail polish is typically sold in toy stores, and the product wears off within a few days. Many will wash off readily with warm water and soap.

14.5 SUMMARY

The nail care market is a mature one with a steady growth rate. Within that market the professional salon environment offers opportunities for higher growth rates, and therefore those products necessary for sanitizing, disinfecting, manicuring, pedicuring, moisturizing, and massaging. Proper hand and foot care is essential for maintaining good nail health, and numerous products are used for that purpose. Future consideration can be given to improvement in drug delivery vehicles and other topical nail treatment products, and surfactants play a central role in the formulation of those products. Surfactant use in nail coatings plays a role in pigment wetting and dispersion, rheology and stability of the product, and flow and leveling of the coating. Surfactants that help to improve those properties also contribute to improved adhesion and lastingness of the nail coating. Major challenges exist for future development of waterborne nail coatings, with special consideration needed for improved adhesion and lastingness.

ACKNOWLEDGMENTS

I thankfully acknowledge the permissions granted by journals, magazines, and publishing firms to reproduce material that originally appeared in their publications. I also wish to recognize Mr. Wayne M. Hoyte and Mr. Raymond C. Smith, Senior Chemists at Coty, Inc., for their review of the original manuscript for content and continuity and for their thoughtful comments in that regard. I also want to recognize Ms. Kim Caufield, Chemist, Coty, Inc., who is a licensed cosmetologist for her review of the manuscript followed by insightful comments from the point of view of a salon professional. Very importantly, I want to thank my wife, Mary, and son, Andrew, for their patience and support.

I am especially thankful to Mitchell L. Schlossman for his vote of confidence in recommending me for this assignment.

REFERENCES

1. Datamonitor report reference code 0199-0114, February 2004, www.datamonitor.com, Datamonitor USA, New York.
2. Datamonitor report reference code 0199-0708, February 2004, www.datamonitor. com, Datamonitor USA, New York.
3. Datamonitor report reference code 0199-0700, February 2004, www.datamonitor. com, Datamonitor USA, New York.
4. http://www.nailsmag.com/home.cfm.
5. Chase, D., *The New Medically Based No-Nonsense Beauty Book*, Henry Holt and Company, New York, 1989, pp. 213–217.
6. *Milady's Art and Science of Nail Technology*, 2nd ed., MILADY, New York 1997, pp. 87–88.
7. Larson, E., Hygiene of the skin: when is clean too clean? *Emerging Infectious Diseases*, 7, 2001, pp. 225–230.
8. Pittet, D., Improving adherence to hand hygiene practice: a multidisciplinary approach, *Emerging Infectious Diseases*, 7, 2001, pp. 234–240.
9. Boyce, J.M. and Pittet, D., in *Guideline for Hand Hygiene in Health Care Settings*, available at http://cdc.gov/mmwr/preview/mmwrhtml/rr5116al.htm.
10. http://www.cdc.gov/elcosh/docs/d0400/d000458/d000458.html.

11. Rosen, M.J. and Dahanayake, M., *Industrial Utilization of Surfactants: Principles and Practice*, AOCS Press, Champaign, IL, 2000, p. 9.

12. Stephan, L.I., Hand Washing Teaching Module (Health Tips: Make Hand Washing a Healthy Habit), Kansas Department of Health & Environment, 1998.

13. Woodward Laboratories, Aliso Viejo, CA, Ingredient Listing for HandClens®, June 2004.

14. http://www.woodwardlabs.com/School_Health_Professionals/school_health_studies.htm.

15. Moadab, A. et al., Effectiveness of a nonrinse, alcohol-free, antiseptic hand wash, *Journal of the American Podiatric Medical Association*, 91, 288–293, 2001.

16. White, C. et. al., Reduction of illness absenteeism in elementary schools using an alcohol-free instant hand sanitizer, *Journal of School Nursing*, 17, 258–265, 2001.

17. Chodosh, D.F., Antimicrobial Compositions and Methods for Using the Same, U.S. Patent 5,661,170, August 26, 1997.

18. Chodosh, D.F., Antimicrobial Compositions and Methods for Using the Same, U.S. Patent 5,827,870, October 27, 1998.

19. International Specialty Products, Refreshing Hand Cream with Vital™ ET and Prolipid® 141, Formula 10890-123-2.

20. Conditioning Hand and Body Lotion, Monasil® PCA Product Data Sheet, 1999, available at www.uniqema.com. Uniqema is a part of the ICI Group of companies.

21. Juliano, A. and Miller, A., Cosmetics Containing Finely Divided Oat Flour, U.S. Patent 4,014,995, March 29, 1977.

22. Wajaroff, T. and Konrad, E., Reducing the Alkali Concentration in Hair Treating Compositions, U.S. Patent 3,975,515, August 17, 1976.

23. Schering Plough Healthcare Products, Inc., Ingredient Listing for Lotrimin Ultra®, Memphis, TN, August 2004.

24. Woodward Laboratories, Ingredient Listing for Mycocide NS®, Aliso Viejo, CA, June 2004.

25. Wadhams, P.S., Griffith, J., Nikravesh, P., and Chodosh, D., Efficacy of a surfactant, allantoin, and benzalkonion chloride solution for onymycosis: Preliminary results of treatment with periodic debridement *Journal of the American Podiatric Association*, 89, 124–130, 1999.

26. Coty, Inc., Research & Development, Morris Plains, NJ.

27. http://www.nailsmag.com/handouts/NAGuide_english.pdf.

28. http://www.nailsmag.com/handouts/NAFootSpa_english.pdf.

29. The previous procedures are from *Milady's Art and Science of Nail Technology*, 2nd ed., MILADY, 1997, pp. 32–33, 117–153.

30. MAXIM, LLC, Ingredient Listing for Pedi Redi Plus, Phoenix, AZ, June 2004.

31. Mittal, K.L., *Adhesion Aspects of Polymeric Coatings*, Plenum Press, New York, 1983, p. 108.

32. Landrock, A.H., *Adhesives Technology Handbook*, Noyes Publications, Park Ridge, NJ, 1985, pp. 4–7.

33. Patton, T.C., *Paint Flow and Pigment Dispersion*, 2nd ed., John Wiley & Sons, New York, 1979, pp. 209–222.

34. Rosen, M.J. and Dahanayake, M., *Industrial Utilization of Surfactants: Principles and Practice*, AOCS Press, Champaign, Illinois, 2000, p. 11.

35. Sauer, F.M., A New Approach to Understanding Rheological Additives, http://www.specialchem4coatings.com/resources/articles/article.aspx?id=1641.

36. Rosen, M.J. and Dahanayake, M., *Industrial Utilization of Surfactants: Principles and Practice*, AOCS Press, Champaign, IL, 2000, p. 11.

37. Schoff, C.K., *Rheology*, Federation of Societies for Coatings Technology, Blue Bell, PA, 1997, pp. 8–13.

38. Lambourne, R., *Paint and Surface Coatings: Theory and Practice*, Ellis Horwood Ltd., Chichester, West Sussex, England, 1987, pp. 226–230.

39. Khamis, A.A., Cosmetic Pigment Coating Composition for Nail Polish, U.S. Patent 5,133,966, July 28, 1992.

40. Socci, R.L. and Ismailer, A., Nail Enamel Compositions Containing Bismuth Oxychloride, U.S. Patent 6,740,314, May 25, 2004.

41. http://www.specialchem4coatings.com/tc/rheology/index.aspx?id=familly.

42. Patton, T.C., *Paint Flow and Pigment Dispersion*, 2nd ed., John Wiley & Sons, New York, 1979, pp. 105–107.

43. Patton, T.C., *Paint Flow and Pigment Dispersion*, 2nd ed., John Wiley & Sons, New York, 1979, pp. 126–157.

44. Patton, T.C., *Paint Flow and Pigment Dispersion*, 2nd ed., John Wiley & Sons, New York, 1979, pp. 192–204.

45. Rodriguez, F., *Principles of Polymer Systems*, McGraw-Hill Book Company, New York, 1970, pp. 107–112.

46. Record ID 183687, Aube Aqua Drop Nail Enamel PK809, available at www.gnpd.com.

47. Record ID 10178500, My Little Pony Nail Polish Set, available at www.gnpd.com.

GENERAL REFERENCES

1. Tsujii, K., *Surface Activity: Principles, Phenomena, and Applications*, Academic Press, New York, 1998.

2. Provder, T., Winnik, M.A., and Urban, M.W., Eds., *Film Formation in Waterborne Coatings*, American Chemical Society, Washington, D.C., 1996.

3. Boxall, J. and Von Fraunhofer, J.A., *Paint Formulation: Principles and Practice*, Industrial Press, New York, 1981.

4. Bennet, H., Bishop, J.L., Jr., and Wulfinghoff, M.F., *Practical Emulsions*, Vol. 1, *Materials and Equipment*, 3rd ed., Chemical Publishing Company, New York, 1968.

5. Bennet, H., Bishop, J.L., Jr., and Wulfinghoff, M.F., *Practical Emulsions*, Vol. 2, *Applications*, 3rd ed., Chemical Publishing Company, New York, 1968.

15 Sunscreens

Steven Harripersad[1] and Linda D. Rhein, Ph.D[2]
[1]Beauty Avenues
[2]Fairleigh Dickinson University

CONTENTS

For sunscreens to provide optimal protection from UV radiation, it is necessary to incorporate several UV filters to cover the entire UV spectrum of potentially harmful radiation. Such sunscreen filters absorb in different regions of the UV spectrum. Filters can be either organic or inorganic. Sun care formulations do challenge formulators:

1. Organic sunscreens that absorb UV radiation often carry incompatibility issues with the base formula.
2. Inorganics produce an intolerable whitening, especially on darker skin.
3. Formulations need to impart water resistance to the filters for protection during beach activities.

To formulate successful sun care products, the chemists must be well informed and must embraced the change from cosmetic products to cosmetic/over-the-counter (OTC) products. Perceptive consumers are becoming aware of the health effects of sun rays and the greenhouse effect, where heat is trapped in the atmosphere and light is allowed in. Most consumers are therefore well versed in the protective effects of sunscreens and are becoming more sophisticated in their selections. They want high sun protection factor (SPF), the broadest-spectrum protection, with water repellency during beach use, yet they want elegant formulations. This goal is not an easy target and has conflicting components.

Change your thoughts and you change your world.

—Norman Vincent Peale (1898–1993)[1]

The focus of this chapter is to provide cosmetic chemists with understanding regarding the harmful effects of sun exposure mechanistically, evidence supporting the need for sunscreens and the role of various sunscreen filters in providing protection from exposure to the sun's rays, and the knowledge required to formulate SPF products that are safe and effective, not misbranded, and also cosmetically pleasing. The chapter also will familiarize the reader with the final U.S. sunscreen monograph and amendments that dictate the permissible sun filters, their doses, and allowable combinations in the U.S., sunscreens available in other parts of the globe, and procedures for testing the efficacy of sunscreens.[2,3]

15.1 SUN EXPOSURE, SUN DAMAGE, AND SKIN CANCER

Most of us are familiar with sunburn. We know it as the visible physiologic response of the skin to overexposure to sunlight. In technical terms, sunburn is an acute cutaneous inflammatory reaction that occurs usually between 1 and 24 h after sun exposure.[4,5] The severity of the sunburn depends on two variables, the intensity of light and the length of exposure to the UV radiation. This all too familiar reaction is characterized by different degrees of erythema and many times by pain, swelling, and presence of blisters.[5–7] If the reaction is severe and covers a large portion of body surface areas, the individual may experience shock, and symptoms such as fever, chills, and weakness may occur.[4,6] If the subject is chronically exposed to solar radiation, the individual is at risk of developing skin cancer in addition to photodamage expressed as wrinkles, elastosis, and hyperpigmentation. [8–10]

Skin cancer is the most prevalent form of human neoplasia. Estimates suggest that in excess of 1 million new cases of skin cancer will be diagnosed this year alone in the U.S. (www.cancer.org/statistics). About 10,200 Americans die annually from skin cancer, and about 8000 of these from melanoma, the most deadly form of skin cancer. The primary cause of skin cancer is the ultraviolet (UV) radiation found in sunlight. The cost of treating nonmelanoma skin cancer is estimated to be in excess of U.S.$700 million each year, and when melanoma is included, the estimated cost of treating skin cancer in the U.S. is estimated to rise to U.S.$3 billion dollars annually.

15.1.1 EPIDEMIOLOGY STUDIES, UV EXPOSURE, AND PHOTOCARCINOGENESIS

The incidence of skin cancers has been rising since the early 1970s, and it is expected that 95% of skin cancers treated in the U.S. occur as a result of sun exposure.[11–14] Many epidemiology studies reported in the literature support this. Most of the skin cancers are basal cell and squamous cell carcinomas[15,16]; however, cutaneous malignant melanoma has also increased by 4 to 5% yearly from 1930 to 1990, and by about 2 to 3% between 1990 to 1995.[17] Nonmelanoma skin cancers occur mainly in the elderly. Roughly 3% of the malignant melanomas occur in children and adolescents, and in Australia it is the most common cancer observed between the ages of 15 and 44 years old.[16,18] The survival rate of malignant melanoma in children is poor.[19,20] In fact, pediatric melanoma is on the rise.

As stated, epidemiology studies have supported long-term UV exposure as a major risk factor of photocarcinogenesis.[4,21–29] In particular family history, the presence of actinic damage and phenotypic factors, combined with excessive sun exposure, plays a role. Studies show that cutaneous carcinomas are particularly common in individuals who were exposed early in life as children and adolescents and in individuals who spend a great deal of time in sunlight.[22,28,30–32] Other epidemiology studies show that the incidence of certain types of malignant melanoma also increases with increasing sun exposure, while other types are related to incidences of sunburn.[4,28,30–37] Thus, conclusions from epidemiology research are that it is the pattern of exposure, rather than total exposure, that is most important and specific for causing different skin cancers. Therefore, circumstances that predispose subjects to risk of developing skin cancer are frequency of sunburns, greater exposure as a child, occupational and nonoccupational (outdoor sports/beach) exposure, behaviors such as intermittent vs. continuous exposure, preexisting nevi/actinic keratoses, fair skin, ethnicity, and also the latitude of residence of the subject.[25,26,30–36] Fair-hair and -skin individuals are more sensitive to sun exposure than individuals with dark skin.[4,23,25] In fact, there is a very low incidence of skin carcinomas in dark-, black-skin individuals. Fair-hair and -skin individuals are therefore at greater risk for the deleterious effects of continuous exposure to the sun.[9,23,25,28] Moreover, the incidence of squamous and basal cell carcinomas of the skin, especially in fair-skin individuals, is directly proportional to the yearly length of time spent in the sun.[30–35] In humans, the reaction to sunlight is different depending on skin type. Various studies[21,22] support the association between melanoma risk and long-term *intermittent* sun exposure, for example, indoor workers, in particular males, have an increased risk of developing melanoma than outdoor workers with chronic sunlight exposure. This finding also suggests that with continued sun exposure, the skin develops a tolerance for UV radiation. Greater childhood exposure, in particular, appears to be a major risk factor. In a survey among 632 subjects, Gallagher et al.[38] showed that there is an increased risk of basal cell carcinomas when children between birth and 19 years were exposed to the sun. This suggests that childhood and adolescence may be critical periods for establishing adult risk for these tumors.[38] While sun protection measures should be adopted at any age, the general consensus is that sun protection will have the greatest impact on prevention of skin cancer if it is practiced as early in life as possible, especially among subjects who experience a high childhood exposure to solar radiation.[31,39]

It is generally accepted that the damaging effects of UV radiation have been attributed primarily to the effects of UVB radiation. However, keep in mind that UVB radiation accounts for only a small fraction of the UV radiation in the Earth's atmosphere (<10%); the large majority of radiation (>90%) is in the form of UVA.[24] Furthermore, UVB skin penetration is largely superficial compared with UVA, which can reach deeper layers of skin.

Because of this, the contemporary research is now focused on profiling the damaging effects of UVA radiation. There is increasing evidence and concern that UVA radiation is responsible for effects, distinct from those of UVB, that are involved in the process of carcinogenesis; however, it is likely that the two are synergistic in their actions.[24] Some epidemiological studies allude to an increased risk of development of melanomatous and nonmelanomatous skin carcinomas specifically associated with excessive exposure to UVA radiation.[21,22,40,41] Increased risk of skin cancer following long-term chemotherapy (PUVA) treatment that involves UVA/psoralen exposure of psoriatic skin[42–44] supports the promoter hypothesis. Studies of the use of alternative tanning methods (i.e., tanning beds and sunlamps), primarily UVA sources, identified a higher incidence of tumors in these patients in body sites not usually exposed to the sun.[45–49] Gallagher's meta-analysis of several studies has overall supported the risk of melanoma from tanning bed exposures.[49] Westerdahl et al.[47] believed that subjects in their epidemiology study were exposed to tanning beds that emit mainly UVA (which were prevalent post-1980), and their finding was a positive association expressed as a significantly higher odds ratio and dose relationship between total sun bed use and melanoma risk.[47] The finding suggested that UVA exposure is a factor in malignant melanoma risk, although Westerdahl acknowledges that other studies are inconclusive.[47]

As previously discussed, long-term exposure to UV radiation, for example, exposure beginning in childhood, has been associated with increased risk of cumulative chronic damage to the skin. It makes sense that the dose of radiation is a key factor in causing skin damage. Therefore, protection from UV exposure beginning early in life, preferably in childhood, may help prevent or reduce the risk of solar-induced conditions, including skin cancers, photodamage, photoaging, and other skin lesions.[3,22,25-31,39,50-56] Numerous epidemiology studies have generally concluded that childhood exposure to UV radiation can lead to greater risk of developing various skin cancers.[31,35,38,56-61] Current epidemiology research is focusing on risk factors in childhood of developing melanoma from exposure to UV radiation and its prevention. Autier and Dore[56] has published epidemiologic research that concluded that avoidance of sun exposure during childhood would have a greater impact on melanoma risk than avoidance during adulthood. Holly et al.[61] similarly reported in her case control study among 1382 women that risk of all types of melanoma increased with increased severity and history of sunburns up to 12 years old. In Holly et al.'s study, the risk also increased with lack of sunscreen use.[61] Whitman et al.,[57] in a systematic review of numerous epidemiologic studies, found that in ecological studies, children who resided in high-UV environments, compared to those in low-UV environments, consistently ran a higher risk of melanoma skin cancer years later.[57] Kennedy et al.[58] found in a study population of 966 cohorts that the recall of high incidences of "painful sunburns" before the age of 20 was associated with increased risk of developing squamous and basal cell carcinoma, malignant melanoma, and actinic keratoses and melanocytic nevi. Frequency of painful sunburns was a more important predictor than total lifetime sun exposure for developing melanoma.[58] In another study, Weinstock et al.[59] found that high incidence of blistering sunburns during the teenage years among women in the study was associated with an increased risk of melanoma. They also found that residence at an equatorial latitude during the teenage years was a factor. Zanetti et al.[60] reported similar findings in a European population-based case control study. In the same study, sunburns after 30 years old were not associated with higher incidence of melanoma.

15.2 Biological Action of Ultraviolet Radiation on Skin

Exposure to excessive doses of solar radiation induces both acute and chronic changes in the skin, including sunburn, edema, immunosuppression, premature skin aging, and skin cancer. At the cellular level, solar radiation can produce adverse structural and functional changes in membrane proteins and lipids, in chromosomal and mitochondrial DNA, and to immunocompetent factors. The increasing awareness of these adverse effects has educated the public to seek and, in fact, demand better photoprotection methods to protect from the sun's damaging rays.

The source of the damaging effects of sunlight is radiation in the ultraviolet (UV) range (290 to 400 nm), more specifically ultraviolet B radiation (UVB) (290 to 320 nm) and ultraviolet A radiation (UVA) (320 to 400 nm).[23] The UV rays penetrate the skin to different depths and, as a result, elicit different biologic effects on the skin.[23] The skin is composed of three layers, which includes the outer dead stratum corneum layer; the living epidermis, which is metabolically active and continuously replaces the stratum corneum; and the thick dermis, which is the support layer of connective tissue (see Figure 1.1 and Figure 1.2, showing the structure of skin). UV radiation around 290 to 320 nm (UVB) penetrates both the skin surface membrane — the stratum corneum — and the upper part of the epidermis and is sufficiently energetic to cause severe burning (erythema) of the skin, especially in fair-skin individuals. Chronic exposure to high-energy UVB causes mutations, leading to skin carcinomas, described later. UVA around 320 to 400 nm penetrates the epidermis and starts penetrating the dermis. In the lower epidermis, actively dividing cells such as keratinocytes and other immune-modulating cells are vulnerable to UV damage. UVA damage to these cells causes immunosupression.[15,16] The lower epidermis also contains melanocytes, which generate the melanin pigment responsible for the color of the skin. Exposure to UVA rays will stimulate the formation of melanin, thus producing a tan that protects the skin from immediate sunburn. Although UVA rays are of lower energy than the UVB rays, the fact that they can penetrate further into the dermis causes elastosis (loss of structural support and elasticity of the skin) and other skin damage, potentially leading to the skin cancers, as discussed earlier.

While UVB comprises only 5% of the UV radiation (UVR) reaching the Earth, it is historically considered the most damaging of the UV rays, a causative agent for development of both melanoma and nonmelanoma types of skin neoplasms.[23,62–64] Ultraviolet A radiation, the most abundant form of UV radiation, penetrating deeper and extending into the growing, proliferative basal layers of the epidermis and also into the dermis, contributes to photodamage and photoaging probably because this deeper penetration reaching the dermis.[8,65–67] It may also potentiate the carcinogenic effects of UVB.[7] Thus, ultraviolet A radiation as well as UVB substantially contributes to chronic skin damage. In addition to its role in skin carcinogenesis, UV radiation also suppresses the immune system. In fact, Ulrich[16] has reviewed studies with both experimental animals and biopsies from proven skin cancer patients, and the results suggest that there is an association between the immune suppressive effects of UV radiation and its carcinogenic potential. Along with this, UV radiation produces numerous known adverse immunologic effects.[24,68,69] The characterization of these effects at the molecular level are detailed next.

UV radiation induces oxidative damage, and this contributes to photocarcinogenesis. Oxidative damage caused by UV induces inflammation, gene mutation, and immunosuppression. Halliday[69] reviews evidence for the hypothesis that UV oxidative damage affects these processes. UVA makes a larger impact on oxidative stress in the skin than UVB by inducing reactive oxygen and nitrogen species that damage DNA, protein, and lipids and that also lead to nicotine adenine dinucleotide (NAD$^+$) depletion, and therefore energy loss from the cell. Lipid peroxidation induces prostaglandin production that, in association with UV-induced nitric oxide production, causes inflammation. Inflammation drives benign human solar keratosis (premalignant skin lesions) to undergo malignant conversion into squamous cell carcinoma, probably because the inflammatory cells produce reactive oxygen species, thus increasing oxidative damage to DNA and the immune system. Reactive oxygen or nitrogen appears to drive the increase in mutational burden as solar keratoses progress into squamous cell carcinomas in humans. UVA is particularly important in causing immunosuppression in both humans and mice, and UV lipid peroxidation-induced prostaglandin production and UV activation of nitric oxide synthase are important mediators of this event. Other immunosuppressive events are likely to be initiated by UV oxidative stress. Antioxidants such as vitamin E have also been shown to reduce photocarcinogenesis. While most of this evidence comes from studies in mice, Halliday[69] reviews supporting evidence in humans that UV-induced oxidative damage contributes to inflammation, gene mutation, and immunosuppression. Available evidence thus implicates oxidative damage as an important contributor to sunlight-induced carcinogenesis in humans.

At the cellular level, following sun exposure or sunburn, most cells are damaged (phototoxicity), including those of the dermal vessels and sweat glands.[4] The epidermis thickens, melanocyte melanin production increases, cell membranes are damaged, and disturbances in synthesis of protein, DNA, and RNA occur.[5–7,69] Likewise, keratinocytes become activated, stimulating production of inflammatory mediators like prostaglandins and interleukins and release of biologic response modifiers, inducing expression of genes at the p53 and NFkappaB locuses, for example, gene products like cycloxygenase-2, all of which lead to inflammation (vascularization and edema).[7,70–73]

At the molecular level, sunburn (primarily a measure of the effect of UVB) is a biochemical reaction that results from damage to specific cellular targets using photochemical mechanisms and generation of reactive oxygen species.[69,70] These effects are believed to be initiated by UV-mediated cellular damage, with proteins and DNA as primary targets due to a combination of their UV absorption characteristics and their abundance in cells (see review by Pattison and Davies[71]). In brief, UV radiation can mediate damage via two different mechanisms: (1) direct absorption of the incident light by the cellular components, resulting in an excited state formation and subsequent chemical reaction, and (2) photosensitization mechanisms, where the light is absorbed by endogenous (or exogenous) sensitizers that are excited to their triplet states. The excited photosensitizers can induce cellular damage by two mechanisms: (1) electron transfer and hydrogen abstraction processes to yield free radicals (type I) or (2) energy transfer with O_2 to yield the reactive excited state, singlet oxygen (type II). Direct UV absorption by DNA leads to dimers of nucleic acid bases, including cyclobutane pyrimidine species and pyrimidine (6-4) pyrimidone compounds, together with their Dewar isomers. These three classes of dimers are implicated in the mutagenicity of UV radiation, which is typified by a high level of CC → TT and C → T transitions. Single base modifications can also occur via sensitized reactions, including the type 1 and type II processes. The main DNA product generated by (singlet) O_2 is 8-oxo-guanine; this is a common lesion in DNA and is formed by a range of other oxidants in addition to UV. The majority of UV-induced protein damage appears to be mediated by (singlet) O_2, which reacts preferentially with Trp, His, Tyr, Met, Cys, and cystine side chains of cellular proteins. Direct photo-oxidation reactions (particularly with short-wavelength UV) and radicals can also be formed via triplet excited states of some of these side chains. The initial products of (singlet) O_2-mediated reactions are endoperoxides with the aromatic residues and zwitterions with the sulfur-containing residues. These intermediates undergo a variety of further reactions, which can result in radical formation and ring-opening reactions; these result in significant yields of protein cross-links and aggregates, but little protein fragmentation.

It is widely accepted that DNA is the principal target of UV-induced damage; the well-known formation of cyclobutane dimers and pyrimidone photoproducts between pyrimidine bases of DNA following exposure to UVR is evidence that the damage occurs at the level of the gene.[25,74] In addition to the photochemically induced covalent bonding between sensitive pyrimidine bases, evidence suggests that damage from reactive oxygen species (strand breakage and abnormal chromosomes) may also, in part, contribute to UV-induced DNA damage.[69,74–81] The different ultraviolet (UV) wavelength components, UVA (320 to 400 nm), UVB (280 to 320 nm), and UVC (200 to 280 nm), have distinct mutagenic properties. A hallmark of UVC and UVB mutagenesis is the high frequency of transition mutations at dipyrimidine sequences containing cytosine. In human skin cancers, about 35% of all mutations in the p53 gene are transitions at dipyrimidines within the sequence 5'-TCG and 5'-CCG, and these are localized at several mutational hot spots. Since 5'-CG sequences are methylated along the p53 coding sequence in human cells, these mutations may be derived from sunlight-induced pyrimidine dimers forming at sequences that contain 5-methylcytosine.[81] Cyclobutane pyrimidine dimers (CPDs) form preferentially at dipyrimidines containing 5-methylcytosine when cells are irradiated with UVB or sunlight. The mutational specificity of long-wave UVA (340 to 400 nm) is distinct from that of the shorter-wavelength UV and is characterized mainly by G-to-T transversions, presumably arising through mechanisms involving oxidized DNA bases.[82]

After damage to DNA strands, the p53 tumor suppressor protein undergoes phosphorylation and translocation to the nucleus and aids in DNA repair or causes apoptosis.[83] Excessive UV exposure overwhelms DNA repair mechanisms, leading to induction of p53 mutations (and to be specific, loss of Fas–FasL interaction). Keratinocytes carrying p53 mutations acquire a growth advantage by virtue of their increased resistance to apoptosis. Thus, resistance to cell death is a key event in photocarcinogenesis, and conversely, elimination of cells containing excessive UV-induced DNA damage is a key step in protecting against skin cancer development. Apoptosis-resistant keratinocytes undergo clonal expansion that eventually leads to formation of actinic keratoses and squamous cell carcinomas. The excellent review by Melnikova and Ananthaswamy[83] details some of the cellular and molecular mechanisms involved in initiation and progression of UV-induced skin cancer.

In this regard, studies have shown that use of sun-blocking agents or organic UV filters, such as those contained in sunscreen products, is capable of reducing

DNA damage as assessed by pyrimidine dimer formation, and thus may be a way of minimizing sun damage.[25,50,55,81,84,85] Sunscreens achieve this by filtering the UV rays that cause the damage.

Continued (chronic) exposure to UV radiation accelerates the aging process of the skin.[8–10,65–67] Wrinkling, elastosis, and pigment alterations (solar lentigines) are the most common consequences of long-term sun exposure.[86–90] Both UVA and UVB are instrumental in eliciting such damage; however, systematic studies of these effects following UVA and UVB exposure in the hairless mouse model demonstrated that UVA is more potent, due to its penetrating power.[8,91] Ultraviolet (UV) irradiation reduces production of type I procollagen, the major structural protein in human skin. This reduction is a key feature of the pathophysiology of premature skin aging (photoaging). Photoaging is the most common form of skin damage and is frequently associated with skin carcinoma. Transforming growth factor (TGF)-beta signaling is the major regulator in formation of collagen and fibrillogenesis associated with the aging and photoaging processes.[92–95] UV-induced downregulation of the TGF-betaRII gene, with attendant reduction of type I procollagen production, is therefore a critical molecular mechanism in the pathophysiology of photoaging. Other studies showed that physiological doses of UVB increase intracellular reactive oxygen species in keratinocytes, which upregulate TGF-beta biosynthesis and activation of TGF-beta through increased activity of matrix metalloproteinases (MMPs) 2 and 9, enzymes that degrade collagen matrix components.[93,94] In addition, application of high-SPF sunscreens to UV-damaged skin in hairless mice showed not only that further damage was expressed as accumulations of elastic fibers, loss of mature collagen, concomitant overproduction of new collagen, and greatly increased levels of glycosaminoglycans prevented, but also that the damage to skin was incurred before sunscreen application was repaired. This appeared as subepidermal reconstruction zones containing normal, mature collagen and a network of fine elastic fibers.[95]

Ultraviolet radiation exposure also results in suppression of both the local and systemic immune system.[4,16,25,68,96,97] Ultraviolet radiation acts on keratinocytes and lymphocytes in the epidermis, stimulating these cells to secrete prostaglandins,[97,98] cytokines, and interleukins.[4,25] Interleukins are one of a variety of biologic response modifiers capable of locally and systemically modulating the immune system.[100–104] Others are also modified by UV radiation, e.g., TNF-alpha.[16,100,105] Following UV exposure, changes in both functionality and distribution of immune cells also occur.[4,25,98–104] For example, after UV exposure, the compositions of local populations of skin cells change; that is, the number of skin Langerhans, Thy1+, and dendritic epidermal T cell populations decrease while T suppressor lymphocytes increase.[4,25] Similarly, UVR may also alter cellular proteins such that once self-antigens are perceived as foreign (photoantigenicity), and consequently precipitate an immune defense reaction.[4]

Suppression of the skin's immune system is one of the mechanisms by which solar ultraviolet radiation induces skin cancer growth.[16,101] Ulrich has provided a review of these mechanisms.[16] An interesting study showed that transfer of UV-induced skin cancers to normal mice resulted in rapid recognition of and destruction of these cancers, suggesting that a major component of UV-induced skin cancer is immunosuppression.[45] An interesting study by Vanbuskirk et al.[106] showed that depletion of CD-4 and CD-8 lymphocytes in mice led to development of UV-induced skin tumors. This likely is why immunosupressed patients are more susceptible to skin cancers. Systemically, suppression of immune surveillance mechanisms is characterized by the production of suppressor T cells and release of soluble immunosuppressive factors, such as TNF-alpha, interleukin-1 and interleukin-10, prostaglandins, and cis-urocanic acid.[4,25,98,99,107,108] It is profoundly evident that sunburned skin lacks the protective immunologic defenses (immunocompetence) present in normal skin.

Several studies show that high UVA protection contributes significantly to and is required for protection against UV-induced damage to the immune system in humans.[109–111] A study by Gueniche and Fourtanier[110] reported inhibition of contact hypersensitivity reactions by UV radiation using a hairless mouse strain (Skh/hr1) model traditionally used in photobiology research. They found that sunscreens containing filters with high UVA protection in addition to SPF 4 filters protected the mice from a contact hypersensitivity response to dinitrochlorobenzene. Schaefer et al.[111] studied the effects of UVR (UVA + UVB, or UVA alone) on local and systemic delayed type hypersensitivity (DTH) reactions in the skin of humans using a battery of recall antigens. He studied the potential of sunscreen filters to block the DTH response. Under conditions of exposure to UVA and UVB radiation, the sunscreen containing UVB filters alone did not provide both local and systemic immune protection, confirming that UVA significantly contributes to UV-induced immune suppression by effectively reducing the DTH response locally and systemically by 60 to 70%. Baron et al.,[109] in a study in humans, showed that an SPF 15 sunscreen containing two different levels of UVA protection — the protection factor A (PFA) of 10 for high-UVA protection and the PFA of 2 for low-UVA protection differed significantly in their immune protection factor (IP), with an IP of 50 for the high UVA and an IP of 15 for the low UVA — measured an *in vivo* contact hypersensitivity response to dinitrochlorobenzene.

The increased risk for development of skin carcinomas clearly depends on the pattern and spectrum of UV exposure as important contributing factors; most of the research has focused on action of UVB.[26,112] Both UVA and UVB are tumorigenic in animals.[113–119] There is an association between UVR and induction of cutaneous malignant melanoma in humans.[120] Carcinogenesis is a multistage process,[121] and in fact, several stages may be influenced by exposure to UV radiation, which is a complete carcinogen, in that it has tumor-promoting actions as well. While the exact mechanisms of action are unknown, scientific research now suggests a variety of genetic and epigenetic effects, some key to UVA radiation. Given both its prevalence and its penetrating power, UVA may conceivably result in damage to skin cells separate from that of UVB. Effects associated with UVA damage are due to oxidative stress mediated through generation of reactive oxygen species,[69,122,123] changes in cellular receptor binding,[124] alteration in phospholipid metabolism,[125] modification of the immune response,[101,126,127] and hot spot mutations in the mammalian genome.[128] In fact, the cellular effects attributed to UVA damage[129-131] are not unlike those of the classic phorbol ester tumor promoter, TPA.[132-135] Induction of melanocytic lesions with UVA wavelengths was shown experimentally in two *in vivo* animal models used to study melanoma, the *Xiphophorus* fish model and the opossum model, *Monodelphis domestica*.[136-138] In the *Xiphophorus* fish, the spectral regions contributing to the development of melanoma were in the long-wave UVA region.[136] A recent study by Agar et al.[139] found that in biopsies of human squamous cell carcinomas and solar keratoses, transformed stem cell keratinocytes isolated from the basal layer harbored more UVA-induced fingerprint mutations than UVB, while the transformed keratinocytes in the suprabasal layers displayed more UVB fingerprint mutations. This suggests that longer (UVA) wavelengths are a more important carcinogen in the lower stem cell compartment because UVA penetrates into the deeper layers of the skin.[139]

15.3 DO WE NEED SUNSCREENS?

Review of all the studies cited above led to the conclusion that there is a need for taking protective and preventive measures to guard against the damaging effects of the complete spectrum of UV light. There is also the continuous need for consumer education regarding the harmful effects of both short- and long-wave UV radiation. Sunburn protection measures should be taken early in life, preferably as children, and continued throughout life so as to prevent the cumulative effects of excessive sun exposure. The best methods of sunburn protection are avoidance during peak hours, protective clothing, including hats, sunglasses, and light-colored tightly woven garments, and the use of topical products containing chemical filters (sunscreens).[24,61,112-116,140-148] Sunscreens, often referred to as sunblocks, are designed specifically to interfere with the skin's normal response to solar radiation. They accomplish this by absorbing, reflecting, or scattering the harmful or burning rays of the sun. The greatest benefit of a sunscreen is achieved through a combination of several active ingredients in order to provide the widest range of sun protection, and they must be applied in adequate amounts as their efficacy is dose dependent. The active sunscreen ingredients, chosen based on their ability to absorb light at different wavelengths throughout the ultraviolet (UVB and UVA) range, act like a series of filters to remove or cancel out the most harmful and damaging rays of the sun. Other characteristics, such as water resistance, enhance or contribute to the overall function of the product.

Most sunscreens currently on the global market contain primarily UVB filters and afford varying degrees of effective sun protection beyond UVB (SPF values) into the UVA region (PFA values). In light of the findings in the literature regarding the potentially damaging effects of UVA, there is need for sunscreens possessing true broad-spectrum action with greater protection in the UVA wavelength regions. Countries with the most aggressive sun protection initiatives, such as Australia, recognize this.[140] Therefore, sunscreens must contain several filters that together provide complete, broad-spectrum UVA and UVB protection, and the protection should be balanced across the UVB and UVA range. In the U.S. there are numerous approved UVB filters that absorb in the region from 280 to 320 nm; many others are approved globally. However, there is only one approved UV filter in the U.S., Parsol 1789, also called avobenzone, which filters in a narrow region of UVA (340 to 400 nm); again, in other parts of the world many UVA filters are used to absorb much more broadly in this UVA region.[2,3] The reason for these issues is that in the U.S., sunscreens are considered drugs and require registration, and this is a costly process. However, without a doubt, U.S. consumers, compared with consumers in other parts of the world, are at greater risk of overexposure to certain damaging sun rays due to the unavailability of UV filters that optimally absorb in the short UVA region.

The U.S. Food and Drug Administration (FDA), in the final U.S. OTC sunscreen monograph, has recommended inclusion of the phrase "limiting sun exposure, wearing protective clothing, and using sunscreens may reduce the risks of skin aging, skin cancer, and other harmful effects of the sun" in sunscreen product labeling.[2] Additionally, it has indicated the use of sunscreens for children 6 months of age and older. Broad-spectrum claims for sunscreens are permitted wherein the sunscreen must include UVA filters to optimize protection against chronic photodamage and resultant photoaging, and most certainly against skin cancer in human subjects.[141–149]

Several key epidemiology studies support the protective effect of sunscreens. Nole and Johnson[150] show that using a sun exposure model predicts that over a lifetime a person will receive tens of thousands of minimal erythema doses worth of UVR through normal, daily, incidental exposure. Therefore, cumulative effect of even casual sun exposure over the years underscores the need for everyday basic UV radiation protection in which even low-level (SPF 4 to 10) sunscreens are shown to offer significant benefit. Analysis shows that daily protection from sun exposure can reduce lifetime exposure by 50% or more. Green et al.[148] reported a randomized controlled trial of an SPF 15 sunscreen with daily skin applications during a 5-year period where the number of squamous cell carcinomas diagnosed among 812 people was reduced by 39% (risk factor of 0.6). Holly et al.[61] reported another study among 1382 women showing that risk of all types of melanoma increased with increased severity and history of sunburns up to 12 years old and also increased with lack of sunscreen use. Stern et al.[144] reported that limiting sun exposure, beginning during childhood and adolescence, through the use of an SPF 15 sunscreen could reduce the lifetime risk of nonmelanoma skin cancers by as much as 78%. Gallagher et al.[145] reported in a pediatric study among over 300 schoolchildren in first through fourth grade that after using a broad-spectrum SPF 30 sunscreen during sun exposure for 3 years, significantly fewer acquired melanocytic nevi were identified on their skin; such nevi are known to be a strong risk factor in later development of melanoma.[145] Thompson et al.[146] and Naylor et al.[147] reported results in two independent studies showing that there was a reduction of solar keratoses (also known to be a risk factor in development of squamous cell carcinoma) by regular sunscreen use. Conclusions from these studies suggest that the use of sunscreens on a regular basis as early in life as possible can reduce the risk of skin cancer caused by exposure to UV radiation.

15.4 ORGANIZATIONS WITH POLICIES ON SUN PROTECTION MEASURES

Several key organizations have issued policies on sun protection measures incorporating specific recommendations for sunscreens and guidelines for prevention and treatment of dermatologic conditions related to excessive sun exposure. The Skin Cancer Foundation is the single most important organization focused completely on prevention using sun protection measures. On its website it is reported that "just one blistering sunburn in childhood is estimated to double the risk of getting melanoma later in life." The American Academy of Pediatrics reports that 80% of lifetime sun exposure occurs before 18 years of age. Such exposure in childhood, especially episodic high exposures, increases the risk of melanoma. The flip side of this is that if we can prevent sunburns in kids, skin cancer and death from skin cancer should decrease. Ninety percent of the nonmelanoma skin cancers are attributed to exposure to UV radiation, and it is the most common malignant neoplasm in the U.S. adult population. Chronic sun exposure without sunscreens can lead to wrinkles and skin thickening and thinning, and it weakens the skin elasticity, resulting in sagging cheeks, deeper facial wrinkles, and skin discoloration later in life. The policy statement reviews many of the other problems with UV exposure discussed above. The academy also recommends a prevention plan that includes use of broad-spectrum sunscreens even on children under 6 months of age in small exposed areas, along with the use of protective clothing and avoidance of direct sunlight. It indicates that these infants have less melanin than at any other time of life and are at greater risk of sunburn than older cohorts.

The Skin Cancer Foundation has the following prevention recommendations:

PROTECT YOURSELF AND YOUR FAMILY ALL YEAR ROUND

1. Seek the shade, especially during the sun's peak hours (10:00 A.M.–4:00 P.M.).
2. Wear a broad-spectrum sunscreen with a sun protection factor (SPF) of 15 or higher.
3. Cover up with clothing, especially a broad-brimmed hat and UV-blocking sunglasses.
4. Avoid tanning parlors and artificial tanning devices.
5. Keep newborns out of the sun. Sunscreens can be used on babies over the age of six months.
6. Teach children good sun-protective practices.
7. Examine your skin from head to toe once every month.
8. Have a professional examination annually.
9. Avoid tanning and especially — **do not burn!** One blistering sunburn doubles your risk of melanoma.

Several other key organizations provide policies and guidelines on sun protection measures. The American Academy of Pediatrics similarly has issued a policy statement on the hazards of UV light to children and has recommended preventive measures.[151] The American Academy of Dermatology has issued recommendations for a sunscreen to be SPF 15 or higher, along with having UVA protection in accordance with its position statement on UVA. Consistent among the Skin Cancer Foundation and the American Academy of Dermatology prevention guidelines mentioned above is the use of sunscreens with *complete* broad-spectrum activity as a key practice for the prevention of photodamage, which leads to photoaging and potentially to skin cancer. Also, several guidelines for caring for patients with dermatologic conditions resulting from excessive exposure to UV radiation are available on the academy's website (www.aadassociation.org). Specific guidelines from the American Academy of Dermatology are "Guidelines for Care of Photoaging and Photodamage," "Guidelines for the Care of Cutaneous Squamous Cell Carcinomas," "Guidelines for the Care of Actinic Keratoses," and "Guidelines for the Care of Basal Cell Carcinomas" (all authored by Dr. Lynn Drake et al. and available on the website). In these guidelines the authors indicate that chronic sun exposure is a major risk factor for all of these cutaneous diseases. These guidelines present the case that there is overwhelming epidemiologic and laboratory evidence that sun exposure and other sources of UV radiation play the major role in causing pigmentation, acitinic keratoses, leathery texture, scaling/ xerosis, sallowness, and telangiectasia, in addition to sunburn. The guidelines also indicate that there is equally compelling evidence that UV radiation exposure is associated with an increased incidence of benign, premalignant, and malignant skin neoplasms. They mention that individuals with fair skin and those living in areas with high exposure to solar radiation are at greater risk. They all consistently recommend use of broad-spectrum sunscreens.

Conclusions from these published reports are that the literature clearly supports the use of sunscreens on a regular basis, beginning as early in life as possible, to reduce the risk of photodamage and skin cancer caused by exposure to UV radiation. The preponderance of available evidence implicates exposure to UVA radiation as equally dangerous as UVB, since UVA is a causative agent in photoaging and a carcinogen in its own accord. Therefore, the broadest protection is advisable. This leads to some challenges, especially in the U.S., where few sunscreens that absorb in the UVA range with a significant extinction are available.

15.5 THE ELECTROMAGNETIC SPECTRUM

Shaath[152] has provided an excellent review of the chemistry and mechanisms of sunscreen action, which is paraphrased in this section. Human skin is constantly exposed to solar radiation each time the subject goes outside. The radiation emitted by the sun is a particular spectrum of electromagnetic radiation and differs from other forms of electromagnetic radiant energy by its specific energy (E), wavelength (w), or frequency (v). Electromagnetic radiation is energy that exhibits

TABLE 15.1
The Electromagnetic Spectrum of Radiant Energy

Short-Wavelength, High-Energy Region			Optical Region			Electrical Region	
Cosmic rays	Gamma rays	X-rays	UV	Visible	Infrared	Microwaves	Radiowaves

UVC	UVB	UVA II	UVA I
200–290 nm	290–320 nm	320–340 nm	340–400 nm

the following relationship:

$$E = h\nu$$

where E = energy (ergs), h = Plank's constant = 6.62×10^{-27} ergs/sec, and ν = frequency (cycles per second (cps) or Hertz (Hz)).

An important physical relationship between the frequency and wavelength that governs the properties of electromagnetic waves is dictated by the following equation:

$$\nu = c/w$$

where w is the wavelength (in cm or m) and c is the speed of light. By substituting the second equation into the first, one arrives at the most significant equation, describing the action of sunlight on humans. In this equation, energy and the wavelength have a reciprocal relationship, as shown below:

$$E = h(c/w)$$

The important take-away from this relationship is that as the wavelength increases, the energy associated with it decreases. Thus, the shorter-wavelength UVB region of the spectrum (290 to 320 nm) will have higher energies associated with it than the longer-wavelength UVA region (320 to 400 nm) (Table 15.1). The significance of this relationship between energy and wavelength was evident in the last section when the detrimental effects of UVA and UVB radiation on the skin were discussed.

Solar radiation in the form of optical rays that are visible to humans is only a very small segment of the total range of the electromagnetic waves, which can be divided into three general regions:

- Electrical rays, which include wireless, Hertzian, radiowaves, and microwaves. These rays are longer wavelengths (measured in meters), and the energies associated with them are much lower than the harmful UV rays.
- Optical rays, which are subdivided into infrared, visible, and UV rays.
- X-rays, gamma rays, and cosmic rays, which have short wavelengths and are obviously high in energy and extremely damaging rays.

In the optical region, the UV rays have the shortest wavelengths and the highest energies associated with them, sufficiently energetic to the cause photochemical reactions, resulting in damage to the skin. The visible part of the optical region comprises the familiar rainbow of colors of the spectrum (violet to red), which we can see every day. The longest-wavelength part of the optical region (hence, lower energy) is the infrared (IR) region, which is responsible for the heat effect. The UV rays, which have been demonstrated to be the most damaging to humans, can be further subdivided into three regions: the UVA, UVB, and UVC.

UVC, also called germicidal region, is the most damaging of the UV radiations because it has the highest energy associated with it (the lower wavelengths, 200 to 290 nm). Fortunately, the harmful rays of the UVC and of course those that are higher energy, namely, x-rays, gamma rays, and cosmic rays, are filtered by the stratospheric ozone layer; thus, none of these rays reach the Earth's surface to any significant degree. As can be seen, damage to the ozone layer will have unfortunate consequences for life on this planet. The depletion of this layer, for example, through continued use of chlorofluorocarbons (CFCs), represents a potential threat to humans. Shaath points out that artificial light sources (tanning salons, mercury arc, or welding arcs) do contain some UVC radiation and should be used only with adequate protection. The UVA and UVB regions that are not completely filtered out by the ozone layer are energetic enough to cause damage to the skin or hair and soft tissue.

The UVB rays, also called the burning or erythemal rays, with wavelengths ranging from 280 to 320 nm, are responsible for most of the immediate damage to the skin, resulting in erythema or sunburn, and subsequent long-term damage if the skin is left unprotected. Such damage has been detailed in the last section. The UVA region extends from 320 to 400 and is further subdivided into UVA I, from 340 to 400 nm, and UVA II, from 320 to 340 nm. UVA radiation, having longer wavelengths, will therefore penetrate deeper.

15.6 AVAILABLE SUNSCREENS AND CRITERIA FOR SELECTION

In the U.S., the recently approved Category I list of sunscreen chemicals lists 16 UV filters, 14 of which are organic UV filters (that absorb UV rays) and 2 inorganic particulates (that both absorb and reflect UV rays).[2] The ingredients, along with their approved percentage in the formulation, the maximum wavelength, and extinction coefficient, are shown in Table 15.2.

This list of UV filters, with the exception of avobenzone and the micronized forms of zinc oxide and titanium dioxide, reflects knowledge that dates back to the early 1970s. They are old technologies in UV filter design. Currently, a company wishing to introduce a new UV filter could submit a New Drug Application (NDA) to the U.S. Food and Drug Administration (FDA). Such a

TABLE 15.2
FDA-Approved U.S. OTC Sunscreens[2]

Sunscreen	Maximum Allowable Dose (%)	Spectral $_{max}$	Extinction Coefficient
Organic Filters			
UVB			
Cinoxate	3	305	11,000
Ensulizole	4	310	26,000
Homosalate	15	306	4300
Octocrylene	10	303	12,600
Ocinoxate	7.5	310	23,300
Octisalate	5	307	4900
Padimate-O	8	307	27,300
PABA (paraminobenzoic acid)	15	290	14,000
Trolamine salicylate	12	298	3000
UVB/partial UVA			
Dioxybenzone	3	327	10,440
Meradimate	5	336	5600
Oxybenzone	6	325	9400
Sulisobenzone	10	324	8400
UVA I			
Avobenzone	3	357	30,500
UVA II			
None			
Inorganic Particulates			
Zinc oxide	25	Broad spectrum	
Titanium dioxide	25	Broad spectrum	

Source: From Shaath, N., Ed., *The Chemistry of Sunscreens in Sunscreens*, 3rd ed., Taylor & Francis, New York, 2005.

submission requires full preclinical toxicology studies, pharmacokinetic (absorption and metabolism) studies in humans, clinical efficacy and long-term safety studies, and full carboxymethyl cellulose (CMC) sections that are costly and time-consuming to prepare, and the NDA covers only *one* formulation. Therefore, each formulation will require a new NDA submission. Alternatively, companies could amend the monograph to include an additional sunscreen, perhaps through a Time and Extent Application, based on the safety profile of a sunscreen marketed outside the U.S. and monitored through pharmacovigilance for at least 5 years in defined marketed combination formulations with other specific UV filters. Unlike treatment pharmaceuticals, for which the return on investment may be in the hundreds of millions of dollars, sunscreen chemicals will not deliver the same level of returns to the companies producing them because their sale is a seasonal business. The cost to obtain an NDA is estimated to be on the order of $100 million with a waiting period exceeding many years to conduct all the toxicology and human safety studies. The waiting period reduces the patent coverage period; however, sometimes 3 to 5 years' exclusivity to market the new sunscreen product can be provided by the FDA if the patent period is about to expire. These limitations are not actionable for most manufacturers embarking on research designed to produce new and innovative UV filters for the U.S. market.

Outside the U.S. there are many other available sunscreens that are more powerful; some of these are tinasorb and mexoryl that absorb strongly in the UVA II region. Tuchinda et al.[153] have published the latest review of emerging sunscreen technologies and their benefits. None of the sunscreens in Table 15.2 absorb to any appreciable extent in this region. Tinasorb has been submitted as a Time and Extent Application and is currently going through the regulatory process in the U.S. for approval in a few years. Table 15.3 displays some of the

TABLE 15.3
New Ultraviolet Filters Not Approved in the U.S.

Type	INCI Name	Trade Name	Spectral max	Approval Status
UVB				
	EHT	Univul T 150	314	Europe, TEA application U.S.
	DBT	Uvasorb HEB	312	Europe
	BMP	Parsol SLX	312	Europe
UVA II				
	TDSA	Mexoryl SX	345	Europe Japan, NDA application?
	DPDI	Neo Heliopan AP	334	Europe
	DHHB	Univul A Plus	354	Europe
UVA and UVB				
	DTS	Mexoryl XL	303 and 341	Europe, Japan, TEA application U.S.
	MBBT	Tinosorb M	305 and 360	Europe, Australia, TEA application U.S.
	BEMT	Tinosorb S	310 and 343	Europe, TEA application U.S.

Source: Tuchinda, C. et al., *Dermatol. Clin.*, 24, 105–117, 2006.[153]

filters approved outside the U.S. and the maximum wavelength at which they absorb UV light. Most of these filters possess a very high extinction coefficient and are very broad and, in fact, absorb at two different wavelengths. Sunscreens containing filters that absorb in the UVA I and II regions appear to be very effective in prevention of polymorphic light eruptions in photosensitive patients and in those patients with lupus erythematosis.[153]

15.6.1 IMPORTANCE OF THE EXTINCTION COEFFICIENT

Shaath[152] provided an excellent premise on the importance of the extinction coefficient of sunscreens, which is summarized herein. Two parameters determine the effectiveness of a sunscreen — the wavelength covered and the numerical size of the extinction coefficient. Therefore, chemicals with a high extinction coefficient are more efficient in absorbing the energy of the harmful UV radiation than chemicals with a lower extinction coefficient. However, if only a part of the spectrum of harmful wavelengths is absorbed, UV radiation may still be harmful to soft tissue.

As reviewed by Shaath, electronic transitions for any compound may be characterized as symmetry allowed or symmetry forbidden; this symmetry depends on the spacial ease of delocalization of electrons in the compound. Symmetry-allowed transitions generally have high extinction coefficients, and symmetry-forbidden transitions have lower extinction coefficients. One can therefore theoretically arrive at a reasonable idea of the extinction coefficients for sunscreen chemicals by examining both the spatial requirements and the electronic transitions responsible for the observed UV spectrum. The number of double bonds and the extent of resonance delocalization in a molecule are the critical factors that give a clear indication as to the maximum wavelength and a qualitative prediction of the extinction coefficient.

The more efficient the electron delocalization in a molecule, the higher its extinction coefficient. Shaath[152] provides a good example by comparing padimate-O with homosalate. In padimate-O, the two substituents on the benzene ring are in a para relation, whereas the two substituents in the homosalate are in a sterically hindered ortho relation. In ortho-disubstituted aromatic compounds, the two groups are close to one another, causing a deviation from planarity. The slightest deviation from coplanarity will significantly reduce resonance delocalization. This results in a lower extinction coefficient for homosalate (= 4300) than for padimate-O (= 27,300). Increased conjugation of double bonds, leading to more efficient resonance delocalization, will also yield higher extinction coefficients. Shaath[152] compares the extinction coefficient of ethylene, which is 15,000, to that of 1,3-butadiene (21,000) and that of 1,3,5-hexatriene (35,000), and for the highly conjugated molecule, B-carotene, it is 152,000. The new UV filters originating in Europe have multiple chromophores, and therefore increased conjugation, resulting in extinction coefficients exceeding 40,000. Some of these are listed in Table 15.3.

15.6.2 THE ULTIMATE UV FILTER

The ultimate sunscreen should, according to Shaath,[152] ideally encompases the following characteristics:

- It should absorb the harmful UV radiation in the region of 280 to 400 nm. Broad-spectrum protection is generally not possible by using a single sunscreen filter; the use of two or more sunscreens that filter the 280- to 320-nm (UVB region) and the 320- to 400-nm (UVA region) radiation may be necessary.
- The individual filters should possess high molar extinction coefficients at their maximum wavelength. Values exceeding 25,000 would be best. This would provide the maximum possible protection for the dose of sunscreens used in the formulations. The new molecules currently designed in Europe with multiple chromophores have unusually high extinction coefficients.
- It should have excellent photostability and be photochemically inert. The lead UVA sunscreen in the U.S. — avobenzone — is known to be photounstable in most formulations. If isomerization such as cis-trans or keto-enol is possible in the molecule, then the degradation quantum yields should be low, indicating that isomerization is reversible. Inorganic particulates are commercially produced with the least amount of photochemical reactivity possible. Therefore, the type of mineral, the specific coating, and the type of dispersant must be carefully selected and studied in the formulation.
- The UV filters should have good solubility in emollients selected. Solid sunscreens such as the benzophenones, avobenzone, and camphor derivatives require special techniques and excipients to solubilize in formulations and ensure that they do not crystallize out on the skin. To ensure the stability of the sunscreen formulation, the UV filter must remain dissolved and uniform throughout the formulation for an acceptable shelf-life and coverage on the skin. The maximum wavelength and the molar extinction coefficient should not be affected by solvents and excipients.
- For water-resistant formulations, the sunscreen should be for the most part insoluble in water. Water-soluble sunscreens will have a role to play in the sunscreen formulations, such as in hair preparations or when boosting the SPF is required.
- It should not be irritating to skin and eyes, comedogenic, sensitizing, or phototoxic.
- It should be compatible with cosmetic vehicles and ingredients, as well as with packaging material, and easy to formulate and manufacture and have patent protection in the various filter combinations.
- UV filters constitute a significant portion of the cosmetic formulation, e.g., sometimes as much as 15% of the formula, and this may impart

moisturizing advantages. However, these filters should not discolor the skin or clothing or produce off-odors when applied to the skin or hair.

- The UV filter substance should be available isometrically pure, be chemically stable during long-term storage, and be chemically inert to other cosmetic ingredients.
- The ideal sunscreen should be cost-effective to use due to the high doses that must be used to produce high efficacy.
- Ultimately, the UV filter should be approved worldwide by the official regulatory agencies with the fewest restrictions on levels used or combinations.

15.7 FORMULAE DEVELOPMENT

Different types of sunscreen formulations are required for color cosmetics, skin care products, lip care, and hair care products. The following section reviews technical requirements for incorporation of sunscreens into formulations for these classes of products and then provides examples of finished formulations for cosmetic and skin and hair care sunscreen products.

15.7.1 FILM-FORMING PROPERTIES

The key step in providing an adequate SPF and UVA PFA protection is the film-forming characteristics of the sunscreen when applied to the skin surface, especially after the water has evaporated. This area is not particularly well studied, however. After the topical product is applied, the water evaporates fairly quickly and the material remaining behind will go through one or more phase changes. The principle of film formation is based on adherence of this oily end product to the semisolid surface — the skin.

Dahms characterizes this in his review, which is briefly discussed herein.[154] As stated above, spreadability is concerned with adhesion forces between two contacting phases — an oily material and a substrate material. Adhesion is defined in terms of the work or energy required to separate unit area of the interface between two phases to create two separate interfaces of each of the phases with a common external medium, e.g., water or air. This is expressed in terms of the work of adhesion.

$$WA = \gamma_{FA} + \gamma_{OA} - \gamma_{FO} \quad \text{Dupré equation} \quad (15.1)$$

Here the γ values represent the relevant surface or interfacial tension, e.g., keratin is the proteinaceous adhesion surface, W_A, where keratin fiber is F, A is the air, and O is the oily liquid emulsion.

When one of the two contacting phases is a liquid, as in the case of an oily droplet at skin temperature, the physical picture becomes much simpler to visualize

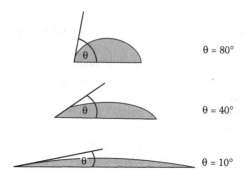

$\theta = 80°$

$\theta = 40°$

$\theta = 10°$

FIGURE 15.1 Effect of contact angle size on spreading of an oil droplet on a solid surface.

and evaluate (Figure 15.1). Resolving horizontal forces (at equilibrium), one has Young's equation:

$$\gamma_{FA} = \gamma_{FO} + \gamma_{OA} \cos \Theta$$

and hence the Young-Dupré equation,

$$WA = \gamma_{OA} (1 + \cos \Theta) \tag{15.2}$$

where Θ is the contact angle the liquid makes with the solid. Young's equation is of fundamental significance, as it allows evaluation of the degree of adhesion in terms of measurable parameters, γ_{OA} and Θ.

To facilitate wetting or adhesion of oil by increasing WA, one should try to reduce γ_{OA} and decrease Θ, i.e., decreasing the contact angle causes wetting of the oily phase. This action represents the well-known role of a wetting agent (Figure 15.1).

Films are formed on the skin by sunscreen emulsions in two steps. For the first, the emulsion is spread over the skin, forming a pure emulsion film. In the second step, the emulsion is physically rubbed further into the skin. The aqueous phase evaporates and the oil film is massaged into the skin. The underlying mechanisms are different for an O/W emulsion than for a W/O emulsion. When a W/O emulsion is applied, it has a continuous external oil phase that first comes in contact with the skin. Thus, it is really the spreading and penetration of the oil phase that dictates the characteristics of the film formed. Dahms indicates that except for silicone emulsifiers, W/O emulsifiers are not capable of reducing the interfacial tension, γ_{OA}. Accordingly, spreading and penetration of the sunscreen can only take place as a result of interfacial tension forces between the sunscreen oil phase and the skin. Dahms suggests that the general rule is that high affinity of the liquid oil phase to the solid phase leads to high spreadability; therefore, only emulsifiers with high affinity for skin are likely to reduce γ_{FO} to a sufficient degree. For this purpose, emulsifiers with hydrophilic amino-functional head groups can be employed. According to Dahms, alkyl-modified PVP derivatives and hydrophobic amino-functional silicones work best. Such compounds form a bridge between the oil phase and the skin, thereby lowering the interfacial tension between the skin and the sunscreen oil phase, permitting spreading ease.

Although the spreading of the oil phase is the basic prerequisite for film formation, the rheology of the oil phase plays a critical role in the formation of a film with a sufficient thickness on the skin. According to Dahms, the general rule is that for higher photoprotection, the film must have a corresponding greater thickness. Therefore, it becomes clear that the viscosity of the film former must also be high to achieve this. However, thicker films with higher viscosity are in direct conflict with spreadability ease of the oil phase. Viscoelasticity therefore comes into play in this case and represents a compromise. The appropriate viscoelastic properties of the oil phase can be achieved by using waxes (according to Dahms[154]). These impart a high viscosity at rest and a low viscosity during spreading. For achieving the required viscoelasticity of the photoprotective film, γ_{FO}, the surface tension between skin and oil or liquid is the only variable available to manipulate to deliver sufficient spreading; hence, the selection of the emulsifier system plays a critical role because these systems help manipulate this variable.

The process of film formation from an O/W emulsion is much more complex than that from a W/O emulsion and is described very nicely by Dahms.[154] During spreading of an O/W emulsion, there is no film formation by the oily photoprotective phase at this stage. This happens after the water evaporates and the critical phase volume is exceeded. After this occurs, Dahms reviews the two things that can happen: either the emulsion breaks and the oil droplets coalesce rapidly to form a homogeneous film with further rubbing, or the emulsion is converted into a single-phase microemulsion wherein the remaining amount of water is present in a stored form. If the microemulsion is further distributed on the surface, it behaves like a W/O emulsion. The viscosity and hence rheological properties of the emulsion are important during distribution on the skin. However, film formation due to spreading begins after the free water evaporates. If some of the water is retained and the microemulsion dominates, with slow evaporation of water, a liquid crystalline structure develops that is easily spreadable and forms a good film as the surface tension, γ_{FO}, drops to zero between that structure and the skin.

Whereas in W/O emulsions the required viscelasticity of the oil phase is regulated by waxes, in most O/W sunscreen emulsions the viscosity is regulated by means of the mixed emulsifier system used; a few are suggested by Dahms in Table 15.4. This is an experimental process to optimize these emulsifiers. These systems will use both micelle-forming hydrophilic emulsifiers and lipophilic coemulsifiers. The gel structure of the sunscreen containing the mixed-emulsifier system can be stabilized by increasing the concentration of the mixed emulsifiers. Hydrocolloids are added to increase the critical temperature above which the emulsion collapses. Only a select few will stabilize the emulsion at higher temperatures and also promote acceptable film formation. To promote film formation, the hydrocolloid must first form a bridging layer between the skin and the sunscreen film with rubbing. Hydrocolloids with amino-functional groups appear to work most effectively. Cross-polymers with carbomers and

TABLE 15.4
Hydrophilic Surfactants and Coemulsifiers That Form Combination Gel Networks as Suggested by Dahms[154]

Hydrophilic Surfactants	Coemulsifiers
Lecithin	Saturated fatty acids (myristic, palmitic, stearic, etc.)
Acyl lactylates	Saturated solid fatty alchohols
Cetyl sulfates and phosphates	Glycerol monostearates
Alkyl polyglycosides	Solid sorbitane esters
PEG surfactants (HLB > 7)	Solid polyglycerine esters
Sugar ester	Solid methyl glucoside esters
Cationic surfactants	Cholesterol, ceramides, etc.

pemulen in combination with linear polymers, like xanthan gum and PVP, also as work effectively.

One of the key issues with sunscreens regards pigment dispersions. With increased rubbing, flocculation occurs on the skin that produces whitening. This is due to the shear forces induced by continued rub in. Continued rubbing can push the oil phase into the pores, thus enriching the concentration of pigment on the surface. If the critical phase volume is approached, then irreversible flocculation, and therefore whitening, occurs. In order to form the appropriate uniform film, micropigments must be dispersed in a manner resistant to shear forces. As you can see, the dispersing agent must be anchored to the pigment surface as well as have good affinity for the skin, so that a homogeneous layer is formed that completely absorbs and reflects UV light. Dahms indicates that PVP and their alkyl-substituted derivatives are good dispersing agents fulfilling these criteria.

15.7.2 GENERAL FORMULA TYPES

The most popular type of vehicle used for sunscreens is the emulsion because it offers the broadest formulation advantages and versatility. If the desire of the formulator is the highest SPF possible at the lowest possible cost, then the emulsion vehicle is the vehicle of choice. Klein and Palefsky[155] reported in their review a synopsis on why emulsions are the best vehicle. They enumerated the factors that lead to consistently high SPFs:

- Uniform sunscreen film
- Thick sunscreen film
- Nontransparent sunscreen film
- Minimum ingredient interaction with the sunscreen's active agent

They[155] report that emulsions exhibit good performance in each of these important areas. Emulsions facilitate incorporation of sunscreen active agents, which are usually oils that can be easily emulsified. Emulsions can be prepared that contain a large percentage of water, making them the more cost-effective vehicle. It is well known that emulsions are cosmetically desirable vehicles that can give the skin a smooth, silky feel without being greasy and can accommodate a wide variety of raw materials; thus, you can tailor the formulation to suit your needs. On the negative side, it is also well known that cosmetic emulsions are thermodynamically unstable (with the exception of spontaneously forming micro-emulsions). Thus, they will always eventually separate. Additionally, emulsions present a perfect medium for microbial contamination and require preservatives.

Emulsions are broadly classified in two categories: oil in water (O/W) and water in oil (W/O). By far, the O/W emulsions are more popular vehicles, but for sunscreen formulations, it is generally known that W/O emulsions are much better vehicles.[155] The reason for this is that W/O emulsions are by design very water resistant and they provide greater efficacy (a higher SPF) for the same concentration of sunscreen activities than O/W emulsions. However, water resistance is not necessary for many formulation types containing sunscreens, like makeups offering daily protection from incidental UV light. Klein and Palefsky offer several explanations for the higher efficacy of W/O emulsions.[155] Since most sunscreens are soluble in the oil phase, in W/O emulsions the oil phase is continuous, and thus when they are applied to the skin, there is no need for agglomeration to occur (as there is with O/W emulsions); as a result, a very uniform sunscreen film is produced during spreading, along with a high SPF.

Another alternate formulation approach discussed by Klein and Palefsky is the use of emulsifiers that promote the formation of liquid crystals.[155] It has been known for many years that emulsions are often stabilized by liquid crystals. Generally, these liquid crystals are lamellar in structure and either form a gel network in the external phase or surround the oil droplets as layers (known to cosmetic chemists as the onion skin effect). In both cases, the liquid crystal structure reduces the tendency to coalesce because of the high viscosity of the lamellar structure, and this facilitates high emulsion stability. Another advantage is that such emulsions are not very hydrophilic and provide water-resistant characteristics for sunscreen formulations. Their lipoidal characteristics facilitate adhesion to the hydrophobic, lipidoidal skin surface, and thus enable formation of a most uniform film.

Oils are generally well-accepted, historic sunscreen vehicles that are most easily formulated. Klein and Palefsky[155] enumerate other benefits. For example, there is only one phase, so they have excellent product stability. Because most sunscreen active agents are lipoidal in nature, they are soluble in the oils employed; because of this, manufacturing processes are more straightforward than the manufacture of emulsions, and in fact, most can even be prepared at room temperature. Oils are easy to apply to the skin, spreading quickly and uniformly to cover a large surface area. Unfortunately, as Klein and Palefsky point out, there are a variety of negatives associated with sunscreen oils. These authors indicate that although they have excellent spreadability, this often results in a very thin, transparent sunscreen film, which will have a lower SPF. It is well known that sunscreen oils yield the poorest SPF performance of any vehicle. Klein and Palefsky explain their poor performance by looking at the interactions between the sunscreen (nonpolar esters) and the very nonpolar oils' vehicles. Nonpolar oils, such as mineral oil, can cause the position of the UV curves to shift to shorter wavelengths, <290 nm, limiting the benefit of the sunscreen *from the claimed labeled SPF perspective.* Klein and Palefsky attribute this shift to stabilization of the ground state by the nonpolar vehicle. Another issue is the spreading ability of the emollients, which can play a major role in determining the SPF of the finished formula; even though the film is uniform, it is too thin. Lastly, the solubility parameter (a measure of stickiness/cohesiveness) determines orientation of the sunscreen within oil (or oil phase of an emulsion). An additional negative for oils relates to limitations in the packaging to minimize interactions and cost, since in this anyhdrous oil system there is no water to lower the cost of expensive raw materials. Sunscreen oils are therefore one of the most expensive systems found.

Various other types of formulations, such as gels, are discussed elsewhere (Klein and Palefsky[155]) and are gaining popularity, but suffer from some of the same issues regarding achieving high SPFs and cost.

Many of the principles described above are applied to the formulations now described below for various cosmetic product applications.

15.7.3 COLOR COSMETICS

Chemists must bear in mind that different skin types will require the use of different sunscreens. There must be adequate tests done on various skin types to determine the optimal blend of sunscreens to be used for all skin types. For example, Formula 1 is a sunscreen foundation with great spreadability and can

FORMULA 1

Ingredients	% Weight
Water	QS
Iron oxides	2.0
Titanium dioxide (USP)	5
Magnesium oxide	1
Zirconium oxide	3
Zinc oxide	6
Talc	4
Titanium dioxide	8
Stearic acid	3
Propylene glycol monostearate	2.5
Lanolin alcohols	1.5
Sorbitan sesquioleate	0.75
Preservatives	As needed
Isopropyl myristate	7
Sodium carboxymethyl cellulose	0.12
Triethanolamine	1.5

be prepared very easily. The use of titanium dioxide, magnesium oxide, zirconium oxide, zinc oxide, and talc will produce "ashiness" on dark skin types. The solution will be to use a formulation similar to Formula 2.

FORMULA 2

Ingredients	% Weight
Water	QS
Nanofine red iron oxides	2.0
Micronized titanium dioxide (USP)	15
Silica	1
Lithium stearate	3
Mica	6
Isostearic acid	1
Stearic acid	3
Propylene glycol monostearate	2.5
Lanolin alcohols	1.5
Sorbitan sesquioleate	0.75
Preservatives	As needed
Isopropyl myristate	7
Sodium carboxymethyl cellulose	0.12
Triethanolamine	1.5

The chalkiness or ashiness is eliminated by using a translucent mica, titanium dioxide, and iron oxides. The use of the lithium stearate helps the powders adhere to the skin. The SPF of approximately 17 is achieved by the use of the microfine titanium dioxide. Formulating pigmented emulsions such as these with one sunscreen is advantageous in that it has a high photostability profile. The downside can be its hydrophobic effect, which may be unstable for the length of a drug stability protocol. In U.S. Patent 5,585,090, Yshioka et al. showed that combining a metal oxide flake and an ultraviolet absorbent-encapsulated polymer resin enhanced SPF efficacy, and also required smaller amounts of both components in formulations. Examples of the polymer resins include vinyl polymers, acrylic resins, polystyrenes, and some others. The ultraviolet resins include salicylic acid, benzophenone derivatives, and aminobenzoic acid derivatives. The metal oxides include zinc oxide, titanium dioxides, and zirconium oxides.

15.7.4 SKIN CARE

Choosing the right vehicle for sunscreens is as important as the effectiveness of the sunscreen system chosen. Sunscreen spray milks contain sunscreens that are water soluble and easily washed off the skin. Carlotti et al.[156] prepared O/W microemulsions using cyclomethicone, menthol, stearyl methicone, and ethylhexyl methoxycinnamate as the sunscreen and surfactant blends. Various surfactants/lipids/sunscreen were characterized by microscopy and laser light scattering. Formula 3 showed the most stable O/W microemulsions that were

---

FORMULA 3[157]

Ingredients	% Weight
Surfactant/lipid	70:30
1:2 hexanediol	30.0
Water	62.11
Decylpolyglucose	2.58
Soya lecithin	2.31
Cyclomethicone	.54
Ethanol	0.25
C12-15 alkyl benzoate	1.01
Ethylhexyl methoxycinnamate	1.2

---

waterproof and had great humectancy. Since microemulsions are one-phase systems, there is no risk of the oil-soluble sunscreens not being adsorbed onto the skin.

Fomulating sun care products means effectively positioning the sun filter to absorb or scatter UV rays. Conventional O/W vehicles fall short in that the sunscreens (mainly lipophilic) are found in the internal phase, as stated previously. W/O vehicles are more effective; that is, sunscreens are more effective at leaving the sunscreen in the external phase and they are more water resistant. The high concentration of the lipophilics, though, means a higher cost of the formula. There are two factors that determine whether an emulsion will be O/W or W/O: (1) phase volume and (2) surfactant used. Formulators can reduce the cost problem by incorporating a polymeric surfactant such as PEG-30 dipolyhydroxystearate. The cost advantage of using this surfactant is that it allows formulating W/O close to the cost of O/W formulations.[158] The incorporation of inorganic sunscreens into the formula is also enhanced due to the dispersing property of the surfactant.

15.7.5 LIP CARE

The lips are rarely seen as an area that needs protection (lips will not tan, no melanin is present here), but lips will burn. As a mucous membrane, lips need to be protected from dehydration as well as from UV. The formulation that will work best on the lips is the anhydrous type, since these types are not easily washed off by saliva and moisture. Formula 4 is a typical SPF lip protectant. Note that the use of dimethicone as a skin protectant also makes the product a

FORMULA 4

Ingredients	% Weight
Petrolatum	35
Carnauba	5
Octyl dodecyl steoryl stearate	15
Paraffin	8
Isopropyl lanolate	6
Dimethicone (USP)	2.00
Castor oil	15.00
Benzophenone-3	3.0
Ethylhexyl methoxycinnamate	7.0
Antioxidants	QS

drug that must follow the FDA's skin protectant monograph.[159] Inorganic sunscreens are typically not used since a minimal SPF of 15 is sufficient and inorganics at high concentrations, above 3%, will show a white residue.

15.7.6 HAIR CARE

Since most sunscreens are not substantive, their use in hair care products is limited. Hair is a nonliving structure. It mainly consists of the following ingredients:[160]

Proteins	91%
Lipids	4.0%
Sulfur (protein bound)	4.7%
Melanin	4.0%
Sugar	1.0%
Ash	0.5%
Zinc	200 ppm

Hair is susceptible to damage by many agents, including sunlight, wind, air pollutants, and chlorine in swimming pools. Although nonliving, these agents can cause damage to the hair fiber, and this must be prevented at great expense, especially treated or relaxed hair. Croda Corporation conducted research on the photoprotection of relaxed hair, and their findings showed irreversible damage caused by UV, mainly observing the change in tryptophan intensity. The use of anionic polymers polyquaternium 59 and butylene glycol significantly increased the sun protection of the hair. Formula 5 is a sunscreen spray formulated especially for the hair. This formula does not contain sunscreens, and the product is not an OTC drug, but a cosmetic, and will not require any OTC testing as long as the claims are carefully thought out.

FORMULA 5

Ingredients	% Weight
Water	90
Butylene glycol (and) polyquaternium 59	2
Preservatives	QS
Hydrolyzed keratin	1
Dimethicone copolyo	15

15.8 EFFICACY TESTING OF SUNSCREENS

As efficacy testing is mandatory, this section shall consider efficacy testing models for different wavelengths of UV light. The methodology is designed for two general categories: UVA ranges from 320 to 400 nm and UVB from 290 to 320 nm. A comprehensive review of sunscreen testing is provided by Gabard[161] and in the final OTC sunscreen U.S. federal monograph.[2]

The effectiveness of a sunscreen depends on many parameters, described earlier. The absorption spectrum of the sunscreen depicts the region of the radiation spectrum where the sunscreen absorbs light. The damaging wavelengths are in the region of 290 to 400 nm. No sunscreen absorbs throughout this entire region. The variety of sunscreens available offer specific absorption characteristics and can be combined to provide the appropriate SPF and UVA protection. The size of the extinction coefficient of the filter, along with the dose, determines the amount of protection provided over time in the sun.

15.8.1 SPF Testing

The sun protection factor measures the length of time a product protects against erythema or skin reddening from UVB, compared to how long the skin takes to redden without protection. If it takes 30 min without protection to begin reddening, using an SPF 15 sunscreen theoretically prevents reddening 15 times longer — about 5 h. Hence,

$$SPF = \frac{SPF = \text{Minimal erythemal dose (protected with sunscreen)}}{\text{Minimal erythemal dose (unprotected skin)}}$$

Minimal erythemal dose (MED) is the least amount of UV radiation that will illicit redness of the skin. This MED number varies from person to person.

The sunscreens available, except zinc oxide, protect from UVB radiation; zinc oxide is a broad-spectrum UV protectant that offers both UVA and UVB protection, but is more effective in the UVB region. Table 15.5 shows some sunscreens and their UV effectiveness.

TABLE 15.5
Sunscreen Effectiveness in the UVA and
UVB Regions

Sunscreen	UVA	UVB
Ethylhexyl methoxycinnamate	+	+
Oxybenzone	+	+
Homosalate	+	+
Avobenzone	+	+
Octyl salicylate	+	+
Zinc oxide	+	++
Titanium dioxide	+	++

SPF effectiveness is determined by radiating the skin of human panelists with a solar ultraviolet simulator. Five methods are currently available according to the intended market in which the SPF product is to be sold:

FDA (U.S.)[2]
COLIPA (EU)
JCCS (Japan)[162]
Australian/New Zealand
ICH (International Harmonized Method)

When choosing human subjects for SPF efficacy, the clinical labs must use the following inclusion and exclusion criteria:

- Skin types I (always burns easily, never tans), II (always burns easily, tans minimally), and III (burns moderately, tans gradually) must be included. Male or female must be included. Ages are usually 18 through 70 years. Signed consent form must be obtained and persons must be in good health.
- Exclusions: Known allergy to sunscreens, UV light, and cosmetics. Any preexisting conditions that could interfere with the test. Pregnant or nursing women, chronic medication dependence, etc.
- The total number of panelists should be no more than 25 human subjects; at least 20 subjects must have valid data.
- Two different SPF determinations are made, called static and water resistant.

15.8.1.1 Static SPF Method (U.S. Regulations)

The static SPF method in accordance with 21 CFR Part 352 Subpart D[2] is run in the following way. One week prior to the start of the study, at least 20 subjects are evaluated for their MED for unprotected skin using this method with an untreated site. On day 1, the investigational drug and reference standard are applied to test sites on the back following a computer-generated randomization scheme. A single topical application (2 mg/cm^2) is applied to an area (~60 cm^2) on the back of each subject. The total dose is 120 mg applied. An untreated control is placed as well. After 15 min, the treated sites are subdivided into seven sites and the untreated sites are subdivided into five sites, each about 1 cm^2 in area, all of which are exposed to increasing doses of UVR. The treated sites are exposed to increasing doses of radiation based on their expected SPFs. The untreated sites are exposed to increasing doses of UVR to determine each subject's inherent MED. The doses selected are a geometric series represented by 1.25^n, where each exposure is 25% greater than the previous one. These provide secondary confirmation values for the MED for unprotected skin that are used to calculate the SPF. Twenty-two to 24 h after irradiation (day 2), all sites are evaluated for edema and erythema. Erythema is graded on a five-point scale of 0, 0.5, 1, 2, and 3. The amount of erythema-effective energy that produces a grade of 1 is used as the MED. A standard 8% homosalate sunscreen is included in the test, which is prepared according to the monograph and must have an SPF of 4 for the test to be valid.[2]

15.8.1.1.1 Calculations and Lamp Characteristics

The SPF can be calculated with a simple formula that depends on a measurement termed the minimal erythema dose (MED). This is the dose of UV irradiation that produces minimal perceptible erythema on the skin 22 to 24 hours after exposure. The SPF is a ratio of the UV dosing time to produce MED on sunscreen-treated skin vs. the dosing time needed to produce MED in untreated skin. The longer the UV exposure before producing erythema, the higher the SPF, but remember that SPF reflects protection against UVB predominantly.

The typical light source for SPF testing is the solar simulator lamp, which emits a spectrum of radiation similar to terrestrial sunlight (within limitations). The exposure dose is expressed in joules per square meter, as show in Equation 15.3:

$$\text{Dose (J/m}^2) = \text{irradiance (W/m}^2) \times \text{time (sec)} \qquad (15.3)$$

$$\text{SPF} = \frac{\text{MED of protected skin}}{\text{MED of unprotected skin}} \qquad (15.4)$$

MED is the minimal erythemal dose of radiation required to produce a barely visible erythema on the site. The irradiance is a constant, and the radiation flow from the lamp is in watts per meter square. The dose of radiation is in joules per meter square. Time of exposure is therefore the variable controlled and measured during the study.

The choice of lamp is an important determinant of the SPF value obtained. Lamps that emit predominantly UVB light will yield a lower SPF value than a lamp that emits predominantly UVA. To minimize variability caused by different light sources, regulatory agencies define specifications for solar simulators.

For example, the U.S. FDA (21 CFR Part 352[163]) requires solar simulations to be filtered so that they provide a continuous emission spectrum from 190 to 320 nm, similar to sunlight at sea level with the sun at a zenith angle of 10°. The simulator has less than 1% of its total energy output contributed by nonsolar wavelengths shorter than 290 nm, and it has not more than % of its total energy output contributed by wavelengths over 400 nm.

Typically, a 1000-W xenon arc solar simulator lamp is suitable with appropriate filters.

15.8.1.2 Water-Resistant SPF Method

This SPF method is also according to 21 CFR Part 352 Subpart D[2] and is a variation of the static method that involves exposure of sunscreen-treated skin to water soaking for a period, followed by determination of SPF as above. Each of at least 20 subjects completed a screening visit within 1 week prior to the start of the study, which included determination of the minimal erythemal dose (MED) for his or her own skin. The quantity of erythema-effective energy that produced a score of 1 was the MED used to calculate the SPF.

On day 1 of the study, the sunscreens and a water-resistant sunscreen (Coppertone Waterproof SPF 15) control were applied to individual areas on the subject's back. A single topical application (2 mg/cm^2) was applied to an area (~60 cm^2) on the back of each subject. The total amount was 120 mg applied. After a waiting period of at least 15 min, the subject entered a whirlpool bath and remained in the circulating water for 20 min. The subject then rested out of the water for 20 min, returned to the whirlpool bath for 20 min, and then exited the bath for the conclusion of the water test, allowing the test sites to air dry. The standard sunscreen control (8% homosalate) was then applied to a designated site on the upper portion of the subject's back. The sites were divided into subsites, about 1 cm^2 in area, each of which was exposed to increasing doses of UVR. The doses selected were a geometric series represented by 1.25^n, where each exposure was 25% greater than the previous exposure. The middle subsite received a dose expected to yield the SPF of the product. The exact series of exposures administered was previously determined by the MED of unprotected skin. The MED for unprotected skin was repeated and used to calculate the SPF as follows: SPF = MED protected skin/MED unprotected skin. On day 2 (22 to 24 h postirradiation), the test sites were evaluated based on the erythema grading scale.

15.8.2 UVA MEASUREMENTS/METHODS

At the present time there is no known marker for assessing damage due to UVA exposure. UVA is most often associated with long-term effects of photodamage and wrinkling of skin rather than the erythematous precursor of sunburn. UVA rays cause immediate and persistent tanning of the skin. While this is a suntan, it can be used as a marker for excessive UVA exposure. There are several ways to measure this, and the method that is used most frequently is persistent pigment darkening (PPD), introduced by the Japan Cosmetic Industry Association (JCIA).[162] It generates a protection factor A (PFA):

$$\text{PFA} = \frac{\text{Minimal PPD (protected skin with sunscreen)}}{\text{Minimal PPD (unprotected skin)}}$$

The determination of the protection factor for UVA (PFA-PA, rated as +, ++, +++; the greater the number of +, the higher the UVA protection) was based on testing procedures proposed by the Japan Cosmetic Industry Association (JCIA).[162] Each of 10 subject's minimal persistent pigment darkening (PPD) dose of untreated, unprotected skin was determined by exposing test sites on the back to UVR. The untreated, unprotected test area from day 0 served as the area for the minimal PPD determination on the actual test day (study day 1). Five subsites were selected within the test site. The UVR doses selected were a geometric series represented by 1.25^n, where each exposure time interval was 25% greater than the previous time. This PPD value was then used in calculating the actual PFA values. The test drug and standard sunscreen control (JCIA two UVA standards (5% avobenzone/3% octinoxate), expected PFA of 3.75) test sites were also divided into five subsites, each about 1 cm^2. Each of the test subsites was subjected to additional doses of UVR, determined using a geometric series of five doses, where the middle dose was placed to yield the expected PFA of the product. Treated and untreated sites were examined for evidence of pigmentation at 3 h ± 1 h after irradiation. Immediate response criteria were graded as present (1) or absent (0). All sites were evaluated for PPD using the scale 0, 0.5, 1, and 2. The quantity of effective energy needed to achieve a score of 1 was considered the minimal PPD value. The PFA was calculated using the minimal PPD of unprotected skin divided into the minimal PPD of protected skin. Label PFA was determined as per JCIA recommended methodology. The rating of PA+ is ascribed to a PFA rating of <4; a PFA rating of PA++ is given if PFA is <8, and a PA+++ rating is given if the PFA is >8.

15.8.3 Lamp Characteristics

Typically a 150-watt xenon arc solar simulator is used. A 1-mm UGA11 and Schott WG345 filter is added to generate a continuous spectrum from 320 to 410 nm.

Several other *in vivo* and *in vitro* methods are available to help determine the efficacy of anti-UVA sunscreens. However, these methods lack a definitive biological endpoint (unlike UVB testing, where much smaller doses are required to induce erythema), and no consensus has formed regarding their use.

Other methods of assessing UVA protection, which have been reviewed elsewhere,[164] include the following:

- The immediate pigment-darkening method (IPD) of assessing UVA sunscreen efficacy involves exposing volunteers to UVA irradiation with an appropriately filtered solar simulator. The threshold dose of IPD, defined as the smallest dose required to produce darkening of the skin with a clearly defined margin, is determined by dosing the skin in 25% increments. Test sunscreens are then applied uniformly to a 15 × 15 cm area (2 mg/cm²), allowing 15 min before irradiation at the test site. The protection factor is the ratio, on treated vs. untreated skin, of the IPD threshold dose. This method has been used to compare sunscreen efficacy,[165] demonstrating that combinations of UVA absorbers may be more effective in reducing exposure, and also that there is no correlation between UVA protection and the UVB sun protection factor.

- UVA-induced erythema measurement (Stanfield et al.).[166]
- Induction of photosensitivity with a 8-methoxypsoralen.[167]
- *In vitro* tests such as the Diffey method,[168] which measures the transmission of UVA through a substrate with and without sunscreen.

15.9 DRUG STABILITY

Due to the high costs of launching a sunscreen product, chemists must do preliminary tests early to ensure ease of transition from product development to the consumers. The following are typical tests done in the industry prior to launch of a SPF product:

- At least 8 weeks of in-house stability testing in the final package (drug substance and physical and microbiological preservation testing).
- A 10% production batch of at least three batches to qualify and validate the method and equipment used for the manufacturing.
- Twelve weeks of accelerated OTC drug substance stability testing under the auspices of cGMPs. The lab will develop and validate a method used to determine the sunscreen active in the formula. This test will determine a tentative 2-year expiration dating (expiration dating is required by 21 CFR Parts 211.137 and 211.166).[169]
- Finally, a 36-month controlled room temperature stability according to FDA approved guidelines. This test includes physical testing as well as assaying of actives at scheduled intervals. The intervals that some companies use are 0, 1, 2, 3, 6, 9, 18, 24, and finally 36 months. The inclusion of effectiveness of preservatives is highly recommended for formulae with a preservative system.

Additionally, the usual tolerability testing is done, photoallergy and phototoxicity if there is a suspected photoallergen, and Draize human repeat insult patch test for irritation and sensitization.

15.10 LAUNCHING THE SPF PRODUCT

The Code of Federal Regulations, Title 21, Volume 5, Parts 300 to 499,[170] lists the conditions necessary for general recognition as safe, effective, and not misbranded; the sunscreen monograph also dictates dose and label for the sunscreen product. Some of these conditions include:

- The product must be manufactured in compliance with current good manufacturing practices, established in 21 CFR Parts 210 and 211.[169]
- The establishments in which the drug product is manufactured are registered and the drug product is listed.
- The product is labeled in compliance with Part 207 of 21 CFR and in accordance with the final OTC sunscreen monograph.[2,169]
- The uses describing the indications must be disclosed in the label as per the monograph.
- The advertising of the product prescribes, recommends, or suggests its use only under the conditions stated in the labeling.
- The products only contain suitable inactive ingredients that are safe and effective in the amounts administered and do not interfere in the final product's standards of identity, strength quality, and purity.
- The product container and container components must meet the requirements of Section 211.94.[169]
- The warning label must state the following: "Keep out of reach of children." Other warnings per the OTC sunscreen monograph must be included.[2]
- Intended dosage amount must be stated in the label.
- The usage of terms in labeling.

The OTC monograph[2] also specifies the sunscreen agents to be used and the maximum allowable, found in Table 15.2.

The permitted combinations of these sunscreens are found in Section 352.20; the testing procedures are found in Section 352.70.[170] Water-resistant determination is found in Section 352.76 of the Code of Federal Regulations.[170]

REFERENCES

1. Norman Vincent Peale (1898–1993).
2. Department of Health and Human Services, Food and Drug Administration, Sunscreen drug products for over-the-counter human use, final monograph, *Federal Register* 1999; 64:27666–27693.
3. Food and Drug Administration, Sunscreen drug products for over-the-counter human use; marketing status of products containing avobenzone; enforcement policy, *Federal Register* 1997; 62:23350–23356,.
4. Taylor CR, Sober AJ, Sun exposure and skin disease, *Ann Rev Med* 1996; 47:181–191.
5. Norris PG, Gange RW, Hawk JLM. Acute effects of ultraviolet radiation on the skin. In *Dermatology in General Medicine*, Fitzpatrick TB, Eisen AZ, Wolf K, Freedberg IM, Austin KF, Eds., McGraw-Hill, New York, 1993.
6. Pandolf KB, Gange RW, Latzka WA, et al., Human thermoregulatory responses during heat exposure after artificially induced sunburn, *Am J Physiol* 1992; 262:610–616.

7. Soter NA, Acute effects of ultraviolet radiation in the skin, *Semin Dermatol* 1990; 9:11–15.

8. Kligman LH, Photoaging. Manifestations, prevention, and treatment, *Dermatol Clin* 1986; 4:517–528.

9. Kligman LH, Kligman MA, The nature of photoaging: its prevention and repair, *Photodermatology* 1986; 3:215–227.

10. Young AR, Cumulative effects of ultraviolet radiation in the skin: cancer and photoaging, *Semin Dermatol* 1990; 9:25–31.

11. Gloeckler-Reis LA, Hankey BF, *Cancer Statistics Review 1973–1988*, National Institutes of Health Publication 91-2789, National Cancer Institute, Bethesda, 1991.

12. Glass AG, Hoover RN, The emerging epidemic of melanoma and squamous cell carcinoma, *JAMA* 1989; 262:2097–2100.

13. Houghton A, Flannery J, Viola MV, Malignant melanoma in Connecticut and Denmark, *Int J Cancer* 1980; 25:95–104.

14. Garland CF, Garland F, Gorham ED, Rising trends in melanoma. An hypothesis concerning sunscreen effectiveness, *Ann Epidemiol* 1993; 3:103–110.

15. Urbach F, Grange R, Eds., *The Biological Effects of UVA Radiation*, Praeger, New York, 1986.

16. Ulrich SE, Mechanisms underlying UV-induced immune suppression, *Mutat Res* 2005; 571:185–205.

17. Setlow R, Spectral regions contributing to melanoma: a personal view, *J Invest Dermatol Symp Proc* 1999; 4:46–49.

18. Almahroos M, Kurban AK, Sun protection for children and adolescents, *Clin Dermatol* 2003; 21:311–314.

19. Silverberg NB, Update on malignant melanoma in children, *Cutis* 2001; 67:393–396.

20. Strouse JJ, Fears TR, Tucker MA, Wayne AS, Pediatric melanoma: risk factor and survival analysis of the surveillance, epidemiology and end results database, *J Clin Oncol* 2005; 23:4735–4741.

21. Gass R, Bopp M, Mortality from malignant melanoma: epidemiological trends in Switzerland, *Schweiz Rundsch Med Prax* 2005; 94:1295–12300.

22. Gandini S, Sera F, Cattaruzza MS, Pasquini P, Picconi O, Boyle P, Melchi CF, Meta-analysis of risk factors for cutaneous melanoma. III. Family history, actinic damage and phenotypic factors, *Eur J Cancer* 2005; 41:45–60.

23. Farmer KC, Naylor MF, Sun exposure, sunscreens, and skin cancer prevention: a year-round concern, *Ann Pharmacol* 1996; 30:662–673.

24. Wang SQ, Setlow R, Berwick M, et al., Ultraviolet A and melanoma: a review, *J Am Acad Dermatol* 2001; 44:837–846.

25. Naylor MF, Farmer KC, The case for sunscreens, *Arch Dermatol* 1997; 133:1146–1154.

26. English DR, Armstrong BK, Kricker A, Fleming C, Sunlight and cancer, *Cancer Causes Control* 1997; 8:271–283.

27. Naylor MF, Erythema, skin cancer risk, and sunscreens, *Arch Dermatol* 1997; 133:373–375.

28. Elmets CA, Anderson CY, Sunscreen and photocarcinogenesis, *Photochem Photobiol* 1996; 63:435–440.

29. Surveillance, epidemiology and end results (SEER), introduction, cancer statistics review, in *Cancer Incidence and Survival among children and Adolescents: U.S. SEER Program 1973–1991*, Vols. 1–16, National Cancer Institute, 1975–1995.

30. Gandini S, Sera F, Cattaruzza MS, Pasquini P, Picconi O, Boyle P, Zanetti R, Melchi CF, Meta-analysis of risk factors for cutaneous melanoma. II. Sun exposure, *Eur J Cancer* 2005; 41:2040–2050.

31. Armstrong BK, Kricker A, The epidemiology of UV induced skin cancer, *J Photochem Photobiol B* 2001; 63:8–18.

32. Richard MA, Grob JJ, Gouvernet J, et al., Role of sun exposure on nevus. First study in age-sex phenotype controlled populations, *Arch Dermatol* 1993; 129:1280–1285.

33. Kelly JW, Rivers JK, MacLennan R, et al., Sunlight: a major factor associated with the development of melanocytic nevi in Australian school children, *J Am Acad Dermatol* 1994; 30:40–48.

34. Rosso S, Zanetti R, Pippione M, Sancho-Garnier H, Parallel risk assessment of melanoma and basal cell carcinoma: skin characteristics and sun exposure, *Melanoma Res* 1998; 8:573–583.

35. Zanetti R, Russo S, Martinez C, Schraub S, Sancho-Garnier H, Franceschi S, Gafa L, Perea E, Tormo MJ, Laurent R, Schrameck C, Cristofolini M, Tumino R, Wechsler J, The multicentre south European study 'Helios'. I. Skin characteristics and sunburns in basal cell and squamous cell carcinomas of the skin, *Br J Cancer* 1996; 73:1440–1446.

36. Rosso S, Zanetti R, Martinez C, Tormo MJ, Schraub S, Sancho-Garnier H, Franceschi S, Gafa L, Perea E, Navarro C, Laurent R, Schrameck C, Talamini R, Tumino R, Wechsler J, The multicentre south European study 'Helios'. II. Different sun exposure patterns in the aetiology of basal cell and squamous cell carcinomas of the skin, *Br J Cancer* 1996; 73:1447–14145.

37. Kopf AW, Kripke ML, Stern RS, Sun and malignant melanoma, *J Am Acad Dermatol* 1984; 11:674–684.

38. Gallagher RP, Hill GB, Bajdik CD, Fincham S, Coldman AJ, McLean DI, Threlfall WJ, Sunlight exposure, pigmentary factors, and risk of nonmelanocytic skin cancer, *Arch Dermatol* 1995; 131:157–163.

39. Truhan AP, Sun protection in childhood, *Clin Pediatr* 1991; 30:676–681.

40. Moan J, Dahlback A, Setlow RB, Epidemiological support for an hypothesis for melanoma induction indicating a role for UVA radiation, *Photochem Photobiol* 1999; 70:243–247.

41. Magnus K, The Nordic profile in skin cancer incidence. A comparative epidemiological study of the three main types of skin cancer, *Int J Cancer* 1991; 47:12–19.

42. Tanew A, Honigsmann H, Ortel B, et al., Nonmelanoma skin tumors in long-term photochemistry treatment of psoriasis, *J Am Acad Dermatol* 1986; 15:960–965.

43. Cox NH, Jones SK, Downey DJ, et al., Cutaneous and ocular side-effects of oral photochemotherapy: results of an 8-year follow-up study, *Br J Dermatol* 1987; 116:145–152.

44. Stern RS, Risks of cancer associated with long-term exposure to PUVA in humans: current status—1991, *Blood Cells* 1992; 18:91–99.

45. Bataille V, Boniol M, DeVries E, Severi G, Brandberg Y, Sasieni P, et al., A multicenter epidemiology study on sunbed use and malignant melanoma, *Eur J Cancer*, 2005; 41:2141–2149.

46. Runger TM, Role of UVA in the pathogenesis of melanoma and non-melanoma skin cancer: a short review, *Photodermatol Photoimmunol Photomed* 1999; 15:212–216.

47. Westerdahl J, Ingvar C, Jonsson N, Olsson H, Risk of cutaneous malignant melanoma in relation to use of sunbeds: further evidence for UVA, *Br J Cancer* 2000; 82:1593–1599.

48. Autier P, Cutaneous malignant melanoma: facts about sunbeds and sunscreen, expert review, *Anticancer Ther* 2005; 5:821–833.

49. Gallagher RP, Spinelli JJ, Lee TK, Tanning beds, sunlamps, and risk of cutaneous malignant melanoma, *Cancer Epidemiol Biomarkers Prev* 2005; 14:562–566.

50. Freeman SE, Ley RD, Ley KD, Sunscreen protection against UV-induced pyrimidine dimers in DNA of human skin *in situ*, *Photodermatology* 1988; 5:243–247.

51. DeRijcke S, Heenan M, Decrease of ultraviolet-induced DNA injury in human skin by p-aminobenzoic acid esters, *Dermatologica* 1989; 179:96–199.

52. Van Praag MCG, Roza BW, Boom C, Out-Luiting J, et al., Determination of the photoprotective efficacy of a topical sunscreen against UVB-induced DNA damage in human epidermis, *J Photochem Photobiol* 1993; 19:129–134.

53. Wolf P, Yarosh DB, Kripke ML, Effects of sunscreens and a DNA excision repair enzyme on ultraviolet radiation-induced inflammation, immune suppression, and cyclobutane pyrimidine dimer formation in mice, *J Invest Dermatol* 1993; 5:523–527.

54. Lowe NJ, Breeding J, Evaluation of sunscreen protection by measurement of epidermal DNA synthesis, *J Invest Dermatol* 1980; 74:181–182.

55. Nohynek GJ, Schaefer H, Benefit and risk of organic ultraviolet filters, *Reg Tox Pharmacol* 2001; 33:285–299.

56. Autier P, Dore JF, Influence of sun exposures during childhood and during adulthood on melanoma risk. EPIMEL and EORTC Melanomas Cooperative Group. European Organization for Research and Treatment of Cancer, *Int J Cancer* 1998; 77:533–537.

57. Whitman DC, Whiteman SA, Green AC, Childhood sun exposure as a risk factor for melanoma: a systematic review of epidemiologic studies, *Cancer Causes Control* 2001; 12;69–82.

58. Kennedy C, Bajdik KC, Willemze R, DeGruijl FR, Bavwes B, Bavinck JN, The influence of painful sunburns and lifetime sun exposure on the risk of actinic keratoses, seborrheic warts, melanocytic nevi, atypical nevi, and skin cancer, *J Invest Dermatol* 2003; 120:1087–1093.

59. Weinstock NA, Colditz A, Willett WC, Stampfer MJ, Bronstein BR, Mihm MC, Speizer FE, Nonfamilial cutaneous melanoma incidence in women associated with sun exposure before 20 years of age, *Pediatrics* 1989; 84:199–204.

60. Zanetti R, Franceschi S, Rosso S, Colonna S, Bidoli E, Cutaneous melanoma and sunburns in childhood in a southern European population, *Eur J Cancer* 1992; 28A:1172–1176.

61. Holly EA, Aston DA, Cress RD, Ahn DK, Kristiansen JJ, Cutaneous melanoma in women, *Am J Epidemiol* 1995; 141:923–933.

62. Robinson ES, VandeBerg JL, Hubbard GB, Dooley TP, Malignant melanoma in ultraviolet irradiated laboratory opossums: initiation in suckling young, metastasis in adults, and xenograft behavior in nude mice, *Cancer Res* 1994; 54:5986–5991.

63. Urbach F, The cumulative effects of ultraviolet radiation on the skin: photocarcinogenesis, in *Photodermatology*, Hawk JLM, Ed., Chapman & Hall, London, 1998.

64. Kusewitt DF, Applegate LA, Bucana CD, Ley RD, Naturally occurring malignant melanoma in the South American opossum (*Monodelphis domestica*), *Vet Pathol* 1990; 27:66–68.

65. Sams WJ, Sun-induced aging. Clinical and laboratory observations in humans, *Clin Geriatr Med* 1989; 5:223–233.

66. Griffiths CE, The clinical identification and quantification of photodamage, *Br J Dermatol* 1992; 127(Suppl 41):37–42.

67. Engel A, Johnson ML, Haynes SG, Health effects of sunlight exposure in the United States, *Arch Dermatol* 1988; 124:72–79.

68. Granstein RD, Photoimmunology, *Semin Dermatol* 1990; 9:16–24.

69. Halliday GM, Inflammation, gene mutation and photoimmunosuppression in response to UVR-induced oxidative damage contributes to photocarcinogenesis, *Mutat Res* 2005; 571:107–120.

70. Hruza LL, Pentland AP, Mechanisms of UV-induced inflammation, *J Invest Dermatol* 1993; 100(Suppl):35S–41S.

71. Pattison DL, Davies MT, Action of UV light on cellular structures, *EXS* 2006; 96:131–157.

72. Marwaha V, Chen YH, Helms E, Arad S, Inoue H, Bord E, Kishore R, Sarkissian RD, Gilchrest BA, Goukassian DA, T-oligo treatment decreases constitutive and UVB-induced COX-2 levels through p53- and NFkappaB-dependent repression of the COX-2 promoter, *J Biol Chem* 2005; 280:32379–32388.

73. Latonen L, Laiho M, Cellular UV damage responses: functions of tumor suppressor p53, *Biochim Biophys Acta* 2005; 1775:71–89.

74. Pence BC, Naylor MF, Effects of single-dose ultraviolet radiation on skin superoxide dismutase, catalase, and xanthine oxidase in hairless mice, *J Invest Dermatol* 1990; 95:213–216.

75. Miyachi Y, Reactive oxygen species in photodermatology, in *The Biological Role of Reactive Oxygen Species in the Skin*, Hayaishi O, Imamura S, Miyachi Y, Eds., University of Tokyo Press, Tokyo, 1987, pp. 37–41.

76. Schellreuter KU, Wood JM, Free radical reduction in the human epidermis, *Free Rad Biol Med* 1989; 6:519–532.

77. Kensler TW, Trush MA, Role of oxygen radical in tumor promotion, *Environ Mutagen* 1984; 6:593–616.

78. Fischer SM, Floyd RA, Copeland ES, Oxy radicals in carcinogenesis: a chemical pathology study section workshop, *Cancer Res* 1988; 48:3882–3887.

79. Reid TM, Loeb LA, Tandem double CC→TT mutations are produced by reactive oxygen species, *Proc Natl Acad Sci USA* 1993; 90:3904–3907.

80. Stewart MS, Cameron GS, Pence BC, Antioxidant nutrients protect against UVB-induced oxidative damage to DNA of mouse keratinocytes in culture, *J Invest Dermatol* 1996; 106:1086–1089.

81. Pfeifer GP, You YH, Besaratinia A, Mutations induced by ultraviolet light, *Mutat Res.* 2005; 571:19–31.

82. van Doorn R, Gruis NA, Willemze R, van der Velden PA, Tensen CP, Aberrant DNA methylation in cutaneous malignancies, *Semin Oncol* 2005; 32:479–487.

83. Melnikova VO, Ananthaswamy HN, Cellular and molecular events leading to the development of skin cancer, *Mutat Res* 2005; 571:91–106.

84. Reinhardt P, Cybulski M, McNamee JP, McLean JR, Gorman W, Deslauriers Y, Protection from solar simulated radiation-induced DNA damage in cultured human

fibroblasts by three commercially available sunscreens, *Can J Physiol Pharmacol* 2005; 8:690–695.

85. Edlich RF, Winters KL, Lim HW, Cox MJ, Becker DG, Horowitz JH, Nichter LS, Britt LD, Long WB, Photoprotection by sunscreens with topical antioxidants and systemic antioxidants to reduce sun exposure, *J Long Term Eff Med Implants* 2004; 14:317–340.

86. Fourtanier A, Berrebi C, Miniature pig as an animal model to study photoaging, *Photochem Photobiol* 1989; 50:771–784.

87. Moloney SJ, Edmonds SH, Giddens LD, Learn DB, The hairless mouse model of photoaging; evaluation of the relationship between dermal elastin, collagen, skin thickness and wrinkles, *Photochem Photobiol* 1992; 56:505–511.

88. Imayama S, Nakamura K, Takeuchi M, et al., Ultraviolet B irradiation deforms the configuration of elastic fibers during the induction of actinic elastosis in rats, *J Dermatol Sci* 1994; 7:32–38.

89. Leyden J, What is photoaged skin? *Eur J Dermatol* 2001; 11:165–167.

90. Herschenfeld RE, Gilchrest BA, The cumulative effects of ultraviolet radiation on the skin: photoaging, in *Photodermatology*, Hawk JL, Ed., Chapman & Hall, London, 1998, pp. 69–87.

91. Kligman L, Zheng P, The protective effect of a broad spectrum sunscreen against chronic UVA radiation in hairless mice: a histologic and ultrastructural study, *J Soc Cosmet Sci* 1994; 45: 21–33.

92. Quan T, He T, Kang S, Voorhees JJ, Fisher GJ, Solar ultraviolet irradiation reduces collagen in photoaged human skin by blocking transforming growth factor-beta type II receptor/Smad signaling, *Am J Pathol* 2003; 165:741–751.

93. Wang H, Kochevar IE, Involvement of UVB-induced reactive oxygen species in TGF-beta biosynthesis and activation in keratinocytes, *Free Rad Biol Med* 2005; 38:890–897.

94. Yin L, Morita A, Tsuji T, The crucial role of TGF-beta in the age-related alterations induced by ultraviolet A irradiation, *J Invest Dermatol* 2003; 120:703.

95. Kligman LH, Connective tissue photodamage in the hairless mouse is partially reversible, *J Invest Dermatol* 1987; 88 (3 Suppl):12s–17s.

96. Hersey P, Haran G, Hasie E, Edwards A, Alterations of T cell subsets and induction of suppressor T cell activity in normal subjects after exposure to sunlight, *J Immunol* 1983; 31:171–174.

97. Nennema K, Cooper K, Baron E, *Dermatol Clin* 2006; 24:19–25.

98. Plummer NA, Hensby CN, Greaves MW, Black AK, Inflammation in human skin induced by ultraviolet radiation, *Postgrad Med J* 1977; 53:656–57.

99. Adams SS, Humphries RG, Mason CG, The relationship between development of ultraviolet erythema and release of prostaglandins in guinea pig skin, *Agent Actions* 1981; 11:473–476.

100. Chung JH, Youn JI, Effect of ultraviolet A on IL-1 production by ultraviolet B in cultured human keratinocytes, *J Dermatol Sci* 1995; 9:87–93.

101. Ulrich US, Photoimmune suppression and photocarcinogenesis, *Front Biosci* 2002; 7:684–703.

102. Murphy GM, Dowd PM, Hudspith BN, Brostoffr J, Greaves MW, Local increase in interleukin 1-like activity following UVB irradiation of human skin *in vivo*, *Photodermatology* 1989; 6:268–274.

103. Bonifati C, Ameglio F, Carducci M, et al., Interleukin-1-beta, interleukin-6, and interferon-gamma in suction blister fluids of involved and uninvolved skin

and in sera of psoriatic patients, *Acta Dermatol Venereol Suppl* 1994; 186:23–24.

104. Wolkenstein P, Chosidow O, Wechsler J, et al., Cutaneous side effects associated with interleukin 2 administration for metastatic melanoma, *J Am Acad Dermatol* 1993; 28:66–70.

105. Skiba B, Neill B, Piva TJ, Gene expression profiles of TNF-alpha, TACE, furin, IL-1beta and matrilysin in UVA- and UVB-irradiated HaCat cells, *Photodermatol Photoimmunol Photomed* 2005; 21:173–181.

106. Vanbuskirk A, Oberyszyn TM, Kusewitt DF, Depletion of CD8 and CD4 lymphocytes enhances susceptibility to transplantatable UV radiation induced skin tumors, *Anticancer Res* 2005; 25: 1963–1967.

107. Kripke ML, Fisher MS, Immunologic parameters of ultraviolet carcinogenesis, *J Natl Cancer Inst* 1976; 57:211–215.

108. Nishigori C, Yarosh DB, Danawho C, Kripke ML, The immune system in ultraviolet carcinogenesis, *J Invest Dermatol Symp Proc* 1996; 1:143–146.

109. Baron ED, Fourtanier A, Compan D, et al., High ultraviolet A protection affords greater immune protection confirming that ultraviolet A contributes to photoimmunosuppression in humans, *J Invest Dermatol* 2003; 121:869–875.

110. Gueniche A, Fourtanier A, Mexoryl® SX protects against photoimmuno-suppression, in *Skin Cancer and UV Radiation*, Altmeyer P, Hoffman K, Stucker M, Eds., Springer-Verlag, Berlin, 1997, pp. 249–262.

111. Schaefer H, Moyal D, Fourtanier A, State of the art sunscreens for prevention of photodermatoses, *J Dermatol Sci* 2000; 23(Suppl 1):S62–S74.

112. International Agency for Research on Cancer, *IARC Monograph of the Evaluation of Carcinogenic Risks to Humans: Ultraviolet Radiation*, No. 55, IARC, Lyon, 1993.

113. Staberg B, Christian W, Poulsen T, et al., Carcinogenic effects of sequential artificial sunlight and UVA irradiation in hairless mice, *Arch Dermatol* 1983; 119:641–643.

114. Staberg B, Christian W, Kemp P, et al., The carcinogenic effect of UVA irradiation, *J Invest Dermatol* 1983; 81:517–519.

115. Van Weedlen H, Gruijl F, Van der Leun J, Carcinogenesis by UVA with an attempt to assess the carcinogenic risks of tanning with UVA and UVB, in *The Biological Effects of UVA Radiation*, Urbach F, Gange R, Eds., Praeger, New York, 1986.

116. Passchier N, Bosnjakovic B, Eds., *Human Exposure to Ultraviolet Radiation: Risks and Regulations*, Exerpta Medica International Congress Series, Amsterdam, 1987, p. 744.

117. Brasch DE, Ziegler A, Jonason AS, et al., Sunlight and sunburn in human skin cancer: p53, apoptosis, and tumor promotion, *J Invest Dermatol Symp Proc* 1996; 1:136–142.

118. Sarasin A, The molecular pathways of ultraviolet-induced carcinogenesis, *Mutat Res* 1999; 428:5–10.

119. Van Kranen HU, Gruijl FR, Mutations in cancer genes of UV-induced skin tumors of hairless mice, *J Epidemiol* 1999; 9(Suppl):558–565.

120. Armstrong BK, Kricker A, Epidemiology of sun exposure and skin cancer, in *Skin Cancer*, Leigh IM, Bishop JAN, Kripke ML, Eds., Cold Spring Harbor Laboratory Press, New York, 1996, pp. 133–153.

121. Weinstein IB, The role of protein kinase C in growth control and the concept of carcinogenesis as a progressive disorder in signal transduction, in *Advances in*

Second Messengers and Phosphoprotein Research, Nishizuka Y, Ed., Raven Press, New York, 1990.

122. Applegate LA, Scaletta C, Labidi F, et al., Susceptibility of human melanoma cells to oxidative stress including UVA radiation, *Int J Cancer* 1996; 6:430–434.

123. D'Angelo S, Ingrosso D, Perfetto B, et al., UVA irradiation induces l-isoaspartyl formation in melanoma cell proteins, *Free Rad Biol Med* 2001; 31:1–9.

124. Matsui M, DeLeo V, Longwave ultraviolet radiation and promotion of skin cancer, *Cancer Cells* 1991; 3:8–12.

125. Hanson D, DeLeo V, Long-wave ultraviolet light induces phospholipase activation in cultured human epidermal keratinocytes, *J Invest Dermatol* 1990; 95:158–163.

126. Moyal DD, Fourtanier AM, Effects of UVA radiation on an established immune response in humans and sunscreen efficacy, *Exp Dermatol* 2002; 11(Suppl 1):28–32.

127. Bestak R, Barnetson RSC, Nearn MR, Halliday GM, Sunscreen protection of contact hypersensitivity responses from chronic solar-simulated ultraviolet irradiation correlates with the absorption spectrum of the sunscreen, *J Invest Dermatol* 1995; 105:345–351.

128. Ikehata H, Masuda T, Ono T, UVA induces CT transitions at methyl-CpG-associated dipyrimidine sites in mouse skin epidermis more frequently than UVB, *Mutagenesis* 2003; 18:511–519.

129. Hanson D, Bodian A, DeLeo V, Ultraviolet-A (320–400 nm) induces phospholipase activation in human keratinocytes in culture, *Clin Res* 1989; 37:731A.

130. Hanson DL, DeLeo V, Long wave ultraviolet radiation stimulates arachidonic acid release and cyclooxygenase activity in mammalian cells, *Photochem Photobiol* 1989; 49:423–430.

131. Matsui MS, DeLeo V, Induction of protein kinase C activity by ultraviolet radiation, *Carcinogenesis* 1990; 11:229–234.

132. Castagna M, Takai Y, Kaibuchi K, et al., Direct activation of calcium-activated, phospholipid-dependent protein kinase by tumor-promoting phorbol esters, *J Biol Chem* 1982; 257:7847–7851.

133. Nishizuka Y, The role of protein kinase C in cell surface signal transduction and tumor promotion, *Nature* 1984; 308: 693–698.

134. Hunter T, Ling N, Cooper JA, Protein kinase C phosphorylation of the EGF receptor at a threonine residue close to the cytoplasmic face of plasma membrane, *Nature* 1984; 311:480–483.

135. Mori T, Takai Y, Minakuchi R, et al., Inhibitory action of chlorpromazine, dibucaine, and other phospholipid-interacting drugs on calcium-activated phospholipid-dependent protein kinase, *J Biol Chem* 1980; 255:8378–8380.

136. Setlow RB, Grist E, Thompson K, Woodhead AD, Wavelengths effective in induction of malignant melanoma, *Proc Natl Acad Sci USA* 1993; 90:6666–6670.

137. Ley RD, Dose response for ultraviolet radiation A-induced focal melanocytic hyperplasia and nonmelanoma skin tumors in *Monodelphis domestica*, *Photochem Photobiol* 2001; 73:20–23.

138. Ley RD, Applegate LA, Padilla, Stuart TD,. Ultraviolet radiation-induced malignant melanoma in *Monodelphis domestica*, *Photochem Photobiol* 1989; 50:1–5.

139. Agar NS, Halliday GM, Barnetson R, Ananthaswamy HN, Wheeler M, The basal layer in human squamous tumors harbors more UVA than UVB fingerprint mutations: a role for UVA in human skin carcinogenesis, *Proc Natl Acad Sci USA* 2004; 101:4954–4959.

140. Woodhead AD, Setlow RB, Tanaka M, Environmental factors in nonmelanoma and melanoma skin cancer, *J Epidemiol* 1999; 9:S102–S114.

141. Seite S, Moyal D, Richard S, et al., Mexoryl® SX: a broad absorption UVA filter protects human skin from the effects of repeated suberythemal doses of UVA, *J Photochem Photobiol* 1998; 44:69–76.

142. Seite S, Colige A, Piquermal-Vivenot P, Montastier C, Fourtanier A, Lapiere C, Nusgens B, A full UV spectrum absorbing daily use cream protects human skin against biological changes occurring in photoaging, *Photoderm Photoimmunol Phototmed* 2000; 16:147–155.

143. Armstrong BK, Kricker A, How much melanoma is caused by sun exposure? *J Clin Epidemiol* 1993; 3:395–401.

144. Stern R, Weinstein M, Baker S, Risk reduction for nonmelanoma skin cancer with childhood sunscreen use, *Arch Dermatol* 1986; 122:537–545.

145. Gallagher RP, Rivers JK, Lee TK, Bajdik CD, Math M, McLean DI, Coldman AJ, Broad spectrum sunscreen use and the development of new nevi in white children: a randomized controlled trial, *JAMA* 2000; 283:2955–2960.

146. Thompson SC, Jolley D, Marks R, Reduction of solar keratoses by regular sunscreen use, *N Engl J Med* 1993; 329:1147–1151.

147. Naylor MF, Boyd A, Smith SW, Cameron GS, Hubbard D, Neldner KH, High sun protection factor sunscreens in the suppression of actinic neoplasia, *Arch Dermatol* 1995; 131:170–175.

148. Green A, Williams G, Neale R, Hart V, Leslie D, Parsons P, Marks GC, Gaffney P, Battistutta D, Frost C, Lang C, Russell A, Daily sunscreen application and betacarotene supplementation in prevention of basal cell and squamous cell carcinomas of the skin: a randomized controlled trial, *Lancet* 1999; 354:723–729.

149. Gasparro FP, Mitchnick M, Nash JF, A review of sunscreen safety and efficacy, *Photochem Photobiol* 1998; 68:243–256.

150. Nole G, Johnson AW, An analysis of cumulative lifetime solar ultraviolet radiation exposure and the benefits of daily sun protection, *Dermatol Ther* 2004; 17 (Suppl 1):57–62.

151. Policy statement — ultraviolet light: a hazard to children. *Pediatrics* 1999; 104:328–333.

152. The chemistry of ultraviolet filters, in Sunscreens, 3rd ed., Shaath N, Ed. Taylor & Francis, New York, 2005, 217–238.

153. Tuchinda C, Lim H, Osterwalder U, Rougier A, Novel emerging sunscreen technologies, *Dermatol Clin* 2006; 24:105–117.

154. Dahms G. The role of surfactants in sunscreen formulations, in *Sunscreens*, 3rd ed., Shaath N, Ed., Taylor & Francis, New York, 2005, 413–448.

155. Klein K, Palefsky I, Formulating sunscreen products, in *Sunscreens*, 3rd ed., Shaath N, Ed., Taylor & Francis, New York, 2005, 353–384.

156. Eugenia M, Carlotti M, Gallarate M, Rossatto V, O/W microemulsion as a vehicle for sunscreens, *J Cosmet Sci* 2003; 54:451–462.

157. Carlotti ME, Gallarate M, Rossatto V, O/W microemulsion as a vehicle for sunscreens, *J Cosmet Sci* 2003; 54:460.

158. Hewitt JP, Rossi P, *Delivering UV Protection Everyday Happi*, September 2003.

159. U.S. federal monograph on skin protectants, *Federal Register* 1983; 48:6820.

160. Robbins C, *Chemistry and Physical Behavior of Human Hair*, 3rd ed., Springer Verlag, New York, 1994.

161. Gabard J, Sunscreens, in *Cosmetics: Controlled Efficacy Studies and Regulations*, Elsner P, Merck HF, Maibach HI, Eds., Springer-Verlag, Berlin, 1999, pp. 116–134.
162. Japan Cosmetic Industry Association (JCIA), Method for UVA Sunscreen Efficacy Testing.
163. Code of Federal Regulations, Title 21, Vol. 5, Parts 200–499.
164. Lowe NJ, Ultrviolet A claims and testing procedures for OTC sunscreens: a summary and review, in *Sunscreens: Development, Evaluation and Regulatory Aspects*, 2nd ed., Lowe NJ, Shaath NA, Pathak MA, Eds., Marcel Dekker, New York, 1997, pp. 527–535.
165. Kaidbey K, Grange RW, Comparison of methods for assessing photoprotection against ultraviolet A *in vivo*, *J Am Acad Dermatol* 1987; 16:346–353.
166. Stanfield JW, Feldt PA, Csortan ES, Krochmal L, Ultraviolet A sunscreen evaluations in normal subjects, *J Am Acad Dermatol* 1989; 20:744–748.
167. Kaidbey KH, Barnes A, Determination of UVA protection factors by means of immediate pigment darkening in normal skin, *J Am Acad Dermatol* 1991; 25:262–266.
168. Diffey BL, A method for broad spectrum classification of sunscreens, *Int J Cosmetic Sci* 1994; 16:47–52.
169. 21 CFR Parts 210 and 211.
170. 21 CFR Parts 300–499.

Part IV

SPECIFIC TECHNOLOGIES FOR PIGMENTED PRODUCTS

16 Formulating with Dihydroxyacetone (DHA)

Ratan K. Chaudhuri
EMD Chemicals, Inc.*

CONTENTS

---

* An affiliate of Merck KGaA, Darmstadt, Germany.

ABSTRACT

There are very few cosmetic ingredients that rely on chemical reactions with the biological surfaces to create more permanent effects; in skin care, these types of ingredients include self-tanning agents. The only approved self-tanning agent is dihydroxyacetone (DHA), which has been used well over 40 years and has unsurpassed safety over sun-induced tanning. Formulation with DHA is often regarded as somewhat challenging due to its instability. Products containing DHA remain stable over a long time if some fundamental rules, such as selection of ingredients, avoidance of high temperature, and adjustment of pH to acidic (3.0 to 4.5), are followed. Experimental and clinical evidence have shown that DHA-containing products provide some photoprotection; however, for better photoprotection, as recommended, always use DHA in combination with non-nitrogen-containing organic sunscreen. This photoprotective property of DHA has been utilized in the treatment of psoriasis. In this chapter, DHA, the primary active for sunless tanners, is reviewed and described at length.

16.1 INTRODUCTION

Despite increasing public awareness of the risks of skin cancer and premature aging associated with sun exposure and the importance of sun protection, the notion that a tan promotes an attractive and healthy appearance remains strong. According to a recent survey[1] by the American Academy of Dermatology, more Americans now recognize that overexposure to ultraviolet (UV) radiation is unhealthy. Yet many younger people fail to implement this knowledge when it comes to modifying sun-seeking behavior. A tanned appearance, however, can be maintained by the use of self-tanning products. The most important and legally allowed self-tanning agent is dihydroxyacetone (DHA). There is no alternative that gives a tanned appearance to the skin as adequately as DHA does, in color, substantivity, and safety. Of course, this is only an artificial coloring reaction, completely different from a true tanning reaction, involving increased production of melanin by melanocytes within the skin and transfer of melanosome to keratinocytes.[2] Nevertheless, the browning effect of DHA application can be useful as a photoprotective tool against UV-induced skin damage.

According to International Union of Pure and Applied Chemistry (IUPAC) nomenclature, DHA is known as 1,3-dihydroxypropanone, which is a triose containing three carbon atoms. Both glyceraldehyde and dihydroxyacetone are trioses. DHA is the simplest of all the ketoses and is the only one that has no optical rotation. DHA is an intermediate in carbohydrate metabolism in higher plants and animals. DHA and its tautomer glyceraldehyde occur in reversible equilibrium in phosphoric acid ester form in carbohydrate metabolism. Fructose-1,6-diphosphate formed from C_6 sugars breaks down into two triose phosphates, dihydroxyacetone phosphate, and glyceraldehyde-3-phosphate. The aldehyde may further react to form pyruvate and enter the citric acid cycle. This chain of reaction is known as Embden–Myerhof degradation. DHA has also been identified[3] in irradiated maize starch.

The browning effect of DHA was discovered by Eva Wittgenstein in the mid-1950s, while she was studying the effect of large oral doses of DHA in children who had glycogen storage disease. Sometimes the children vomited some of the sweet concentrated material, and it splashed on their skin. Dr. Wittgenstein noticed that the children had brown spots on their skin where stray splashes had not been wiped off. Wittgenstein was able to do something with her observation other than berate the staff for not getting those kids cleaned up. She prepared aqueous solutions of varying concentrations of DHA and was able to reproduce the pigmentation on her own skin; she turned her skin brown.[4] This was the beginning of self-tanning products based on DHA. Commercially, DHA is produced from glycerol by *Acetobacter* sp. under aerobic conditions.[5] Optimization of the microbial synthesis of DHA from glycerol with *Gluconobacter oxydans* has recently been reported.[6] There are three reviews available on this subject.[7–9]

16.2 GENERAL PROPERTIES OF DHA

16.2.1 Molecular and Crystal Structure

Research has shown that pure DHA occurs as a mixture of one monomer and four dimers (Figure 16.1), in which the dimers predominate.[10] The monomer is formed by heating or melting dimeric DHA or by dissolving it in water. One can observe the conversion process in water by measuring the UV spectrum of a freshly prepared solution. During the first half hour, the absorption increases constantly until reaching the endpoint, indicating the presence of monomeric DHA. The monomeric crystals revert to dimeric forms within a month of storage at room temperature.[11] Only the monomeric form undergoes the Maillard reaction that leads to tanning.

A detailed x-ray crystallographic analysis of the three crystalline forms of the DHA dimer (α, β, γ), as well as the DHA monomer, has been reported recently by Slepokura and Lis.[12] The DHA molecule is present in an extended conformation, with both hydroxyl groups being *synperiplanar* to carbonyl O atom. The two hydroxyl groups are involved as donors in medium strong and weak intermolecular O–H ... O hydrogen bonding.

Because the different crystal structures have different spectra, and various mixed forms of modifications occur, it is not possible to use infrared (IR) measurements as an unequivocal quality control criterion for DHA. IR spectroscopy

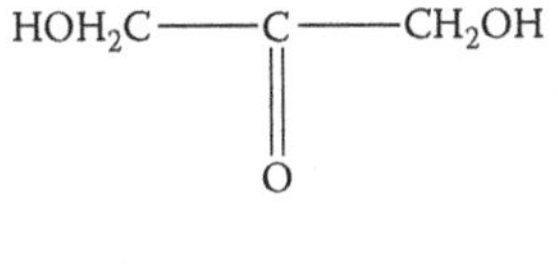

$$HOH_2C\text{——}\underset{\underset{O}{\|}}{C}\text{——}CH_2OH$$

FIGURE 16.1 Structure of dihydroxyacetone.

can, however, be used for identification purposes if all possible spectra are taken into account. The monomer and several dimers can be detected by examining nuclear magnetic resonance (NMR) spectra of DHA.

16.2.2 BEHAVIOR IN AQUEOUS AND ANHYDROUS SYSTEMS

The investigation of DHA structure in solution was made by Davis in 1973, who established that the commercial DHA is present predominantly in dimeric forms and dissociates into a mixture of two monomeric forms, the free carbonyl and hydrated gem-diol form in a ratio of 4:1.[13] In aqueous solution, DHA monomer can gradually tautomerize into glyceraldehyde (Figure 16.2). The equilibrium is shifted according to the pH of the solution (Figure 16.3).

Under alkaline conditions, starting from glyceraldehyde, various isomerization and condensation reactions occur, which ultimately lead to the formation of brown-colored oligomers. Glyceraldehyde itself can also play a role in the Maillard reaction chain.

When assessing the stability of DHA, one must distinguish between DHA content, pH value, and the occurrence of by-products. The pH value of solutions drops over time to about pH 3 to 4 due to the formation of organic acids. At pH ~5, DHA is in equilibrium with the isomer glyceraldehyde. Approximately 10% of the DHA is converted into the isomer at this pH. At pH ~2.5, no glyceraldehyde is observed. The major degradation product, however, is pyruvaldehyde, which is converted into pyruvic acid and most importantly to pyruvaldehyde polymers. It is estimated that at pH 5 at 40°C for 3 weeks, approximately 20 to 30% of the DHA is converted into pyruvaldehyde polymers. Storage at room temperarature of a DHA solution at pH 5.0 (buffered with acetic acid/acetate buffer) leaves only 60% DHA (5 to 3%), whereas at pH 4.0 (buffered with acetic acid/acetate buffer), about 90% DHA is left (5 to 4.4%). The concentration of formic acid is kept at a minimum when DHA is formulated at pH 3.0 to 4.5. At the same time, a low

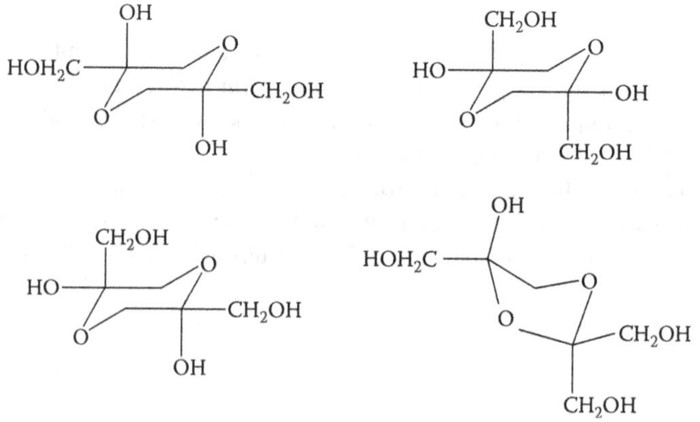

FIGURE 16.2 Structures of dihydroxyacetone dimers.

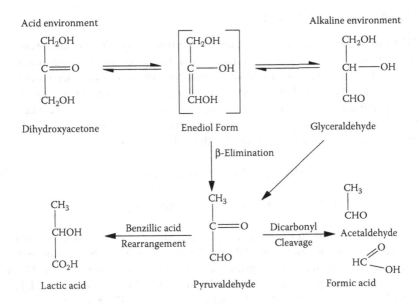

FIGURE 16.3 Chemistry of DHA in aqueous solution.

pH prevents isomerization to glyceraldehyde and, to a lesser extent, also degradation to pyruvaldehyde and pyruvaldehyde polymers.

Solubility of DHA in glycerol (74% soluble) is slightly higher than in water (70% soluble). Propylene glycol is also a very good solvent for DHA (53% soluble). Unfortunately, neither solvent provides any increased stability to DHA, especially at elevated temperature. Furthermore, these DHA solutions provide only very slight tanning when used as is because DHA remains in an ineffective dimeric form and water is required to convert DHA dimers to the reactive DHA monomer for self-tanning.

16.2.3 STORAGE AND HANDLING

DHA content can be dramatically reduced by improper storage conditions or by processing at elevated temperatures. Aldehydes and ketones, e.g., methylglyoxal, can be formed via decomposition or rearrangement reactions. Some of them have a tanning effect, but produce a more orange coloration. When assessing the stability of DHA, one must distinguish between DHA content, pH value, and the occurrence of by-products.[14]

DHA is a slightly hygroscopic material that should be shipped and stored in tightly closed containers under refrigeration (<6°C). Heating the material to above 40°C for long periods should be avoided. In manufacturing finished products, DHA should be added to the process at or below 40°C. Also, DHA is subject to microbial degradation in aqueous solution. Microbial decomposition reactions are often characterized by an accompanying pungent odor resulting from the formation of a variety of organic acids and aldehydes. DHA can be stored well over 1 year under refrigeration.

16.2.4 Analytical Methods

DHA can be analyzed by either thin layer chromatography (TLC) or an enzymatic test method. The TLC method works well with a precoated high-performance (HP) TLC plate silica gel (without fluorescent indicator) using acetone/water (95:5) as an eluent. A DHA spot can be visualized by spraying a solution of 2',7'-dichlorofluorescein and lead tetra-acetate in ethanol, drying the plate at 105°C, and observing under UV light (366 nm). DHA can be assayed enzymat-ically using glycerol dehydrogenase by the following reaction:

$$DHA + NADH + H^+ \rightarrow glycerol + NAD^+$$

(NADH = reduced nicotinamide adenine dinucleotide)

The reaction is allowed to continue to the endpoint and is measured at 340 nm (coefficient of absorbance of NADH = 6.3 cm^2/μmol) or 365 nm (coefficient of absorbance of NADH = 3.4 cm^2/μmol). The decrease in absorbance at 340 or 360 nm, induced by the NAD formed, is proportional to the quantity of DHA. There is no influence of higher glycerol contents on the DHA assay.

A gas chromatography (GC) method has been reported to determine DHA in self-tanning formulations using a DB-5 or OV-101 column with flame ioniza-tion detector (FID). This method requires a pretreatment of samples with acetic anhydride.[14] DHA content as well as trace amounts of impurities can also be determined directly in self-tanning products as reported by Ostrovskaya et al.[15]

16.3 MECHANISM OF SKIN TANNING

The site of action of DHA in the skin is the stratum corneum.[16] Tape stripping removes the color[17] as does mechanical rubbing. Deeper staining of the palms and soles and no tanning of mucous membranes have been noted. Microscopic study of stripped stratum corneum demonstrates pigment masses distributed irregularly in the keratin layer. Intradermal injection of DHA produces no pigmentation.

The first step in the self-tanning reaction is the conversion of DHA to pyru-valdehyde with the elimination of water. Then the keto or aldehyde function reacts with the amine functionality of skin keratin to form an imine. Subsequent steps of this reaction are a complex chain of reactions and are not fully understood.[4] However, it is well known that the resulting products are cyclic and linear polymers having yellow or brown color.[18,19]

The self-tanning process takes place in the outer layers of the epidermis and is similar to the Maillard reaction, also known as nonenzymatic browning. The Maillard reaction is defined as the reaction of the amino group of amino acids, peptides, or proteins with the glycosidic hydroxyl group of sugars.[20] The brown products formed have been referred to as melanoidins (Figure 16.4). They are polymeric compounds, which are linked by lysine side chains to the proteins of

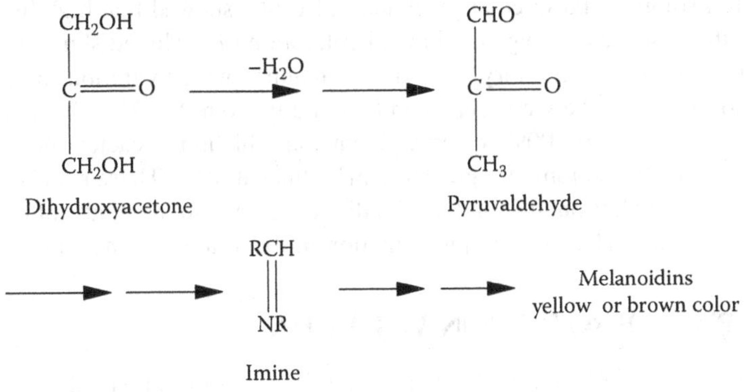

FIGURE 16.4 Self-tanning reaction of dihydroxyacetone.

the stratum corneum. Although the formation of melanoidins is different from that of melanin, some of their properties are similar, especially their absorption spectra.[21] Melanins consist of indoles (eumelanins) or benzothiazinyl alanines (pheomelanins) and are derived from the aromatic amino acid tyrosine. Melanoidins, on the other hand, consist mainly of an aliphatic moiety with very few aromatic functionalities in the side chains.

The reaction of DHA and an amino group of proteins leads to polymeric products on the skin within about 4 h, the first tan appearing within 2 to 3 h. DHA reacts only with the amines of the stratum corneum. The polymers have a brown color that comes near to the hue of a natural suntan. As the polymers are anchored to the proteins of the horny layer, the tan is substantive. It diminishes only when the dead cells of the horny layer flake off, which usually takes 5 to 10 days.

The role of pH in tanning is very important. To achieve a uniform tan, exfoliation is recommended before application to remove loose skin scales. The optimum pH for the Maillard reaction is from 5 to 6, which is the normal pH of the healthy skin. When formulations with a higher or lower pH are applied, the skin buffer adjusts the pH on the skin to the optimal tanning pH. Tests showed that unbuffered formulations with a pH from 2 to 6 always led to the same coloring results. The browning intensity is reduced significantly only when the pH was above 6. The intensity of tanning, varying from a light to dark orange-brown, depends on the concentration of DHA and the frequency of its application. Usually three to five applications give rise to a golden-brown color, stimulating a tanning reaction.

Recently, Nguyen and Kochevar have examined the influence of hydration and oxygen on the development of DHA-induced pigmentation *in vivo* using an occlusive dressing and *ex vitro* on human epidermal preparations.[22] Two spectroscopic techniques, diffuse reflectance and fluorescence emission, were used to monitor the extent of pigment development. The optimal relative humidity for DHA-induced pigmentation was assessed on the epidermal preparations. The formation of products from reactions between DHA and nine amino acids was studied in solutions buffered at pH 5 and 7. Results showed that high hydration, but not the absence of oxygen, inhibited coloration of occluded skin. The extent of pigmentation did not vary in a simple manner with hydration, as pigment formation was positively correlated with humidity from 0 to 75%, but negatively correlated from 75 to 100%. Lysine, glycine, and histidine reacted most rapidly with DHA, with reaction rates greater at pH 7 than at pH 5. These results indicate that extent of hydration, pH, and availability of certain amino acids influence the development of DHA-induced pigmentation in the stratum corneum.

16.4 PHOTOPROTECTION WITH DHA

In addition to DHA's ability to elicit an artificial tan on human skin, it is also known that the reaction product of DHA and the skin protein that produces the tan color is an effective sunscreen agent. However, this is not a U.S. Federal Drug Agency (FDA)-approved claim. In particular, this reaction product is known to absorb UV light in the 300- to 600-nm range, with a peak of about 350 nm, thus protecting the skin from damage to exposure to UVA radiation.[23,24] In fact, this property has been utilized in protecting uninvolved skin by DHA during psoralene–UVA (PUVA) treatment of psoriasis.[25] By preferentially protecting uninvolved skin, DHA allows higher UVA doses to be tolerated and delivered to the psoriatic plaques with acceleration in clearing.

Previous studies have also shown that DHA induces concentration-dependent photoprotection against UVA and visible light.[26] Commercial products containing DHA are often labeled as having no sun protection. However, studies have shown that DHA does absorb UVB and delays photocarcinogenesis in hairless mice[27] and offers modest protection against erythema in humans.[28] Durability of the sun protection factor provided by dihydroxyacetone has recently been demonstrated in humans by Faurschau and Wulf.[29]

The photoprotective effect has also been demonstrated *in vivo* in patients suffering from erythropoietic protoporphyria (EPP), in which the skin reactions are mainly elicited by exposures to wavelengths around 400 nm. It has been shown that patients with EPP tolerated a fourfold increased dose of visible radiation when treated with DHA lotions.[30,31] The photoprotection afforded by DHA against long-wave UV has also been reported in patients with polymorphous light eruption (PLE), a very common idiopathic photodermatose characterized by the appearance of itching papules 24 to 48 h after sun exposure. The lesions occur on light-exposed skin areas and are known to be provoked by ultraviolet light, especially UVA.

Riccio et al.[32] have studied the effectiveness of topical sunscreens associated with 5% DHA in a cream on 20 females affected by PLE. The result showed a skin response, characterized by erythematous papules, on the control areas daily irradiated with UVA. No response was elicited by repeated exposure to UVA on skin areas treated with the cream containing 5% DHA plus sunscreens. Similar results were obtained by Stege et al.[33] on five of eight patients with PLE. They showed that creams containing DHA and sunscreens decrease the expression of KC ICAM-1 (a proinflamatory molecule in epidermis) in experimentally induced PLE lesions.

16.5 REGULATORY STATUS

Neither the National Institute for Occupational Safety and Health (NIOSH) nor Occupational Safety and Health Organization (OSHA) has set a standard or guideline for occupational exposure to workplace-allowable levels of DHA. DHA is not on the American Conference of Governmental Industrial Hygienists (ACGIH) list of compounds for which recommendations for a threshold limit value (TLV) or biological exposure index (BEI) are made.

The FDA has approved DHA as a permanently listed colorant (21 CFR §73.2150), which is exempt from certification for drugs and cosmetics. It may only be used in externally applied drugs and cosmetics intended solely or in part to impart a color to the human body. A monograph for DHA has been included in the ninth supplement of the U.S. Pharmacopeia (USP) 23.

There is no limitation according to the EEC Cosmetics Directive (76/768/ EEC). The Japanese Cosmetic Ingredient Dictionary (JCID-II-80) includes DHA as a cosmetic ingredient.

No other ingredients are legally allowed for use as sunless tanners. Tanning boosters or enhancers are also not legally allowed ingredients for inclusion in sunless tanning products.

16.6 SELF-TANNING FORMULATIONS WITH DHA

16.6.1 TYPES OF FORMULAS

Tanning products fall loosely into two categories: wash-offs and wear-offs. Wash-offs (also known as bronzers) are cosmetic tanning products in cream or gel formulas, without DHA, that give the appearance of a tan, but are not substantive to skin and wash off in the shower at the end of the day. Wear-off formulations containing DHA are the true self-tanning products; these are available in creams, lotions, milks, gels, foams, sprays, or airbrush (for in-house application). These products, when applied onto skin, develop tan over a matter of hours and wear off over a period of 5 to 10 days.

By far the most popular of all vehicles used for self-tanning products, the emulsion offers almost unlimited versatility. DHA is most often formulated in oil-in-water (O/W) emulsions. Lotions are more popular than creams owing to their ease of spreadability on the skin and dispensability from bottles. Creams can lead to a more intense tan than lotions because the applied film is thicker. From an aesthetic viewpoint, emulsions are an elegant medium that can give the skin a smooth, silky feel without being greasy or tacky. They can accommodate a wide variety of raw materials. Due to the high water solubility of DHA, aqueous or aqueous-alcoholic lotions and gels can be prepared easily. By appropriate control of viscosity, spray lotions or gels can also be developed.

A novel patented technology introduced in 1999 is the sunless tanning booth, which employs misters to apply an even coat of sunless tanning solution to the consumer's bare skin.[34] The technique is promoted as the means to a perfect tan and healthy skin. In this mode of application, DHA is used as a solution in water or alcoholic water containing 8 to 15% DHA with other ingredients. The tanning booths employ misters that are either mobile or stationary, which helps apply a uniform amount of tanning solution to all parts of the body. Tanning sessions range from 6 to 60 sec and, in most cases, end with the evacuation of mist from the booth. Towel buffing is a critical part of this method of tanning and helps get a uniform and darker tan. Sunless tanning booths appear to be becoming the most commonly offered sunless tanning application modality.[35]

16.6.2 Formulation Do's and Don'ts

The content of DHA in tanning products depends on the desired browning intensity on the skin and is normally in the range of 4 to 8%. Depending on the type of formulation and skin type, a tanning effect appears on the skin in approximately 2 to 3 h after use. During product storage, the pH of a DHA-containing formulation will drift over time to about 3 to 4. At this pH, DHA is quite stable. In order to ensure end-product stability, the following factors must be considered before developing new formulations containing DHA.

16.6.2.1 Temperature

Heating DHA above 40°C for a long period must be avoided, as it causes rapid degradation of DHA (>40% within 3 months). During manufacturing processes involving heating, as in the case of emulsions, DHA should not be added until the formulation has been cooled to below 40°C. Products containing DHA should be stored in an opaque and resealable package.

16.6.2.2 pH

When DHA is incorporated in a formulation, the pH of the formulation drops to 3 to 4 within about 2 days from the date of preparation. In the past, buffering was recommended to keep the pH at a level of 4 to 6. Recent investigations in our laboratories revealed that storage stability of DHA could be increased when the formulations are kept at pH 3.0 to 4.5. Buffering at a higher pH is counterproductive, as it enhances degradation of DHA, thereby reducing its storage stability.

16.6.2.3 Buffers

Use of buffers to maintain the pH of a formulation above 4.5 is not recommended. The pH of the formulation may be adjusted to approximately 3 to 4 by using a small amount of citric acid or using acetate buffer, because they do not affect DHA stability.[7] Phosphate buffers are not recommended. At pH values above 7, brown-colored compounds are produced via isomerization and condensation reactions, and tanning efficacy is reduced.

16.6.3 SELECTION OF INGREDIENTS

In order to have a stable DHA formulation, one must carefully select appropriate ingredients for each formula because there is always a potential for ingredient interaction. Certainly, all ingredients selected must be cosmetically acceptable, have a good safety record, be stable, and must not interfere with the efficacy of DHA in any way. The following are some comments on how to select ingredients.

16.6.3.1 Emulsifers

The use of nonionic emulsifiers is recommended over ionic emulsifiers because of improved stability of DHA in the formulations. Typical nonionic emulsifiers or emulsifier systems used in commercial products are glyceryl stearate, PEG-100 stearate, polysorbate 60, laureth-7, ceteareth-20, ceteareth-15, cetearyl glucoside, etc.

16.6.3.2 Emollients

Emollients represent one of the most important classes of emulsion components. They provide a silky skin feel on application. There are many types of emollients: esters, waxes, fatty alcohols, mineral oils, and silicone materials. Esters are the most common classes of emollients used in self-tanning products. Silicone-based oils have also enjoyed an increase in popularity. Dimethicone and cyclomethicone are the widely used materials of this type. All these emollients are compatible with DHA.

16.6.3.3 Thickeners

Thickening a formulation containing DHA, especially to produce a clear gel, is relatively difficult because many conventional cosmetic thickeners are not compatible with DHA. Scientists at Merck KGaA, Darmstadt, Germany, screened a wide variety of thickeners in the early 1990s. The simple method used for this study called for a solution of 5% DHA and a thickener, storing at room temperature and at 40°C for 3 months, and analyzing for DHA content and solution colors.

Based on this and other studies, they determined that three good choices for thickeners are hydroxyethylcellulose, methycellulose, and silica. Additionally, xanthan gum and polyquaternium-10 may also be used for thickening emulsions. Carbomers, sodium carboxymethylcellulose, PVM/MA decadiene cross-polymer, and magnesium aluminum silicate are not acceptable thickeners because they cause a rapid degradation of DHA at 40°C.

16.6.3.4 Moisturizers

The natural water content of stratum corneum is not sufficient to cause the tanning reaction; therefore, water-free systems are not at all useful for formulating tanning products. Moisturizers, like sorbitol or propylene glycol, at a level of approximately 20% (w/w of formulation) help increase the tanning intensity.

16.6.3.5 Preservatives

An aqueous solution or emulsion of DHA is susceptible to microbial attack. For this reason, preservation of the final product as well as hygienically clean manufacturing and packaging procedures are particularly important. Parabens and phenoxyethanol, alone or in combination, are recommended preservatives.

16.6.3.6 Compounds Containing Nitrogen

Amines or other nitrogen-containing compounds should be avoided in the final formulation. These compounds include collagen, urea derivatives, amino acids, and proteins. The reactivity of DHA toward these nitrogen-containing compounds can lead to gradual breakdown of DHA, and thus to a loss of efficacy in use. However, many of the available commercial formulations include amino acids. This combination gives a perceptual advantage; customers begin to see a tanning effect within about 45 min due to the reaction between DHA and the amino acids. Only glycine and histidine provide brown color. However, this tan is not substantive, and part of it is easily washed off.[7] In order to prevent the reaction from occurring before application, Suares has patented a two-compartment dispenser; the amino acids are in one compartment and the DHA in the other.[36]

16.6.3.7 Sunscreens

It must be noted that a tan achieved with DHA alone does not offer sun protection comparable to that resulting from natural melanin production during sunbathing. It is, however, possible to combine DHA with non-nitrogen-containing sunscreens, such as ethylhexyl methoxycinnamate (octinoxate), ethylhexyl salicylate (octisalate), homosalate, benzophenone-3, octocrylene, and avobenzone. Avobenzone requires a stabilizer, as it has limited photostability. Diethylhexyl syringylidene malonate (Oxynex® ST) has recently been shown to provide significant improvement in photostabilization of avobenzone.[37] The combination with sunscreens delivers self-tanning products with an additional sun protection effect. Inorganic sunscreens, such as titanium dioxide, zinc oxide, and other metal oxides, must be avoided because they induce rapid degradation of DHA.

16.6.3.8 Fragrance Oils

The choice of a proper fragrance can enhance the aesthetics of self-tanning formulations. However, their use level must be kept as low as possible because fragrance oils can be irritating. They can also discolor formulations or degrade DHA. Their breakdown products can be photosensitizers. Thus, great care must be taken in choosing them.

16.6.3.9 Tinting

To achieve a makeup effect with self-tanning products, we suggest combining DHA with organic compounds such as carotene and D&C Blue 4, staining dyes such as D&C Red 21, and other approved dyes. The use of iron oxides must be avoided, because DHA will degrade rapidly.

16.6.3.10 Tonality

A DHA-induced sunless tan can often lie outside the realm of the natural tan; it is possible to improve this tonality to a more natural look by adding strong antioxidants to the DHA formulations.[38]

16.7 SUMMARY

With the new profound popularity of self-tanning products and a year-round market to sell in, the array of sunless products and their benefits continue to rise. Some products include sunscreen or multifunctional aspects, while others stick to the task of providing color or both. The self-tanning market continues to develop and grow as self-tanning products have become easier to apply, greaseless in texture, and odorless, and most importantly, they offer a natural-looking color. No matter whether the reasons are vain or protective, sunless tanners will continue to evolve into a year-round skin care regimen for many consumers.

REFERENCES

1. People Aware of the Dangers of the Sun, Protection Not Practiced, news release, American Academy of Dermatology, April 29, 2003.
2. Prota G, Melanins, melanogenesis and melanocytes: looking at their functional significance from the chemist's viewpoint, *Pigment Cell Res* 2000; 13:283–293.
3. Raffi JJ, Agnel JP, Frejaville CM, Saint-Lebe LR, Radoinduced products in maize starch: glyceraldehydes, dihydroxyacetone, and 2-hydroxymalonaldehyde, *J Agric Food Chem* 1981; 29:548–550.
4. Wittgenstein E, Berry HK, Staining of skin with dihydroxyacetone, *Science* 1960; 132:894–895.
5. Ohrem HL, Westmeier F, Microbial Process for the Preparation of Dihydroxyacetone with Recycling of Biomass, U.S. Patent 5,770,411, 1998.
6. Hekmat D, Bauer R, Fricke J, Optimization of the microbial synthesis of dihydroxyacetone from glycerol with *Gluconobacter oxydans*, *Bioprocess Biosyst Eng* 2003; 26:109–116.
7. Kurz T, Formulating effective self-tanners with DHA, *Cosmet Toil* 1994; 109:55–61.
8. Chaudhuri RK, Hwang C, Self-tanners: formulating with dihydroxyacetone, *Cosmet Toil* 2001; 116:87–96.
9. Chaudhuri RK, Dihydroxyacetone: chemistry and applications in self-tanning products, in *The Chemistry and Manufacture of Cosmetics*, Vol. III, Book 1, Schlossman M, Ed., Allured Publishing, Carol Stream, Illinois, 2002, pp. 383–402.
10. Kobayashi Y, Igarashi T, Takahashi H, Higasi K, Infrared and Raman studies of the dimeric structures of 1,3-dihydroxyacetone, d(+)- and dl-glyceraldehyde, *J Mol Struct* 1976; 35:85–99.

11. Spoehr HA, Strain HH, The effect of weak alkalies on the trioses and on meth-ylglyoxal, *J Biol Chem* 1930; 89:503–525.
12. Slepokura K, Lis T, Crystal structures of dihydroxyacetone and its derivatives, *Carbohydrate Res* 2004; 339:1995–2007.
13. Davis L, Structure of dihydroxyacetone in solution, *Biorg Chem* 1973; 2:197–201.
14. Hild J, GC-determination of dihydroxyacetone in cosmetics, *Dtsch Lebens* 1993; 89:48–49.
15. Ostrovskaya A, Rosalia AD, Landa PA, Maes D, Stability of dihydroxyacetone in self-tanning cosmetic products, *J Soc Cosmet Chem* 1997; 47:275–278.
16. Goldman L, Barkoff J, Blaney D, Nakai T, Suskind R, Investigative studies with the skin coloring agents dihydroxyacetone and glyoxal, *J Invest Dermatol* 1960; 35:161–164.
17. Maibach HI, Kligman AM, Dihyroxyacetone: a suntan-simulating agent, *Arch Dermatol* 1960; 82:505–507.
18. Angrick M, Rewicki D, Die Mailardreaction, *Chemie Unserer Zeit* 1980; 14:149.
19. Severin T, Hiebl J, Popp-Ginsbach H, Investigations relating to the Maillard reaction. XX. Identification of glyceraldehyde dihydroxyacetone and other hydro-philic sugar degradation products in caramel mixtures, *Lebensm Unters Forsch* 1984; 178:284–287.
20. Ellis GP, The Maillard reaction, *Adv Carbohydr Chem* 1959; 14:63–134.
21. Meybeck A, A spectroscpic study of the reaction products of hydroxyacetone with amino acids, *J Soc Cosmet Chem* 1977; 28:25–35.
22. Nguyen BC, Kochevar IE, Factors influencing sunless tanning with dihydroxyac-etone, *Br J Dermatol* 2003; 149:332–340.
23. Gilles R, Kollias, Noninvasive *in vivo* determination of sunscreen ultraviolet A protection factor using diffuse reflectance spectroscopy, in *Sunscreens: Develop-ment, Evaluation, and Regulatory Aspects*, Lowe N, Shaath NA, Pathak MA, Eds., Marcel Dekker, New York, 1997, pp. 601–610.
24. Johnson JA, Dihydroxyacetone for protection against long wavelength UVA radi-ation and blue light, *Br J Dermatol* 1992; 126:94.
25. Taylor CR, Kwangsukstith C, Wimberly J, Kollias N, Anderson RR, Turbo-PUVA: dihydroxyacetone-enhanced photochemotherapy for psoriasis: a pilot study, *Arch Dermatol* 1999; 135:540–544.
26. Fusaro RM, Johnson JA, Protection against long ultraviolet and/or visible light with topical dihydroxyacetone: implications for the mechanism of action of the sunscreen combination, dihydroxyacetone/napthoquinone, *Dermatologica* 1975; 150:346–351.
27. Petersen AB, Na R, Wulf HC, Sunless skin tanning with dihydroxyacetone delays broad-spectrum ultraviolet photocarcinogenesis in hairless mice, *Mut Res* 2003; 542:129–138.
28. Faurschau A, Janjua NR, Wulf HC, Sun protection effect of dihydroxyacetone, *Arch Dermatol* 2004; 140:886–887.
29. Faurschau A, Wulf HC, Durabililty of the sun protection factor provided by dihydroxyacetone, *Photodermatol Photoimmunol Photomed* 2004; 20:239–242.
30. Fusaro RM, Johnson JA, Dihydroxyacetone napthoquinone sunscreen, *JAMA* 1972; 222:1651–1657.
31. Fusaro RM, Runge WJ, Erythropoietic protoporphyria IV: protection from sun-light, *Br Med J* 1970 1:730–731.

32. Riccio G, Masturzo E, Del Dorbo A, Riccardo AM, Piccirillo M, Monfrecola G, Dermatite polimorfa solare: prevenzione mediante filtri UV e diidossiacetone, *G Ital Dermatol Venereol* 1999; 134:197–200.

33. Stege H, Ahrens C, Billman-Eberwein C, Ruzicka T, Krutman J, Rougier A, Pretreatment of Human Skin with a Sunscreen or Dihydroxyacetone (DHA) Prevents Photo-Provocation-Induced Polymorphous Light Eruption (PLE) and Keratinocytes (KC) ICAM-1 Expression, poster presented at the 19th World Congress of Dermatology, Sydney, 1997.

34. Laughlin TJ, System for Automatically Coating the Human Body, U.S. 5,922,333, July 13, 1999.

35. Fu JM, Dusza SW, Halpern AC, Sunless tanning, *J Am Acad Dermatol* 2004; 50:706–713.

36. Suares AJ, Self-Tanner Cosmetic Composition, EP 0547864 B1, September 9, 1998.

37. Chaudhuri RK, Puccetti G, Design of a Photostabilizer Having Built-In Antioxidant Functionality and Its Utility in Obtaining Broad-Spectrum Sunscreen Formulations, poster presented at the 23rd IFSCC Congress, Orlando, 2004.

38. Muizzuddin N, Marenus KD, Maes DH, Tonality of suntan vs. sunless tanning with dihydroxyacetone, *Skin Res Technol* 2000; 6:199–204.

17 Hydrocarbons in Pigmented Products

Gina Butuc and David S. Morrison, Ph.D.
Penreco

CONTENTS

17.1 INTRODUCTION AND BACKGROUND

Color cosmetics are substances designed to enhance the beauty of the human body apart from simple cleansing. Their use is widespread, especially among women in Western countries, but women in other parts of the world have their fair share of cosmetic usage.

The role of modern cosmetics is to simulate youthfulness, health, and, to an extent, arousal. The various forms of color cosmetics include lipstick and lip gloss (used to color and add shine to the lips); foundation, powder, and rouge (used to color the face, while also lightening and removing flaws to produce an impression of health and youth); mascara (used to enhance the eyelashes — larger eyes are perceived as an indication of youth); eyeliner (used to color the eyelids); and nail polish (used to color the fingernails and toenails).

The first use of color cosmetics is estimated to have occurred around 4000 B.C. by the Egyptians.[1] Apparently, the affluent women of those days applied a bright green paste of copper minerals to their faces to provide color and definition of features. They used perfumed oils and painted eyebrows on themselves with cream made from sheep's fat, lead, and soot. It is thought that perfumed oils were used because of the odor from the animal fat-based facial makeup. (Soaps, which could be used for cleaning the skin, were not available until sometime around 1000 B.C.)

Other ancient cultures also mention the use of color cosmetics. The Chinese, Japanese, Greeks, and Romans all used henna products for dyeing the skin and hair.[2] Other practices of using color on the body existed as well. For example, the Chinese would dye their teeth black or gold, and the Romans would frequently dye their hair blond. When Greek women wanted a little color, they chose ochre clays laced with red iron for lipstick. In 100 A.D. in Rome, Platus wrote, "A woman without paint is like food without salt."[3]

By the Middle Ages, Western European aristocrats were using cosmetics on a regular basis. Italy and France became the chief centers of cosmetics manufacturing. The French perfected the art of creating new fragrances and cosmetics, primarily by blending various ingredients. However, poisonous compounds were still being used in the manufacture of cosmetics: in eye shadow, lead and antimony sulfide; as lip reddeners, mercuric sulfide; and to make one's eyes sparkle, Belladonna, also known as deadly nightshade (which contains the alkaloid atropine).

Although color cosmetics were popular due to their ability to enhance the wearer's beauty, their history was not without some pitfalls. Jessica Pallingston points out in her book *Lipstick* that in the 1800s, Queen Victoria publicly declared makeup impolite.[4] Thus, the use of makeup was drastically reduced, and paleness became vogue for almost a century.

In the 19th century, France was the stage for a turning point in the cosmetic industry: chemical processing began replacing fragrances made by natural methods. Zinc oxide became widely used as a facial powder, replacing the mixtures of lead and copper that were previously used. Also, the first commercially successful lipstick was produced by Guerlain in about 1880.[5]

During and after World War I, cosmetics and fragrances were manufactured on larger scales and began to be marketed to the masses. It was now okay for women to drop the Victorian image and to dress up and use cosmetics. The wide appeal and market for cosmetics was ensured with the advent of the dime store (later replaced by department stores and chain stores), which proliferated during the first part of the 20th century.

Between the 1930s and 1960s, Hollywood stars began having a large influence on the use of color cosmetics.

In the 1970s, certain animal-based ingredients were banned from use in cosmetics to protect endangered species. In addition, testing on animals by cosmetics manufacturers began to be questioned. This age of environmental concern fostered the start of many movements demanding more disclosure from the cosmetics industry. This was a major turning point in the industry; fewer animal-derived ingredients were used in cosmetic products, and testing of the products on animals also fell out of favor.

More recently, multiple functionalities have begun to be required from products that previously were just decorative. We want our color cosmetic products not only to beautify us, but also to protect us against harsh UV rays that lead to premature skin aging, to have added moisturization, and to fill in the fine lines on the skin, for example. Currently, a lipstick should have not only pigments to color our lips, but also sunscreens, moisturizers, film formers that translate into added UV protection, lip plumpness benefits, and transfer resistance.[6]

17.2 CHEMISTRY

17.2.1 PETROLEUM PRODUCTS

Formed over millions of years, petroleum (often called crude oil) has a very complex composition. Due to this complexity and the variety seen in petroleum from different source locations around the world, no exact composition of petroleum can be defined. Simply stated, it is a naturally occurring mixture of hydrocarbons, usually including nitrogen-, sulfur-, and oxygen-containing compounds.[7]

Upon extraction, the crude oil goes through a series of refining processes. Refinery products include transportation fuels, lubricants, waxes, asphalt, and specialty hydrocarbon products. The materials used by the cosmetic, personal care, and pharmaceutical industries are extremely purified specialty hydrocarbon products, such as white mineral oil, petrolatum (petroleum jelly), waxes, and solvents. These products have been highly refined to meet the stringent requirements of their end-use applications in these industries.

Separation and isolation techniques of the components of petroleum involve an enormous effort and have led to the identification of only about 200 individual compounds.[8] However, even with such draconian efforts, the petroleum does not give up the identity of many of its components. Once petroleum has been refined to remove the aromatic components, the remainder generally consists of saturated hydrocarbons: normal alkanes (paraffinics), isoalkanes (isoparaffinics,) and cycloalkanes (naphthenics). Classifying compounds within refined petroleum is extremely difficult, if not impossible, especially since most of the components are combinations of these structures. Since most of the components are not purely paraffinic, isoparaffinic, or naphthenic in nature, the molecule is classified by what is predominant in its structure. Take, for example, a compound whose structure contains both isoparaffinic and naphthenic moieties; if its isoparaffinic structure is predominant, then it will be characterized as an isoparaffinic product.

Paraffins found in petroleum-based products vary from C_5 through C_{44}, but other studies have found that the carbon chain can be up to C_{78}. *Isoparaffins* are more difficult to isolate and identify than paraffins, due to their multitude of branches. Chromatographic analysis has given a common range of C_5 to C_{35} for isoparaffinic materials in petroleum. *Naphthenics* isolated from petroleum products typically contain five, six, or seven carbon atoms in their rings.

17.2.2 PIGMENTS AND DYES

Pigments used in color cosmetics can be both inorganic and organic compounds. Although most pigments are inorganic, many organic compounds are also used as pigments, while dyes are almost entirely organic compounds. There is no well-defined division between pigments and dyes in terms of chemical structure, and some of them have dual functions. In many cases, a pigment will be made by precipitating a soluble dye with a metallic salt; the resulting compound is called a "lake." However, pigments and dyes differ in solubility characteristics and in the method of application. Pigments and dyes are used as colorants in cosmetic products, but some of the white pigments are also used as fillers and sunscreen ingredients.

17.2.2.1 Inorganic Pigments

In the coloring of a cosmetic formulation, a pigment is a dry colorant, usually an insoluble powder. Pigments work by selectively absorbing some parts of the visible light spectrum, while reflecting others. The vast majority of cosmetic pigments are metal oxides, but other metallic salts can also be used as pigments, such as carbonates, chromates, phosphates, silicates, and sulfides.[9] Chemical composition is not the only property that determines a pigment's properties — features such as particle size, particle shape, particle size distribution, and the nature of the pigment surface also play an important role in the coloring process.

Table 17.1 lists a few examples of inorganic pigments that are approved for color cosmetic use in the U.S.

17.2.2.2 Organic Pigments

Similar to inorganic pigments, organic pigments can impart color to a formulation, but they are insoluble in the medium. For organic compounds, color is associated with the presence of multiple bonds. These groups of multiple bonds are called chromophores.[10] Examples of chromophores include azo, azomethine, azoxy, carbonyl, ethenyl nitro, nitroso, and thiocarbonyl groups. Besides chromophores, auxiliary groups can also enhance or modify the color. Such groups are called auxochromes. Examples of auxochromes include alkylamino, amino, dialkylamino, hydroxy, and methoxy substituents.

Organic pigments can be classified as azo and nonazo pigments. The azo pigments are the most important class of organic pigments used in color cosmetics.

TABLE 17.1
Inorganic Pigments Approved for Color Cosmetic Use in the United States

Pigment	Lip Products	Body and Face Products	Eye Products
Bismuth oxychloride	Approved	Approved	Approved
Chromium oxide	Not Approved	Approved	Approved
Copper chromite black	Approved	Approved	Approved
Ferric ammonium ferrocyanide	Not Approved	Approved	Approved
Iron oxide red	Approved	Approved	Approved
Iron oxide yellow	Approved	Approved	Approved
Mica	Approved	Approved	Approved
Talc	Approved	Approved	Approved
Titanium dioxide	Approved	Approved	Approved
Zinc oxide	Approved	Approved	Approved

Important features of the azo pigments are their light, heat, and acid stabilities. Monoazo (one chromophore group) and diazo (two chromophore groups) pigments are formed by successive diazotization and coupling reactions. The azo pigments are hydrophobic, but some of them have a tendency to bleed in oil and organic solvents. These are the stainers sometimes used in transfer-resistant lipstick products. Probably the most commonly used azo pigments in lipsticks are Red 7 Calcium Lake and Red 6 Barium Lake.

17.2.2.3 Dyes

Dyes are substances used for the coloration of a substrate. They differ from pigments not by chemical composition, but by their solvency on a substrate. The art of dyeing goes back 5000 years ago to textile dyeing. Natural dyes, such as indigo, alizarin, and logwood, were used for thousands of years before the first synthetic dye — mauveine — was obtained in 1856 by W.H. Perkin.[11,12] Optical properties of dyes are determined by electronic transmissions between the various molecular orbitals of the molecule, which absorb some but not all of the incident radiation.

17.3 MINERAL OIL, PETROLATUM, AND WAXES

Through the end of the 1800s, vegetable or animal oils and fats were key ingredients used in cosmetic formulation. While suitable cosmetics can be produced using these materials, they also have a major disadvantage: their stability is very limited. Vegetable or animal oils and fats are prone to rancidity after short time, usually 6 to 12 months, they show signs of discoloration, and probably the most noticeable aspect — unpleasant odors — can easily develop.[13] The shelf-life of a cosmetic product containing unadditized vegetable or animal oils and fats can be increased by careful control of raw materials and by the elimination of trace impurities, along with cleanliness in preparation and packaging, but it is still quite difficult to go beyond a shelf-life of 12 months. By increasing the amount of antioxidants, one can prolong the shelf-life of a cosmetic product containing vegetable or animal oils and fats, but high levels of antioxidants may be undesirable in the finished formulation.

As the 20th century approached, hydrocarbons, such as petrolatum, mineral oil, paraffin wax, and ceresin wax, were introduced for use in cosmetics and have been used ever since. The major advantage of these types of oils and fats is their superb stability (no rancidity), resulting in an odorless and tasteless material even after years of storage. Many cosmetic products and raw materials now have an expected shelf-life of 2+ years, owed, in part, to the availability of mineral hydrocarbons and improved preservation and stabilization techniques. The globalization of cosmetic products was also made possible, so that products can be shipped around the world, to a variety of climates, without concerns over product rancidity and instability.

In the majority of color cosmetic products that use hydrocarbons, these materials act as inert ingredients, while pigments and dyes are really the performance ingredients. However, more sophisticated cosmetics are being demanded by consumers. Therefore, added features are welcome, such as moisturization and emolliency, and this is when hydrocarbons behave as more than just a carrier or filler in the formulation.

17.3.1 MINERAL OIL

Mineral oil is a liquid — a mixture of saturated hydrocarbons, odorless and tasteless, with a high chemical, thermal, and light stability.[14] Its unique lubricity, ready availability, extraordinary stability, and low cost are just a few of the features that make white mineral oil (pharmacopoeia quality) attractive for color cosmetic products.

In lipstick manufacturing, oil absorption plays an important role. Oil absorption is defined as the weight of oil in grams absorbed by 100 g of pigment to produce a paste of specific consistency.[15] This is particularly important for different shades of the same lipstick formulation, where varying levels of oil absorption can affect the product's texture and its feeling on the lips.

17.3.1.1 Rheology

The science that studies the way in which liquids and solids behave under the application of shear stress is called rheology.[16] The term *viscosity* is used to describe the resistance that a fluid exhibits when any attempt is made to change its shape. The dynamic viscosity (η) for an ideal liquid can be determined from the following relationship:

$$\tau = \eta D$$

where τ = shear stress and D = shear rate.

The kinematic viscosity of a fluid, v, is related to the dynamic viscosity as follows:

$$v = \eta/\sigma$$

where σ = density. The units of kinematic viscosity are m^2sec^{-1}.

Based on their rheological behaviors, fluids can be classified as Newtonian or non-Newtonian.

17.3.1.2 Newtonian Behavior

Mineral oils exhibit Newtonian flow characteristics. This flow is only exhibited by ideal, or Newtonian liquids, and describes a linear increase in shear stress with increasing shear rate. For this type of liquid flow, the value of the dynamic viscosity (η) is independent of shear rate. Therefore, a Newtonian flow curve follows a mathematically straight-line relationship, as illustrated in Figure 17.1.

The dynamic viscosity can therefore be calculated from the following equation:

$$\text{Dynamic viscosity } (\eta) = \tan \alpha = \tau_1/D_1$$

17.3.2 PETROLATUM

Petrolatum is an amorphous, semisolid mixture of saturated hydrocarbons and is odorless and tasteless. It is one of the oldest petroleum-based ingredients still in use today, and it is used in both personal care and color cosmetic products. The composition of petrolatum is extremely complex, due to the wide variety of molecular structures present.[17]

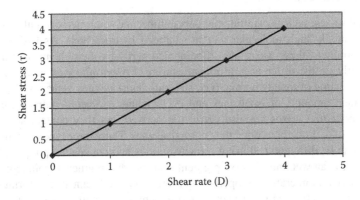

FIGURE 17.1 Shear stress vs. shear rate of a Newtonian fluid (mineral oil).

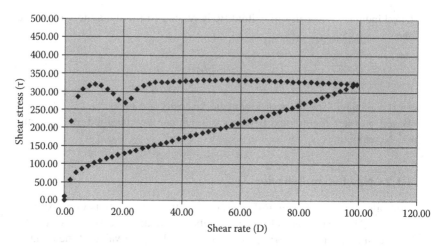

FIGURE 17.2 Shear stress vs. shear rate of a nonNewtonian shear thinning material (petrolatum).

17.3.2.1 Rheology

Because of its colloidal nature, petrolatum has a non-Newtonian behavior. For non-Newtonian fluids, viscosity is constant at all shear rates. The viscosity can decrease with constant shear (thixotropic behavior), or it can increase with constant shear (dilatant behavior). *Thixotropic* liquids exhibit a time-dependent response to the shear strain rate over a longer period than that associated with changes in the shear strain rate. They may liquefy on being shaken and then solidify (or not) when this has stopped. The thixotropic behavior of a typical petrolatum is clearly shown in Figure 17.2.

17.3.3 MINERAL WAXES

Mineral waxes, such as paraffin, microcrystalline, and semimicrocrystalline waxes, are essentially high molecular weight saturated hydrocarbons. As hydrocarbon-based products, these waxes are differentiated partly by their chemical structures and partly on the differences in manufacturing.[18] A *paraffin* wax is a petroleum wax consisting of mainly normal (i.e., straight-chain) alkanes, typically C_{18} to C_{36}, with small amounts of isoalkanes and cycloalkanes.[19] *Semimicrocrystalline* and *microcrystalline* waxes are also petroleum derived, but they contain substantial amounts of hydrocarbons other than normal alkanes. These three types of petroleum waxes can be differentiated using refractive index and congealing point analyses.

Waxes can wet and disperse pigments and prevent pigments from agglomeration or reagglomeration, properties that are very important in the formulation of color cosmetics. Mineral waxes tend to remain rigid under mild stress, but behave similarly to Newtonian fluids under greater stresses. This is called "plastic flow" and allows the waxes to disperse high levels of pigments while minimizing settling. This characteristic makes waxes valuable in high-gloss cosmetic lip products. Petroleum-derived waxes also improve a product's resistance to mechanical impact, along with increasing the hardness and softening point properties of color cosmetic preparations.

17.3.3.1 Formulations

Most color cosmetic products benefit from having hydrocarbons as ingredients, due to both functionality and price. Hydrocarbon-based products can make up to 60% (by weight) of a color cosmetic product.[14] Table 17.2 shows several examples of color cosmetic products that often contain hydrocarbon ingredients.

17.3.3.2 Lipstick

Among color cosmetics, lipstick is one product that uses a significant amount of hydrocarbon in its composition. According to Maison G. de Navarre, "Lipstick is a molded, solid fatty base containing dissolved and suspended colorants having

TABLE 17.2
Color Cosmetic Products

Facial Makeup
Vanishing creams
Powder creams
Loose facial powder
Compressed facial powder

Eye Makeup
Compressed eye shadow
Emulsion eye shadow
Mascara
Eyeliner
Eyebrow pencil
Eye cream
Eye fix

Lip Products
Lipstick
Lip gloss
Lip fix
Lip contour pencil

Nail Products
Nail polish
Nail lacquer

a number of technical prerequisites."[15] A good lipstick should be easy to apply and it should color the lips for several hours without the color being transferred to objects coming in contact with the lips. While having a defined shape, it should be nongreasy and must not bend or break during usage or transportation. Although an appealing taste is a very important feature, a uniform distribution of pigment and dyes throughout composition is probably the first characteristic observed by the cosmetic consumer.

What types of hydrocarbons can be found in lipstick formulations? These products can contain:

- Waxes for binding and molding properties and to raise the melting point of the entire composition. Microcrystalline and paraffin waxes provide mechanical strength thanks to their high melting points.[20]
- Mineral oil for added lubrication and shining properties. Usually higher molecular weight and straight-chain hydrocarbons are preferred.
- Petrolatum, which often provides a combination of the properties of both wax (high molecular weight) and mineral oil (low molecular weight). Obviously, the highly refined grades of petrolatum are preferred for purity reasons.

Table 17.3 lists a lipstick formulation containing petrolatum, mineral oil, and waxes. This lipstick applies easily and gives the lips a soft feel. Mineral oil and petrolatum help add moisturization, while the waxes add rigidity.

TABLE 17.3
Lipstick 1

Ingredient	Weight %
Ricinus communis (castor) seed oil	41.90
Red 40 lake	5.70
Red 27 lake	2.40
Mica (and) titanium dioxide	1.90
Titanium dioxide	0.95
Caprylic/capric triglyceride	11.75
Petrolatum	7.45
Propylene glycol dicaprylate/dicaprate	6.20
Copernicia cerifera (Carnauba) wax	5.70
Euphorbia cerifera (Candelilla) wax	5.70
Beeswax	4.30
Mineral oil	2.85
Microcrystalline wax	2.65
Tocopheryl acetate	0.50
BHT	0.05
Fragrance	q.s.
	100.00%

TABLE 17.4
Lipstick 2

Ingredient	Weight %
Ricinus communis (castor) seed oil	44.00
Octyldodecyl stearoyl stearate	10.80
Mineral oil	10.00
Ethylhexyl palmitate	10.00
Beeswax (and) *Euphorbia cerifera* (Candelilla) wax (and) hydrogenated soy glyceride (and) paraffin (and) *Copernicia cerifera* (Carnauba) wax (and) stearic acid	7.50
Euphorbia cerifera (Candelilla) wax	5.50
Petrolatum	4.00
Copernicia cerifera (Carnauba) wax	4.00
Propylparaben	0.10
BHT	0.10
Red 6 lake	3.30
Red	360.70
Fragrance	q.s.
	100.00 %

Another formulation example for a lipstick is shown in Table 17.4. This lipstick contains high levels of liquid emollients for added smoothness during application. Mineral oil and petrolatum provide moisturization to keep lips soft and supple.

17.3.3.3   Lip Gloss

A lip gloss formulation typically is not used to color the lips like lipsticks, so its consistency is different, meaning it will be applied to the lips differently as well. Lip gloss formulations are usually fluid (liquids or semisolids), so waxes are generally not needed, but petrolatum and mineral oil can be key ingredients.

Table 17.5 contains an example of a lip gloss formula. This product glides on smoothly, and the mineral oil provides high shine to the lips. Petrolatum helps moisturize the lips and prevents chapping.

17.3.3.4   Makeup

In general, makeup helps address small irregularities of the skin while imparting a natural appearance and freshening pale skin.[13] Makeup products can use low levels of mineral oil, usually below 10 wt%. As in many lipsticks, the mineral oil is considered an inert material and is used as a binder and/or carrier for the

TABLE 17.5
Lip Gloss

Ingredient	Weight %
Petrolatum	50.00
Mineral oil	31.60
Ricinus communis (castor) seed oil	15.00
Lanolin oil	2.00
Simmondsia chinensis (jojoba) seed oil	1.00
Tocopheryl acetate	0.10
Retinyl palmitate	0.10
Propylparaben	0.10
BHT	<u>0.10</u>
	100.00 %

pigments, talc, zinc oxide, titanium dioxide, and other fine particles in the formulation. These solid particles are usually present in high concentrations.

Table 17.6 contains an example of a makeup formulation. This rich, creamy liquid spreads very easily and dries without a tacky or shiny residue. Mineral oil provides moisturization due to its occlusivity.

TABLE 17.6
Liquid Facial Makeup

Ingredient	Weight %
Deionized water	69.60
Magnesium aluminum silicate	0.75
Citric acid	0.20
Methylparaben	0.20
Xanthan gum	0.15
Titanium dioxide	7.50
Glycerin	3.00
Iron oxides	2.10
Talc	1.10
Mineral oil	6.25
C12-15 alkyl benzoate	4.75
Stearyl alcohol (and) ceteareth-20	2.50
Myristyl alcohol	1.00
Polysorbate 85	0.50
Propylparaben	0.10
Imidazolidinyl urea	0.30
Fragrance	<u>q.s.</u>
	100.00%

17.3.3.5 Eye Makeup

Using makeup around the eyes is an ancient procedure, practiced by the Egyptians, Hebrews, and Greeks. Several categories of eye makeup exist, including:

- Eyelash products that color, thicken, and lengthen (e.g., mascara)
- Eyebrow products that darken and define (e.g., eyebrow pencils)
- Eye products that highlight and accentuate the eyes (e.g., eyeliner)
- Eyelid products that tint and color (e.g., eye shadow)

All these products contain high loads of pigments (particularly eye shadow) and sometimes high loads of hydrocarbon products. Mascaras can contain waxes for enhancing the length of the eyelashes and volatile hydrocarbon solvents to carry the pigments, then quickly evaporate. Eye shadows can contain small amounts of mineral oil, which acts as a binder.

17.4 PATENTS

Mineral oil, petroleum waxes, and petrolatum are well known for their versatility in cosmetic formulations, as well as their extraordinary stability. That is why these products are still extremely attractive to cosmetic formulators. In addition to the well-known and frequently used color cosmetic products, many types of novelty products are being created using hydrocarbon products as major ingredients in both anhydrous products and emulsions. Within the past 4 years, numerous patents[21–32] have been issued to various individuals or cosmetic companies on lipstick or other lip product formulations containing hydrocarbon solvents, mineral oil, petroleum waxes, or petrolatum. Eye cosmetic products such as eye shadow, mascara, and eyeliners are also well represented in the newly issued patent arena.[28,33–37]

REFERENCES

1. Ragas MC, Kozlowski K, Vienne V. *Read My Lips: A Cultural History of Lipstick.* San Francisco: Chronicle Books, 1998:1–16.
2. Johnson R. Lipstick. *Chem Eng News* 1999; 77:31–33.
3. Chronological History of Cosmetics from FragranceWholesale.com. Available at http://storm.prohosting.com/cezumoto/cosmetichistory.html. Accessed July 28, 2004.
4. Motischke L. Facial-make-up (general). In *Cosmetics and Toiletries: Development, Production and Use,* Umbach W, Ed. Chichester, U.K.: Ellis Horwood, 1991:5–78.
5. Barone S, Corrigan A, Mody M, Baustita M, Macchio R, Veltry L. Cosmetic Formulation. U.S. Patent 6,649,151 (November 18, 2003).
6. Thompson J. Innovations in lipstick technology. *Cosmet Toil* 2003; 118:96.
7. Barker C. Origin of petroleum. In *Kirk-Othmer Encyclopedia of Chemical Technology,* 3rd ed., Vol. 17, Grayson M, Exec. Ed., Eckroth D, Assoc. Ed. New York: John Wiley & Sons, 1982:113.

8. Elliott JJ. Petroleum (composition). In *Kirk-Othmer Encyclopedia of Chemical Technology*, 3rd ed., Vol. 17, Grayson M, Exec. Ed., Eckroth D, Assoc. Ed. New York: John Wiley & Sons, 1982:119–131.

9. Schiek R. Pigments (inorganic). In *Kirk-Othmer Encyclopedia of Chemical Technology*, 3rd ed., Vol. 17, Grayson M, Exec. Ed., Eckroth D, Assoc. Ed. New York: John Wiley & Sons, 1982:788–838.

10. Fytelson M. Pigments (organic). In *Kirk-Othmer Encyclopedia of Chemical Technology*, 3rd ed., Vol. 17, Grayson M, Exec. Ed., Eckroth D, Assoc. Ed. New York: John Wiley & Sons, 1982:839–871.

11. Bannister DW, Olin AD, Stingl HA. Dyes and dye intermediates. In *Kirk-Othmer Encyclopedia of Chemical Technology*, 3rd ed., Vol. 17, Grayson M, Exec. Ed., Eckroth D, Assoc. Ed. New York: John Wiley & Sons, 1982:159–212.

12. Rzepa H. Mauveine: The First Industrial Organic Fine-Chemical. Available at http://www.ch.ic.ac.uk/motm/perkin.html. Accessed November 4, 2004.

13. Jellinek JS. The composition of cosmetic preparations. In *Formulation and Functions of Cosmetics*. New York: Wiley Interscience, 1970:108–201.

14. Morrison DS, Schmidt J, Paulli R. The scope of the mineral oil in personal care products and its role in cosmetic formulations. *J Appl Cosmetol* 1996; 14:111–118.

15. de Navarre MG. Lipstick. In *The Chemistry and Manufacture of Cosmetics*, 2nd ed., Vol IV, de Navare MG, Ed. Wheaton, IL: Allured, 1988:767.

16. Knowlton J, Pearce S. Rheology of cosmetic systems. In *Handbook of Cosmetic Science and Technology*, 1st ed. Oxford: Elsevier Science, 1993:1–10.

17. Morrison DS. Petrolatum: conditioning through occlusion. In *Conditioning Agents for Hair and Skin*, Schuller R, Romanowski P, Eds. New York: Marcel Dekker, 1999:57–93.

18. Hamilton RJ. Waxes: chemistry, molecular biology and functions. In *Commercial Waxes: Their Composition and Applications*, Hamilton RJ, Ed. Glasgow: The Oily Press, 1995:277.

19. Letcher CS. Waxes. In *Kirk-Othmer Encyclopedia of Chemical Technology*, 3rd ed., Vol. 17, Grayson M, Exec. Ed., Eckroth D, Assoc. Ed. New York: Wiley, 1982:473–474.

20. Hamilton RJ. Waxes: Chemistry, molecular biology and functions. In *Commercial Waxes: Their Composition and Applications*, Hamilton RJ, Ed. Glasgow: The Oily Press, 1995:290.

21. El-Nokaly M, Walling DW, Vatter ML, Leatherbury NC. Lipstick Composition Containing Association Structures. U.S. Patent 6,325,995 (December 4, 2001).

22. La Bras-Roulier V, Miguel-Colomber D, Pradier F. Cosmetic Composition in the Form of a Soft Paste and Process for Preparation of the Same. U.S. Patent 6,344,187 (February 5, 2002).

23. Rabe TE, Drechsler LE, Smith III ED. Transfer-Resistant Lip Compositions. U.S. Patent 6,482,398 (November 19, 2002).

24. Dorf P. Cosmetic Composition for Adding Fullness to the Lips and Surrounding Area. U.S. Patent 6,514,505 (February 4, 2003).

25. Sakuta K. Lipstick Composition Containing Hydrophilic Crosslinked Silicone. U.S. Patent 6,585,985 (July 1, 2003).

26. Suzuki K, Miyagawa S, Inagawa K, Watanabe S, Naito N. Cosmetic Composition. U.S. Patent 6, 759,052 (July 6, 2004).

27. Yoshida K, Nanba T. Solid Cosmetics. U.S. Patent 6,740,328 (May 25, 2004).

28. Zoltowski CE, Gilley JM, Scott AA. Pseudoplastic, Film Forming Cosmetic Composition. U.S. Patent 6,716,419 (April 6, 2004).
29. Heider L, Loch M, Schupp N, Kniess H. Colored Interference Pigments. U.S. Patent 6,719,838 (April 13, 2004).
30. Jose N, Ureneck AM. Color Cosmetic Compositions Containing Organic Oil and Silicone Mixture. U.S. Patent 6,620,417 (September 16, 2003).
31. Jacks T, Mattox B. Solvent-Based Non-drying Lipstick. U.S. Patent RE 38,441 (February 24, 2004).
32. Calello JF, Opel JE, Ordino RJ, Sandewicz RW, Jose NR. Method for Treating Chapped Lips. U.S. Patent 6,086,859 (July 11, 2000).
33. Cavazzuti R, Mattox R, Swanborough M. Moisturizing and Long-Wearing Make-Up Composition. U.S. Patent 6,444,212 (September 3, 2002).
34. Van Liew T, Alonzo O, Smith M. Make-up Composition Containing a Blend of Waxes. U.S. Patent 6,503,516 (January 7, 2003).
35. Schoen S, Vogt R, Schul N, Osterried K, Munz J. Pigment Mixture. U.S. Patent 6,773,499 (August 10, 2004).
36. Brieva H, Russ JG, Sandewicz IM. Cosmetic Compositions. U.S. Patent 6,780,422 (August 24, 2004).
37. Toumi B. Cosmetic Composition Comprising a Particle Dispersion. U.S. Patent 6,793,916 (September 21, 2004).

18 Meadowestolide and Meadowlactone: Unique Materials for Skin Care and Pigmented Products

Alan Wohlman, Ph.D.
The Fanning Corporation

CONTENTS

18.1 INTRODUCTION AND BACKGROUND

The formulation of pigmented products requires the proper selection of ingredients that not only contribute to the product's aesthetics, but also provide benefit to the skin. The optimum product provides not only decorative color in a manner that is pleasing to apply, but also treatment that is needed to improve the condition of the skin. These multifunctional raw materials are becoming more and more important in the formulation of high-end products, providing aesthetic and functional benefits. The integrity of the skin depends upon the continued production and maintenance of structural and active biological materials whose configuration and function are largely dependent upon the local environment in which they exist. This environment can be defined, in part, by the quantitative balance of oil and water in the tissue. One of the primary challenges for those of us who strive to provide effective skin care is the development of ingredients and formulations that facilitate the preservation of the correct balance of lipid and aqueous components in the complex layers that comprise the epidermal surface. Frequent use of surfactants can strip away a significant amount of protective lipids, enabling evaporative loss of water and consequent dehydration of the skin. Estolides and lactones are unique new functional ingredients derived from natural sources such as Meadowfoam seed oil, which provide dual properties in pigmented products. These materials are spatially oriented compounds that can help reestablish a physiologically correct balance of oil and water in epidermal tissue, and thereby restore skin to a healthy, youthful morphology.

18.2 CHEMISTRY

As seen in Figure 8.1, Meadowestolide and Meadowlactone are prepared by the acid-catalyzed condensation of Meadowfoam fatty acids, forming a dimeric ester (Meadowestolide) and the delta lactone (Meadowlactone). The delta lactone is an anhydride formed by the removal of a water molecule from the hydroxyl and carboxyl groups of hydroxy fatty acids. Meadowlactone is an amphoteric compound whose isomeric structures can shift between oil and water solubility as a function of pH. These materials have highly desirable properties when applied to skin.

It has been observed that Meadowestolide and Meadowlactone, when applied to skin in reasonably low concentrations, produce marked sensory improvement in both feel and appearance. Even after a single application of as little as 1 to 5%, panelists note a significant improvement in skin tone and texture. This has been verified on a tissue level and relates this bioactivity to the dynamic molecular structure and amphoteric nature of these compounds. These properties make Meadowestolide and Meadowlactone highly desirable additives to pigmented products, providing both superior aesthetics and treatment benefits.

Meadowestolide and Meadowlactone were synthesized from Meadowfoam fatty acids by a complex acid-catalyzed condensation reaction process. Significant posttreatment steps are required to obtain a cosmetically acceptable product. These steps include filtration and high-vacuum distillation. The purified materials are controlled and quantified by infrared spectroscopy and

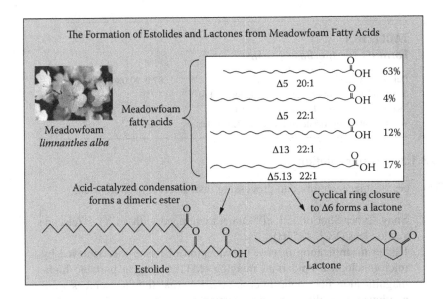

FIGURE 18.1 Synthesis and structures of Meadowestolide and Meadowlactone.

high-performance liquid chromatography (HPLC) coupled with an evaporative light-scattering detector.

18.3 MATERIALS AND METHODS

18.3.1 MOISTURIZATION

18.3.1.1 Protocol Control and Test Formulations

Since moisturizing creams are the most popular form of commercial products used as skin conditioners, a very simple cream base, containing no conditioning agents other than the test material, was chosen as the preferred vehicle for these studies. The specific concentration of active material used in any given study is clearly labeled on the photographic Figures 18.4, 18.5, and 18.6.

18.3.1.2 Subjects and Application Procedure

The formulation in Table 18.1 was tested on a panel of subjects consisting of both males and females, ranging from 20 to 35 years of age. Initial applications and instructions for subsequent applications were supervised by a professional aesthetician. A variety of application procedures were employed in an attempt to reflect actual market usage of these types of products, as well as to determine the extent to which observed results were a function of duration or frequency of use. Results are see in Figures 18.4, 18.5, and 18.6.

TABLE 18.1

Formula for the Base Cream

Deionized water	87.0–90.0% (by weight)
Self-emulsifying wax national formulation (N.F.)	7.75%
Methyl paraben/propyl paraben (preservative)	0.25%
Water (control) or Meadowestolide or Meadowlactone	2.0

18.3.1.3 Instrumentation

Two types of image capture and processing instrumentation were used:

1. Sony Cyber-Shot digital still camera equipped with an X1.4 Teleconversion lens (VCL-1452H).
2. Higher-magnification *in vivo* visualization of tissue was achieved by microtopological epidermal imaging (MTEI) using a portable high-magnification fiber-optic microscope. External lighting sources were employed to facilitate the visualization of epidermal surface topography. In some instances, optical shadow-casting techniques were used to better define surface topology.

18.3.1.4 Transepidermal Water Loss (TEWL) and Tissue Hydration Studies

This phase of the study was conducted to assess and compare the moisturizing efficacy of Meadowestolide and appropriate controls on human skin using the NOVA Dermal Phase Meter^{Æ} and the ServoMed Evaporimeter^{Æ}. Twenty subjects completed the TEWL/hydration study.

The NOVA Technologies Dermal Phase Meter 9003 (DPM) was used to quantify moisture content in the stratum corneum (SC) by an electrical capacitance method. The measurement has no units, but is proportional to the dielectric constant of the surface layers of the skin, and increases as the skin becomes more hydrated. The DPM numbers are directly related to the skin's electrical capacitance measured as picoFarads (pF). The ServoMed Evaporimeter was used to measure transepidermal water loss (TEWL). The handheld probe samples the relative humidity at two points above the skin surface, allowing the rate of water loss to be calculated from the humidity gradient. The measurement is recorded as $g/m^2/h$. Each TEWL measurement was taken after 45 sec of site stabilization. The instrument operator wore a surgical mask over the nose and mouth to minimize the effects of breathing, and a padded, well-insulated glove to minimize the influence of body temperature on the probe. The combined use of these instruments assessed the moisturizing and barrier enhancement properties of topically applied materials. Typically, good moisturizers will exhibit the classical inverse relationship with an increased tissue hydration, as recorded by electrical capacitance and decreased TEWL (Figure 18.3).

18.4 MEADOWESTOLIDE

18.4.1 *In Vitro* Water Binding Activity

I have postulated that owing to the structure of the estolide, wherein the carboxylic acid function and ester linkage are in juxtaposition to one another, a considerable degree of hydrogen bonding and consequent water binding should be evident. Comparative controls were carefully selected to include the oil from which the estolide was derived (Meadowfoam seed oil), the fatty acid from which the estolide was formed (Meadowfoam fatty acid), and jojoba oil, which has no carboxylic acid functions. The results of this study can be seen in Figure 18.2. It was observed that a measurable amount of water can partition into the estolide where it would be expected to bind to the polar hydrophilic center.

18.4.2 *In Vivo* Water Binding Activity

Similar studies were conducted *in vivo* using appropriate comparative controls. In this case, the triglyceride oil (Meadowfoam seed oil), a C-40 Guerbet ester of the fatty acid, and the estolide were compared for TEWL and tissue hydration. The Guerbet ester was chosen since it is consistent in size to the estolide but does not contain the carboxylic acid/ester binding site (Figure 18.3).

The TEWL and tissue hydration studies were designed to evaluate the moisture retention properties of the estolide compared to relevant oil and a nonpolymerized ester. For these studies, the natural oil to select was Meadowfoam seed oil, since it was the precursor oil from which the estolide was derived. The results of the *in vivo* studies can be seen in Figure 18.3. The ester selected for comparison was the Guerbet ester of Meadowfoam fatty acid (labeled Meadowester GME in Figure 18.3), since it has approximately the same molecular weight as the estolide and, owing to the branched chain, is quite fluid at room temperature.

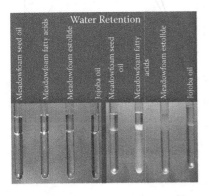
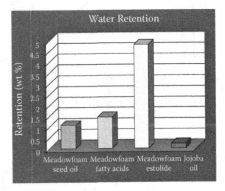

FIGURE 18.2 *In vitro* water binding activity.

Comparative Structures (*In Vivo* Water Retention Studies)

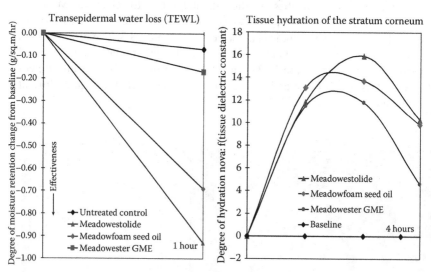

FIGURE 18.3 *In vivo* water retention activity.

The results of TEWL and tissue hydration clearly show that Meadowfoam estolide is very efficient in preventing water loss and retaining water in the epidermal tissue. The decrease in TEWL and improved hydration vs. Meadowfoam seed oil indicate that more than simply occlusivity accounts for the results. It is likely that the hydrophilic center of the estolide is actively holding on to water through hydrogen bonding. Since the estolide structure is oriented in a manner that concentrates polarity at one end of the molecule, and therefore presents multiple sites for H-bonding, it is not surprising that its hydration capability exceeds that of a simple ester, even when the molecular sizes are reasonably equivalent.

18.4.3 SKIN CARE APPLICATION AND IMAGING

A total of 20 clients completed the topical application study. Each member of the panel applied Meadowestolide or Meadowlactone, plus an appropriate control to their face, hands, or forearms. The application protocols varied, as noted on the figures. In every case there was a noticeable improvement in skin feel and texture for the area treated with the active product, compared to the control site treated with the base cream alone or base cream plus glycerin or petrolatum.

Figure 18.4 presents a client who applied the Meadowestolide formulation, containing 2% of the active ingredient, and the appropriate control to her face

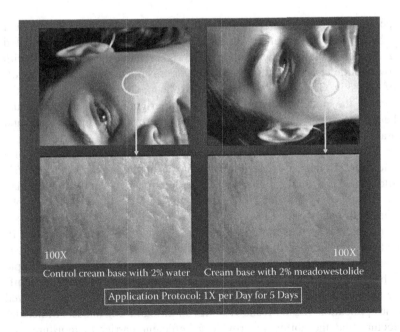

FIGURE 18.4 Skin moisturization and toning following multiple applications of Meadowestolide.

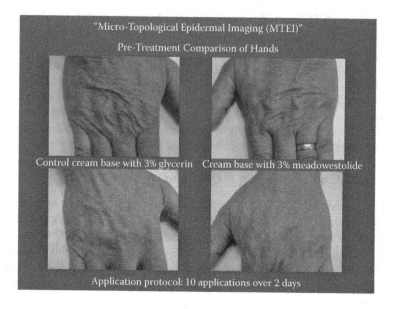

"Micro-Topological Epidermal Imaging (MTEI)"

Pre-Treatment Comparison of Hands

Control cream base with 3% glycerin   Cream base with 3% meadowestolide

Application protocol: 10 applications over 2 days

FIGURE 18.5 Comparison of skin toning achieved with 3% Meadowestolide vs. 3% glycerin in the same base.

once per day for 5 days. The right side of her face received the active product while the left side was treated with the control (same cream base formulated with 2% water in place of the estolide). The right side of the face treated with Meadowestolide clearly shows a significant improvement in the surface topology of the skin. The aesthetician observed "a marked improvement in the condition of the epidermal tissue, noting that the right side was smoother and had better tone than did the left side." The improved condition, tone, and appearance of the skin were clearly obvious to the client.

An even greater challenge is faced when one tries to moisturize skin of a geriatric client. In this case, Meadowestolide was applied to the hands of a 63-year-old man. The application protocol called for five applications a day (approximately every 3 h) for 2 days. In Figure 18.5 the two top photographs represent both hands prior to any application of the products. The bottom set on Figure 18.5, as well as those in Figure 18.6, show the same hands after 10 applications. Each succeeding set is at a higher level of magnification. It is quite evident that while the control product containing 3% glycerin in a simple cream base improved the overall appearance and texture of the hands, a significantly greater degree of moisturization, toning, and elasticity was achieved with the application of 3% Meadowestolide in the same cream base. Molecular architecture and the ability to provide an efficient barrier to moisture loss suggests that Meadowestolde may be a functional analogue for ceramide as shown in Figure 18.7.

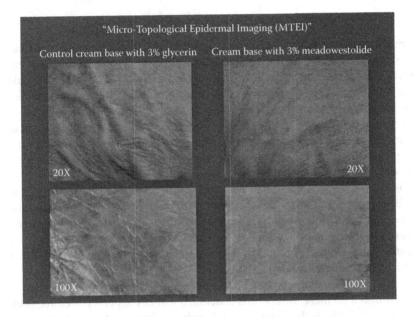

FIGURE 18.6 Comparison of skin toning achieved with 3% Meadowestolide vs. 3% glycerin in the same base—at higher magnification.

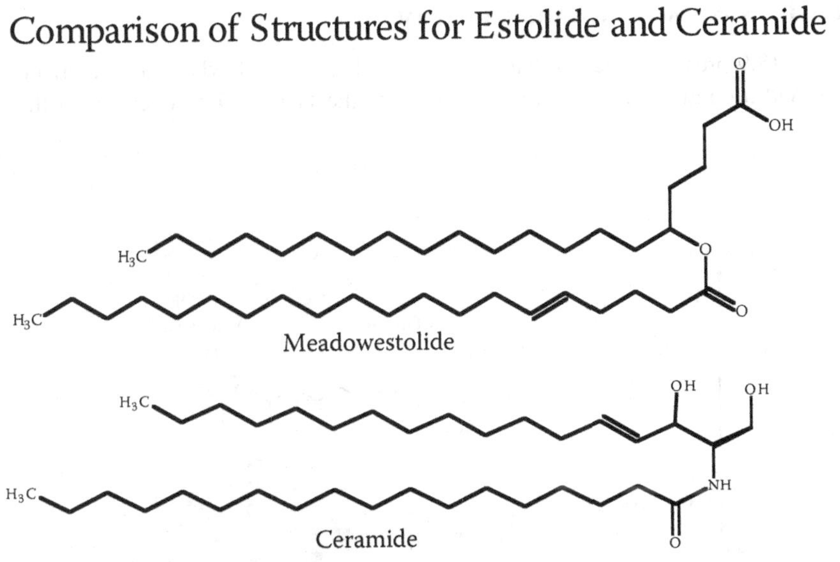

Comparison of Structures for Estolide and Ceramide

Meadowestolide

Ceramide

FIGURE 18.7 Comparison of molecular structures for Meadowestolide and a common ceramide. Both compounds exhibit similar barrier properties.

18.5 MEADOWLACTONE

The chemical nature of Meadowlactone has biological significance. Initial use trials of skin creams containing Meadowlactone indicated that the compound provided very effective skin moisturization that seemed to last for a longer period than one would expect from simple topical applications. In an attempt to better understand the bio-chemical mechanisms underlying the ability of this material to have such a pronounced effect on epidermal tissue, a series of physical chemistry studies was conducted to examine the structural configuration of the lactone under conditions simulating those likely to occur in tissue. The results of these studies and their implications with respect to moisturizing or conditioning tissue are described in Figure 18.8.

Meadowlactone is an amphoteric compound whose isomeric structures can shift between oil and water solubility as a function of pH. When acidic, the lactone exists as a closed-ring structure. As the pH is raised, the ring opens and the resulting intermediate is quickly hydrated to form a 5-hydroxy fatty acid. This transition is physiologically significant since the lactone is oil soluble and the 5-hydroxy fatty acid is water soluble

Solubility of Meadowlactone as a function of pH was determined in aqueous systems. Based on these tests, it was concluded that at the pH reported for skin, (pH 4.5 to 5.5), both the lactone and 5-hydroxy fatty acid exist together in equilibrium. Both oil-soluble and water-soluble forms are present in the skin to facilitate maintenance of a physiologically correct balance of oil and water within the treated epidermal tissue.

18.5.1 Skin Care Application and Imaging

Figure 18.9 presents a pair of hands treated with 2% Meadowlactone in a cream base and a control with 2% water in place of the lactone. Improvement in the

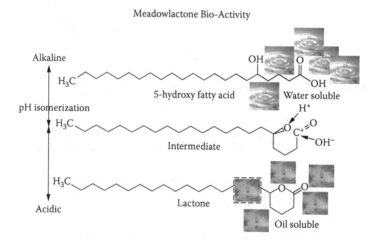

FIGURE 18.8 Dynamic equilibrium between water-soluble and oil-soluble forms of Meadowlactone.

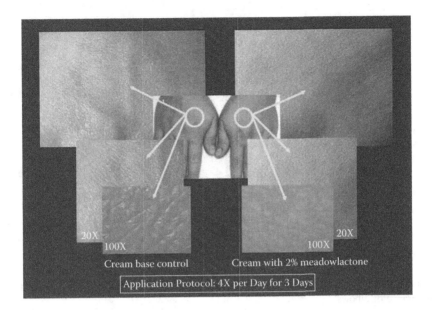

FIGURE 18.9 Application of 2% Meadowlactone vs. control (same base emulsion).

surface topology, observed as reduced irregularities and wrinkling, is visually more evident in the lactone-treated hand.

In the case of the next pair of hands, seen in Figure 18.10, petrolatum at a level of 3% was used as the comparative control.

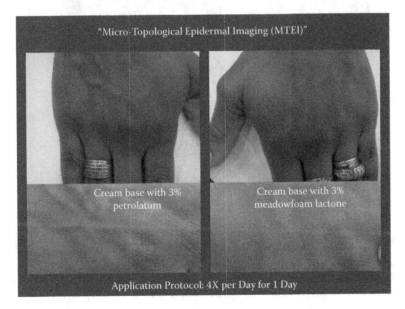

FIGURE 18.10 Application of 3% Meadowlactone vs. 3% petrolatum.

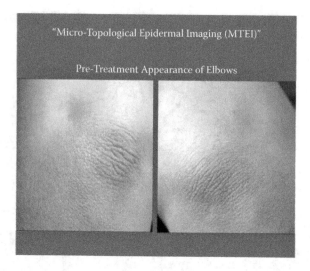

FIGURE 18.11 Intensive moisturization of dry elbows with Meadowlactone. Pre-treatment appearance of elbows.

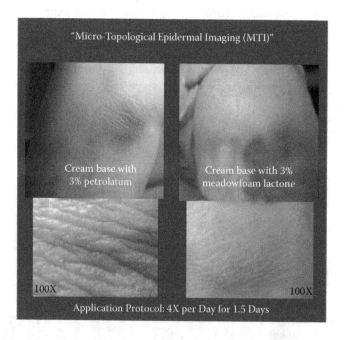

FIGURE 18.12 Intensive moisturization of dry elbows with Meadowlactone. Following treatment with 3% Meadowlactone vs. 3% petrolatum control.

Dry elbows are a very common complaint, and therefore represent a good test system for moisturization and conditioning. Figure 18.11 and Figure 18.12 depict the elbows of a 40-year-old female who indicated difficulty in keeping her skin moisturized. Figure 18.11 shows both elbows prior to any treatment. Figure 18.12 compares the results of six applications of 3% petrolatum to the control elbow vs. 3% Meadowlactone to the other elbow. This technique of microtopological epidermal imaging (MTEI) clearly shows improved skin tone after use of Meadowlactone. The benefits are most obvious at the higher magnifications.

18.6 SUMMARY AND CONCLUSIONS

1. Meadowestolide and Meadowlactone are unique new functionally active ingredients for the effective treatment of skin that should be incorporated into pigmented products.
2. The molecular configuration of these materials is quite dynamic, accounting for their ability to actively participate in tissue rehydration and conditioning.
3. Meadowestolide may be functioning as a bioactive analogue of ceramides.
4. Meadowlactone may be functioning as a pH-sensitive isomer with dual lipophilic-hydrophilic character.
5. Following the application of 2 to 3% Meadowestolide or Meadowlactone in a simple cream emulsion base, microphotographic images of skin provide clear visualization of improved tone, texture, and overall appearance.

19 Polyesters in Pigmented Products

Carter LaVay
Zenitech LLC

CONTENTS

19.1 INTRODUCTION

In color cosmetics, the pigments and fillers are critical ingredients that influence the integrity and performance of the final cosmetic. Wetting, grinding, and dispersing of pigments are key processes in the manufacture of all pigmented products. In order for each process to run efficiently, careful attention needs to be paid to selection of the optimum oil in which that process is to be run.

Pigment wetting and dispersion stability determine the acceptability of a pigmented cosmetic product. There are several wetting-related factors to consider in making products. First, since the mass tone of the pigmented product (that is, the appearance in the bottle) needs to match the skin tone when applied, pigments need to be preferentially wet in the external phase of the finished product. Second, following application, after evaporation of volatiles, the pigment should be adequately

371

wet by the film that remains on the skin, which is often very different from the starting composition. This ensures both uniformity of the film and proper setting of the color. Third, the pigments in anhydrous systems should wet well into the oleaginous product base, dispersing without flotation during processing, and should have no negative effect on the wax/oil matrix upon setup. As with emulsions, good correlation between mass tone and skin tone is an indicator of good pigment wetting.

19.1.1 PIGMENT INCORPORATION[1]

There are three steps in all dispersed systems in the successful incorporation of insoluble dry ingredients:

- Wetting
- Dispersion
- Disperlsion stabilization

Wetting refers to the spreading of a liquid over the surface of a solid, displacing the air; it is the first step in the incorporation of solids into liquids. Measurement of the contact angle (the angle between the tangent to the liquid surface and the substrate) of a drop of the liquid on the solid is a means to quantify the ability of a liquid to wet a solid. The greater the affinity of a liquid for a solid, the lower the contact angle. A contact angle of <90° indicates spontaneous wetting.

Wetting is influenced by the physical properties of raw materials, so it can be manipulated through careful selection of ingredients. The selection of a proper polyester can dramatically improve the wetting, dispersion, and stabilization of pigmented systems.

Dispersion is the reduction of pigment and filler agglomerates and their subsequent homogenous distribution throughout a liquid vehicle by mechanical means. As supplied, most pigments are in an agglomerated state, thus requiring some type of high-shear agitation to be adequately dispersed. Mass tone/skin tone and batch-to-batch shade reproducibility cannot be achieved without control of the degree of pigment dispersion. For cosmetic purposes, <25 μm is usually adequate for foundations, eye shadows, and blushers. For lipsticks, however, <10 μm is necessary because of the sensitivity of the lips, and even lower values are needed for high-gloss nail lacquers. Equipment is chosen based on vehicle characteristics and the degree of dispersion required.

19.1.2 POLYESTERS

Polyesters are a class of compounds that have multiple repeating ester groups. The ester is made by reaction of an organic acid and an alcohol. In order to have polyesters, the alcohol and acid each need to have more than one acid or alcohol group. Polyesters can have many different structures, for example:

$$HO—(CH_2—CH_2O)—(\overset{\overset{O}{\|}}{C}—CH_2—CH_2—\overset{\overset{O}{\|}}{C}—O—CH_2—CH_2—O)_x—H$$

The above polyester is made by the reaction of the following:

HO—CH$_2$CH$_2$—OH   Ethylene glycol (a diol)

$$HO—\underset{\underset{O}{\|}}{C}—CH_2CH_2—\underset{\underset{O}{\|}}{C}OH \qquad \text{Succinic acid (a di-acid)}$$

The polyester has two ends, the hydroxyl terminated end and the carboxyl terminated end.

$$HO—(CH_2—CH_2O)—(\overset{\overset{O}{\|}}{C}—CH_2—CH_2—\overset{\overset{O}{\|}}{C}—O—CH_2—CH_2—O)_x—H$$

Hydroxyl terminated end   Carboxyl terminated end

In addition, the polyester and a salient property of polyesters have an internal repeating group, shown underlined below.

$$HO—(CH_2—CH_2O)—\underline{(\overset{\overset{O}{\|}}{C}—CH_2—CH_2—\overset{\overset{O}{\|}}{C}—O—CH_2—CH_2—O)_x}—H$$

Hydroxyl terminated end   Carboxyl terminated end

The specific diol and diacid used to make the polyester determines the polyester's physical properties. Branching introduced into the molecule lowers viscosity. Consequently, Polyester A has as a higher viscosity than Polyester B.

$$HO—(CH_2—CH_2O)—(\overset{\overset{O}{\|}}{C}—CH_2—CH_2—\overset{\overset{O}{\|}}{C}—O—CH_2—CH_2—O)_x—H \quad \text{Polyester A}$$

$$HO—(CH_2—CHO)—(\overset{\overset{O}{\|}}{C}—CH_2—CH_2—\overset{\overset{O}{\|}}{C}—O—CH_2—CH—O)_x—H \quad \text{Polyester B}$$

              CH$_2$CH$_3$ CH$_2$CH$_3$

The x value, referred to as the degree of polymerization (dp), is a critical value, as it defines how many groups are linked together. This also has an impact upon viscosity and physical properties.

Since the selection of a polyester in which a pigment is wet, dispersed, and solubilized depends upon the polyester's polarity, viscosity, and other physical attributes, selection of the proper polyester is critical.

19.1.3 CASTOR POLYESTERS

Castor oil has been used in pigmented products, most importantly lipsticks, for many years. It is well accepted and effective. It has also been found to be an excellent raw material from which to make polyesters. Just as aspirin has recently been rediscovered, providing new benefits in addition to the relief of pain, so too has castor oil been rediscovered as a raw material for making polyesters for pigmented products. The chemical twist that allows for this rediscovery is the polymerization and functionalization of classic castor oil into polyesters.

19.2 CASTOR OIL *(RICINUS COMMUNIS)*[2]

19.2.1 SOURCE

Castor oil is a unique, naturally occurring triglyceride derived from *Ricinus communis* L. The castor plant grows wild in many subtropical and tropical areas. Today Brazil, China, and India provide over 90% of this oil. Castor oil contains a large content of hydroxy-containing compounds that are unsaturated.

This versatile material is a clear, light-colored, viscous, free-flowing fluid that is nondrying and quite stable. The purity of composition of castor oil occurs with remarkable uniformity. Regardless of its country of origin or the season in which it is grown, the composition and chemical properties remain within a very narrow range. Castor oil has broad compatibility with oils, waxes, natural resins, and gums.

19.2.2 CARBON DISTRIBUTION

Component	Typical % Weight
C16:0	1
C18:0	1
C18:1-OH	89
C18:1	3
C18:2	6

CAS number: 8001-79-4
INECS number: 232-293-8
Titer point: 2°C
Iodine value: 85

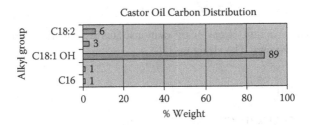

FIGURE 19.1 Castor oil carbon distribution.

Castor oil is a high-purity oil in terms of the carbon chain distribution provided by nature. This makes castor oil both compositionally pure and natural. In spite of its unsaturation, castor oil has outstanding oxidative stability. We can demonstrate this by looking at color formation at 200°C. Refined oils were held at this temperature and color change monitored.[3] The results are shown in Figure 19.2.

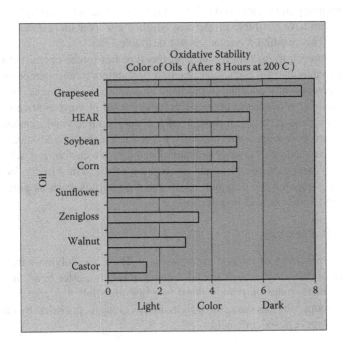

FIGURE 19.2 Oxidative stability color of oils.

19.2.3 CHEMICAL STRUCTURE

The chemical structure of castor oil demonstrates its importance in the making of a suitable polymer. The structure is

$$
\begin{array}{l}
\quad\quad\quad\; OH \quad\quad\quad\quad\quad O \\
\quad\quad\quad\; | \quad\quad\quad\quad\quad\quad\; \| \\
CH_3\text{---}(CH_2)_5\text{---}CHCH_2CH\text{=}CH(CH_2)_7\text{---}C\text{---}O\text{---}CH_2 \\
\quad\quad\quad\quad\quad\quad\quad\quad\quad\quad\quad\quad\quad\quad | \quad\quad O \\
\quad\quad\quad\quad\quad\quad\quad\quad\quad\quad\quad\quad\quad\quad | \quad\quad \| \\
\quad\quad\quad\quad\quad\quad\quad\quad\quad\quad\quad H\text{---}C\text{---}O\text{---}C\text{---}(CH_2)_7CH\text{=}CHCH_2CH\text{---}(CH_2)_5\text{---}CH_3 \\
\quad\quad\quad\quad\quad\quad\quad\quad\quad\quad\quad | \quad\quad\quad\quad\quad\quad\quad\quad\quad\quad\quad\quad\quad OH \\
CH_3\text{---}(CH_2)_5\text{---}CHC_2CH\text{=}CH(CH_2)_7\text{---}C\text{---}O\text{---}CH_2 \\
\quad\quad\quad\; | \quad\quad\quad\quad\quad\quad\quad\quad \| \\
\quad\quad\quad\; OH \quad\quad\quad\quad\quad\quad O
\end{array}
$$

$$
\quad\quad\quad\quad\quad\quad\quad\quad\quad O \\
\quad\quad\quad\quad\quad\quad\quad\quad\quad \|
$$

The OH is a hydroxyl group, CH=CH is an alkene, and C–O is an ester.

The castor polyesters of interest use the 3-hydroxyl groups to make the polymer and to incorporate functional groups onto the polymer.

Many polymeric materials are formed by the free radical polymerization of vinyl-containing monomers and become high molecular weight polymers. These polymers can have desirable properties, but they also contain residual unreacted monomer. This residual monomer is not desirable.

The approach to making products of this type has forced chemists to look at new raw materials, processes, and reaction parameters in an attempt to make a suitable, cosmetically acceptable product. This approach continues, but another has worked that is not based upon the polymerization of vinyl-containing mono-mers. This approach results in products that contain no free vinyl monomers. The polymers are based upon the naturally occurring castor oil and succinic acid. They can be made to varying molecular weights, for customized selection of viscosity, playtime on the skin, and penetration of the skin. Finally, by placing functional groups on the polymer, a variety of properties, such as gloss, conditioning, and hardness, can be affected.

19.2.4 POLYESTERS

The castor polymers of interest are polyesters. These are polymers that contain a number of castor oil groups linked together through a ester bond. In order to make polymers, there must be at least two raw materials that contain multiple reactive groups.[4] In this case, the polyhydroxyl group is provided by castor oil, and the polyacid is succinic acid.

19.2.4.1   Castor Succinate Polyester: The Backbone for Functional Polymers[5]

The reaction of castor, with its 3-hydroxyl groups, and succinic acid, with its 2-hydroxyl groups, is the first step in the creation of the polyester. Structure 19.1 shows the reaction. The first step is reaction of one carboxyl group with one hydroxyl group.

Structure19.1
Polyester Reaction

$$CH_3-(CH_2)_5-\overset{\overset{\displaystyle OH}{|}}{C}HCH_2CH=CH(CH_2)_7-\overset{\overset{\displaystyle O}{||}}{C}-O-CH_2$$

$$H-\overset{|}{C}-O-\overset{\overset{\displaystyle O}{||}}{C}-(CH_2)_7CH=CHCH_2\overset{|}{C}H-(CH_2)_5-CH_3$$

$$CH_3-(CH_2)_5-\overset{|}{C}HCH_2CH=CH(CH_2)_7-\overset{|}{C}-O-\overset{|}{C}H_2 \qquad OH$$

Castor oil
(a tri-hydroxy compound)

+   HO–C(O)–(CH$_2$)$_2$–C(O)–OH   --------→

Succinic acid   –H$_2$O
(a dicarboxylic acid)

$$CH_3-(CH_2)_5-\overset{\overset{\displaystyle OH}{|}}{C}HCH_2CH=CH(CH_2)_7-\overset{\overset{\displaystyle O}{||}}{C}-O-CH_2$$

$$H-\overset{|}{C}-O-\overset{\overset{\displaystyle O}{||}}{C}-(CH_2)_7CH=CHCH_2CH-(CH_2)_5-CH_3$$

$$CH_3-(CH_2)_5-\overset{|}{C}HCH_2CH=CH(CH_2)_7-\overset{|}{C}-O-\overset{|}{C}H_2 \qquad OH$$

C(O)–(CH$_2$)$_2$–C(O)–OH

19.2.4.2   Castor Succinate Diester

It should now be clear why there is no free vinyl monomer in the product. There is simply none used in the reaction. The monomers are castor oil and succinic acid. This carboxylated castor oil still has a free carboxylic group, which in turn reacts with another hydroxyl group on another castor oil to make a diester, as shown in Structure 19.2.

Structure 19.2
Diester

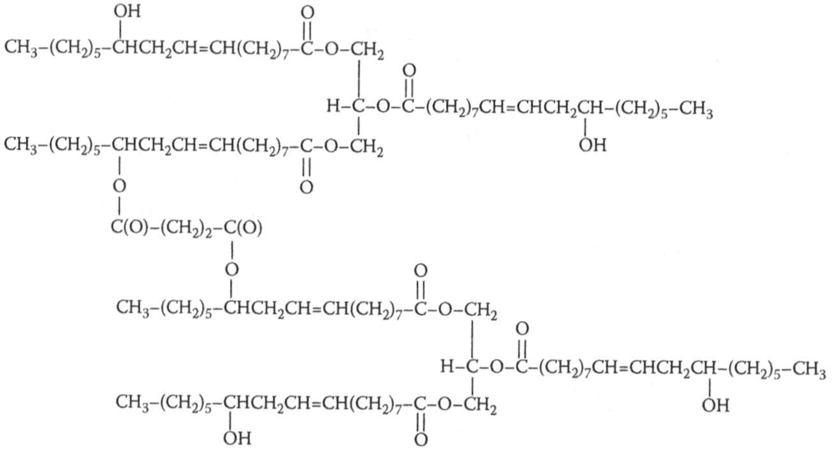

Castor succinate diester

Given the correct catalyst and processing conditions, if only one succinic acid is added per castor, the above product results. The diester product has no free acid groups and has four free hydroxyl groups. The degree of polymerization (dp) is 2. The molecular weight of the material more than doubles, and the polarity decreases compared to castor oil.

If one continues to add succinic acid, the polymer will grow, that is, the dp will increase.

The lowest molecular weight polyester has a dp of 3, has three castor oils linked together, and has five of its original nine hydroxyl groups. As the formulator increases the amount of succinic relative to castor, the dp increases and more of the central castor groups are added (Figure 19.3).

Structure 19.3
Polyester

OH   O
| ||
CH₃–(CH₂)₅–CHCH₂CH=CH(CH₂)₇–C–O–CH₂
                                      | O
                                      | ||
                                 H–C–O–C–(CH₂)₇CH=CHCH₂CH–(CH₂)₅–CH₃
                                      | |
CH₃–(CH₂)₅–CHCH₂CH=CH(CH₂)₇–C–O–CH₂ | OH
                      | ||
                      O   O
                      |
                 C(O)–(CH₂)₂–C(O)
                      |
                      O   O
                      | ||
     CH₃–(CH₂)₅–CHCH₂CH=CH(CH₂)₇–C–O–CH₂
                                      | O
                                      | ||
                                 H–C–O–C–(CH₂)₇CH=CHCH₂CH–(CH₂)₅–CH₃
                                      | |
     CH₃–(CH₂)₅–CHCH₂CH=CH(CH₂)₇–C–O–CH₂   OH
                          | ||
                          O   O
                          |
                     C(O)–(CH₂)₂–C(O)
                          |
                          O   O
                          | ||
CH₃–(CH₂)₅–CHCH₂CH=CH(CH₂)₇–C–O–CH₂
                                      | O
                                      | ||
                                 H–C–O–C–(CH₂)₇CH=CHCH₂CH–(CH₂)₅–CH₃
                                      | |
CH₃–(CH₂)₅–CHCH₂CH=CH(CH₂)₇–C–O–CH₂   OH
                      | ||
                      OH   O

Castor succinate polyester (dp = 3)

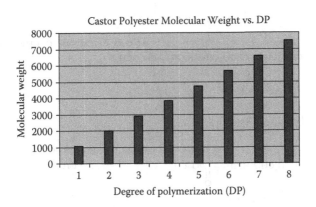

FIGURE 19.3 Castor polyester molecular weight vs. DP.

19.2.4.3 Polymer Capping[6]

The introduction of a monohydroxy compound into the reaction mixture will result in the capping of the molecule and initiates functionality. One such capping group is ricinoleylamidopropyl trimethyl ammonium chloride:

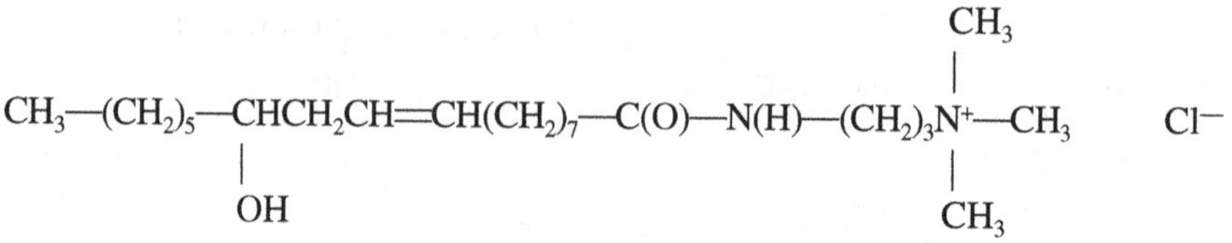

$$CH_3-(CH_2)_5-\underset{\underset{OH}{|}}{C}HCH_2CH=CH(CH_2)_7-C(O)-N(H)-(CH_2)_3\underset{\underset{CH_3}{|}}{\overset{\overset{CH_3}{|}}{N^+}}-CH_3 \qquad Cl^-$$

If the proper ratio and reaction conditions are employed, the simple polyester, illustrated below, is the result:

Structure 19.4

Cationic Polyester

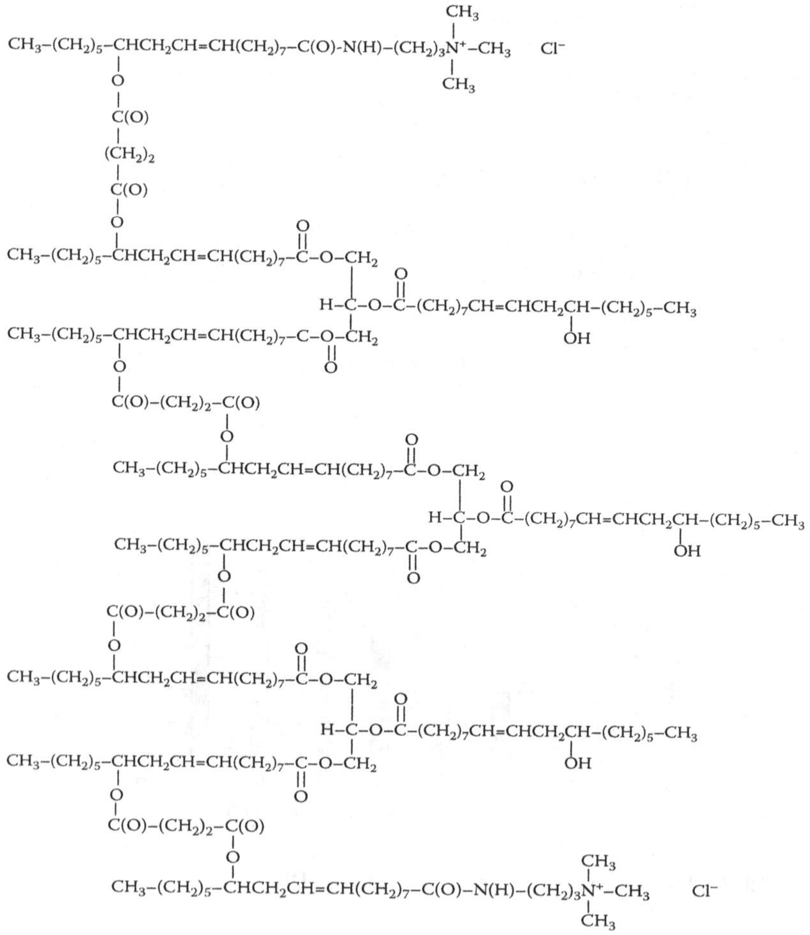

The resulting polymer is cationic (with two cationic sites) and thus provides substantive conditioning and gloss to hair.

19.3 FUNCTIONALIZATION OF THE BACKBONE

If the free hydroxyl groups on the polyester are esterified with fatty acid, a glossing compound results. The exact properties of the compound, like gloss, playtime, and viscosity, are determined by the dp of the particular polyester. The higher the dp of the polyester, the higher the molecular weight, viscosity, and playtime, and the lower the penetration. If the acid used to cap is saturated and has 18 or more carbon atoms, a solid polyester will result. The specific fatty acid chosen will determine both the melting point and the hardness of the polyester (Table 19.1).

Uses/Applications

1. Eyeliner pencils	4. Liquid makeup remover	6. Lipsticks
2. Lip gloss stick	5. Lip gloss pots	7. Makeup pencils
3. Makeup remover spray		

TABLE 19.1
Castor Succinate Polyester

Feature	Benefit
1. 100% active	1. High total performance product; fully functional
2. Pigment wetter	2. Improves color brightness
3. Versatile	3. Hair, skin, sun, and color applications
4. Natural organic ingredients	4. No petroleum base or phenyl groups; biodegradable
5. High molecular weight	5. High substantivity and high gloss; little penetration of the skin
6. High oxidative solubility	6. Retards discoloration in finished formula
7. Known ingredient (castor oil and succinic acid)	7. Easy to formulate product

19.4 FORMULATIONS

The formulations in Tables 19.2–19.10 demonstrate the use of the various castor succinate polyester compounds. The names are the official INCI names given by CTFA.

TABLE 19.2
Lip Gloss Stick

Ingredient	% by Weight
Castor oil	28.7
Carnauba	2.0
Candelilla	7.5
Ceresin	3.5
Triisostearin	20.0
Octyldodecanol	6.0
Castor isostearate	25.0
Succinate beeswaxate	
Polyglyceryl-3 diisostearate	5.0
Silica dimethyl silylate/castor oil	2.0
Methyl paraben	0.2
Propyl paraben	0.1
	100.0

Manufacturing instructions:

1. Prewet the silica dimethyl silylate/castor oil in the castor oil.
2. Mill until homogenous, using a three-roll mill.
3. Combine all ingredients.
4. Heat to 85 to 90°C with stirring until clear.
5. Stir and allow to cool down to 70 to 72°C and fill.

TABLE 19.3
Solid Lip Gloss

Ingredient	% by Weight
Castor oil	30.25
Carnauba	0.80
Candeliila	4.00
Ceresin (m.p. 75°C)	1.60
Triisostearate	9.00
Castor isostearate succinate beeswax (solid castor polymer)	25.00
Octyl hydroxystearate	10.00
Octyldodecanol, quaternium-18 hectorite, and propylene carbonate (bentone EUG)	6.00

TABLE 19.3 (Continued)
Solid Lip Gloss

Ingredient	% by Weight
Methyl paraben	0.20
Propyl paraben	0.10
Color Grinds	
35% CI 15820 (Red 7 Lake)/castor oil	0.55
25% CI 17200 (Red 33 Lake)/castor oil	1.30
40% CI 77491 (iron oxides)/castor oil	0.80
20% CI 42090 (Blue 1 Lake)/castor oil	0.40
Mica and titanium dioxide (flamenco red)	10.00
	100.00

Procedure:

1. Prepare color grinds in advance, using a three-roll mill.
2. Combine all ingredients.
3. Heat and stir to 85°C, until homogenous.
4. Cool, stirring down to 58°C, and fill pans or jars.

TABLE 19.4
Lip Gloss Stick

	Ingredient	Function	% by Weight
1.	Castor oil	Wax solvent, emollient	28.70
2.	Carnauba	Structure-forming wax	2.00
3.	Candelilla	Structure-forming wax	7.50
4.	Ceresin	Structure-forming wax	3.50
5.	Triisostearin	Wax solvent, emollient	20.00
6.	Octyldodecanol		6.00
7.	Castor isostearate beeswax succinate	Gloss agent, emollient	25.00
8.	Polyglyceryl-3 diisostearate	Wax solvent	5.00
9.	Silica dimethyl silylate/castor oil	Gellant	2.00
10.	Methyl paraben	Preservative	0.20
	Propyl paraben	Preservative	0.10
	Total		100.00

Manufacturing instructions: Prewet the Aerosil 972 in the castor oil. Mill until homogenous, using a three-roll mill. Combine all ingredients. Heat to 85 to 90°C while stirring until clear. Stir down to 70 to 72°C and fill.

TABLE 19.5
Gloss Lipstick

	Ingredient	Function	% by Weight
1.	Castor oil	Wax solvent, emollient	25.10
2.	Candelilla	Structure-forming wax	8.50
3.	Carnauba	Structure-forming wax	2.10
4.	Ozokerite, m.p. 75°C	Structure-forming wax	2.00
5.	Microcrystalline wax, m.p. 72°C	Structure-forming wax	3.50
6.	Octyldodecanol	Co-solvent	6.00
7.	Isostearyl stearoyl stearate	-	
8.	Hydroxylated lanolin	Wetting agent	1.00
9.	Triisostearin	Wax solvent, emollient	24.50
10.	Castor isostearate succinate	Gloss agent, emollient	15.00
11.	Methyl paraben	Preservative	0.20
12.	Propyl paraben	Preservative	0.10
13.	Mearlmica SV (Mica)	Filler	4.00
14.	Color grind		8.00

Color Grinds

e19-011 (Sun) D&C Red 7 Ca Lake
e19-012 (Sun) D&C Red 7 Ba Lake
e33-5138 (Sun) red iron oxide
Castor oil

Total			100.00

TABLE 19.6
Emollient Lipstick

	Ingredient	Function	% by Weight
1.	Pale pressed castor oil	Wax solvent, emollient	23.10
2.	Candelilla	Structure-forming wax	7.00
3.	Carnauba No. 1 flakes	Structure-forming wax	2.10
4.	Ozokerite, m.p. 75°C	Structure-forming wax	2.00
5.	Microcrystalline wax, m.p. 72°C	Structure-forming wax	3.50
6.	Octyldodecanol and beeswax[7]	Creamy emollient	15.00
7.	Hetester ISS	Wax solvent, emollient	15.00
	Isostearyl stearoyl stearate		
8.	Eutanol G	Co-solvent	6.00
	Octyldodecanol		
9.	OHlan	Wetting agent	1.00
	Hydrogenated lanolin		
10.	Triisostearin	Wax solvent, emollient	9.50

TABLE 19.6 (Continued)
Emollient Lipstick

	Ingredient	Function	% by Weight
11.	Methyl paraben		0.20
12.	Propyl paraben		0.10
13.	35% Red 7 Lake/castor oil	Color grind	5.50
14.	30% Blue 1 Lake/castor oil	Color grind	2.00
15.	40% red iron oxide/castor oil	Color grind	4.00
16.	Mearlmica SV (Mica)	Filler	23.10
	Total		100.00

Manufacturing instructions: Premill pigment grinds using a three-roll mill. Combine waxes, oils, and preservatives. Heat to 85°C with propellor agitation until clear. Adjust temperature to 75 to 80°C. Add pigment grinds and mica, stirring until homogeneous. Fill into molds at 70°C.

TABLE 19.7
Gloss Lipstick

	Phase	Ingredient	Function	% by Weight	Batch Size, 500.00
1.	A	*Ricinus communis* seed oil	Wax solvent, emollient	16.55	
2.	A	*Euphorbia cerifera* wax	Structure-forming wax	6.00	
3.	A	*Copernicia cerifera* wax	Structure-forming wax	1.80	
4.	A	Ceresin	Structure-forming wax	2.00	
5.	B	Microcrystalline wax	Structure-forming wax	3.00	
6.	B	Octyldodeconal	Solvent	6.00	
7.	B	Hydroxylated lanolin	Wetting agent	1.00	
8.	B	Trisocetyl citrate		15.00	
9.	C	Castor isosteareate succinate		15.00	
10.	D	Cetyl dimethicone, beeswax		10.00	
		Total		100.00	500.00

TABLE 19.8
Water-Resistant Mascara

	Ingredient	Function	% by Weight
1.	Deionized water		41.60
2.	Polyvinylpyrrolidone	Dispersant, film former	2.00
3.	Hydroxyethylcellulose	Thickener	0.30
4.	Triethanolamine 99%	Neutralizer	1.00
5.	Black iron oxides	Color	10.00

TABLE 19.8 (Continued)
Water-Resistant Mascara

	Ingredient	Function	% by Weight
6.	(Fumed) silica	Thickener	0.20
7.	Butylene glycol	Humectant	4.00
8.	Methyl paraben	Preservative	0.20
9.	Stearic acid	Emulsifier (with tea)	3.50
10.	Glyceryl stearate, potassium stearate	Co-emulsifier	3.00
11	White beeswax	Film-forming wax	4.50
12.	Candelilla	Film-forming wax	2.80
13.	Carnauba	Film-forming wax	3.50
14.	Castor isostearate succinate	Plasticizer	1.00
15.	Propyl paraben	Preservative	0.10
16.	PPG-17/IPDI/DMPA copolymer	Film former	20.00
17.	Deionized water		2.00
18.	Diazolidinyl urea	Preservative	0.30
			100.00

TABLE 19.9
Gloss Lipstick

Ingredient	INCI Name	%
Castor oil	*Ricinus communis* seed oil	16.55
Candelilla	*Euphorbia cerifera* wax	6.00
Carnauba	*Copernicia cerifera* wax	1.80
Ozokerite, m.p. 77°C	Ceresin	2.00
Microcrystalline wax		3.00
Octyldodecanol		6.00
Hydroxylated lanolin		1.00
Triisocetyl citrate		15.00
Zenigloss UP		15.00
Zenibee Cream[7]		10.00
PPG-3 myristyl ether adipate		5.00
Methyl paraben		0.20
Propyl paraben		0.10
35% Red 7 (15850) in castor oil		1.50
35% Red 6 (15850) in castor oil		1.50
40% titanium dioxide (77891) in castor oil		2.00
50% (Red) iron oxides (77492)		12.00
Mica, titanium dioxide (77492)		5.00
Ascorbyl palmitate		0.05
		100.00

TABLE 19.10
Cream Foundation

	Ingredient	Function	% by Weight
1.	**Water phase**		51.81
2.	Deionized water		0.10
3.	Dimethicone copolyol	Wetting agent	10.00
4.	80% titanium dioxide/talc	Color	0.80
5.	80%yellow iron oxide/talc	Color	0.80
6.	80% red iron oxide	Color	0.40
7.	80% black iron oxide	Color	0.08
8.	French talc		2.72
9.	10% potassium hydroxide	Neutralizing agent	0.84
10.	Butylene glycol	Humectant	4.00
11.	Magnesium aluminum silicate	Thickener	0.80
12.	Butylene glycol	Humectant	2.00
13	Celloluse gum (CMC7H3SF)	Thickener	0.12
14.	Sucrose cocoate	Emulsifier	1.00
15.	Methyl paraben	Preservative	0.20
16.	Disodium EDTA	Preservative	0.05
17.	**Oil phase**		
18.	Propylene glycol Dicaprylate/dicaprate	Emollient	7.00
19.	Isostearyl stearoyl stearate	Emollient	5.00
20.	Octyldodecanol and beeswax[7]	Creamy emollient skin conditioner	4.00
21.	Sorbitan stearate	Emulsifier	3.00
22.	Cetearyl alcohol, dicetyl phosphate, ceteth-10 phosphate	Emulsifier	4.00
23.	Propyl paraben	Preservative	0.10
24.	Deionized water		1.00
25.	DMDM hydantoin	Preservative	0.18
	Total		100.00

Manufacturing instructions: Combine oil phase ingredients. Heat to 75 to 80°C with stirring. Combine water and dimethicone copolyol. Begin heating to 75°C and add premilled pigment extenders while homomixing at low speed, avoiding aeration. Add KOH. Combine and add butylene glycol and MgAl silicate. Homogenize for 15 min. Combine butylene glycol and CMC. Homogenize for 15 min. Add remaining water phase ingredients. When homogenous, add oil to water phase with homogenization. Maintain temperature and agitation for 15 min. Cool to 45°C with side sweep agitation. Combine and add water and DMDMH. Cool to 30°C.

REFERENCES

1. Karleskind, A. (Ed.), *Oils and Fats Manual*, Intercept Ltd., 1996, p. 212.
2. O'Lenick, A.J., Steinberg, D., and Klein, K., *Primary Ingredients*, 1998, available for download at www.zenitech.com.
3. Zenitech Technical Bulletin 2001-5, p. 4
4. O'Lenick, A.J., *Surfactants Chemistry and Properties*, Allured Publishing, Carol Streams, IL, 1999, p. 77.
5. U.S. Patent 6,342,527, Polymeric Castor Polyesters, January 29, 2002.
6. U.S. Patent 6,521,220, Polymeric Castor Polyester Quaternary Compounds, February 18, 2003.
7. U.S. Patent 6,630,134, Guerbet Wax Esters in Personal Care Applications, October 7, 2003.

20 Alkyl Dimethicone in Pigmented Products

Rick Vrckovnik and Anthony J. O'Lenick, Jr.
Siltech Corporation

CONTENTS

20.1 BACKGROUND AND INTRODUCTION

The long history of silicone use in the personal care industry can be traced in part to the distinctive aesthetics these materials provide to hair.[1-5] Silicone fluids are one class of materials that were among the first to gain acceptance in personal care products. These materials offer desirable, unique aesthetics, but they are not soluble in either oil or water. This lack of solubility presented a conundrum to the formulator, namely, How can silicone fluid be incorporated into products in which it is insoluble? Fortunately, a series of products that are hybrids has been developed. One such hybrid is silicone waxes. These materials are also called alkyl dimethicone. They are silicone molecules in which oil-soluble groups have been incorporated, rendering the final product oil soluble and, consequently, easier to incorporate into a formulation. Another hybrid is the PEG/PPG dimethicone. These products incorporate water-soluble polyoxyethylene (PEG) or polyoxypropylene (PPG) groups into the molecule and allow the formulator an opportunity to incorporate silicone into water-based systems.

David Floyd, a pioneer in the silicone industry, has stated, "In addition to their solubility in hydrocarbon, alkyl dimethicone compounds provide moisturization, substantivity, and highly desirable aesthetics."

There are several instances in which the formulation of pigmented products is simplified by incorporating silicone compounds. These include as an oil phase for pigment grinding and to minimize syneresis in formulation. Both applications can be accomplished by selecting a very specific class of silicone compounds, called alkyl dimethicone.

The growing interest in this class of silicone compounds is based on the fact that silicone fluids, mineral oil, and water are not soluble in each other. This mutual lack of solubility has resulted in the need to expand the concept we generally think of as hydrophobicity. A new series of terms have been introduced[6] that allow for a more accurate description of the term *hydrophobic*. Classically, the term *hydrophobic* was used to describe a material that was insoluble in water. The term did little to describe if such insolubility was due to the material being soluble in oil (oleophillic) or soluble in silicone oil (siliphillic). The difference is very important since both oil and silicone are insoluble in each other.

20.2 GROUP OPPOSITES

If a compound is:	It may be either:
Water insoluble (hydrophobic)	Oil soluble (oleophillic) Silicone soluble (siliphillic)
Oil insoluble (oleophobic)	Silicone soluble (siliphillic) Water soluble (hydrophilic)
Silicone insoluble (siliphobic)	Oil soluble (oleophillic) Water soluble (hydrophilic)

Because of these insolubilities, a class of materials that have both an alkyl group and a silicone group have been attracting increasing attention in the formulation of many pigment products. Alkyl dimethicone is a class of compounds that is neither a classical oil nor a classical silicone. Silicone oils conform to the following structure:

$$CH_3\text{--}Si\text{--}(O\text{--}Si\text{--})_x\text{--}O\text{--}Si\text{--}CH_3$$

with CH_3 groups on each silicon   silicone fluid (a silicone fluid)

A typical hydrocarbon oil conforms to the following structure:

$$CH_3\text{--}(CH_2)_{10}\text{--}CH_3 \qquad \text{dodecane (an oil)}$$

Alkyl silicones have elements of both and conform to the following structure:

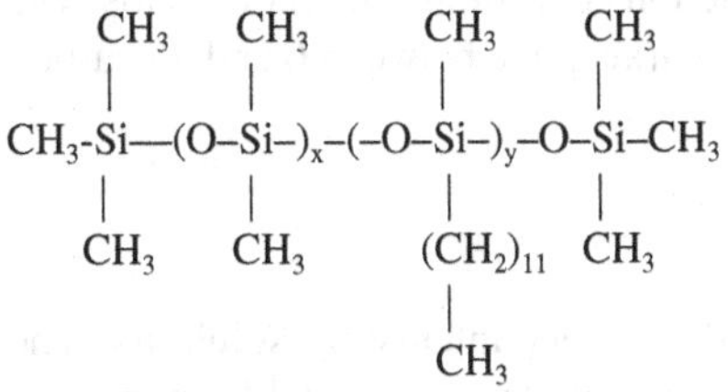

$$
\begin{array}{cccc}
CH_3 & CH_3 & CH_3 & CH_3 \\
| & | & | & | \\
\end{array}
$$

CH_3-Si—(O-Si-)$_x$–(–O-Si-)$_y$–O-Si–CH$_3$ lauryl dimethicone (an alkyl dimethicone)

$$
\begin{array}{cccc}
| & | & | & | \\
CH_3 & CH_3 & (CH_2)_{11} & CH_3 \\
& & | & \\
& & CH_3 &
\end{array}
$$

This marriage of alkyl and silicone into a molecule results in a product that, despite its silicone nature, is soluble in mineral oil. This dichotomy results in materials that minimize syneresis and improve the properties of many formulations that contain both oil and silicone.

Most of today's pigments are coated. The coating that improves the hydrophobicity of the pigment is either an oil-based or silicone-based product. Most of today's pigmented products contain an oil phase, silicones, and water. The selection of the proper alkyl dimethicone results in a stable pigmented product and minimization of syneresis.

Most long-wear lipsticks contain a silicone resin and many oils, and esters. To prevent these phases from separating from each other, a rather messy situation, called syneresis, silicone couplers are employed. Couplers allow the oil phase and silicone phase to stay together and provide a cosmetically acceptable product. Alkyl dimethicone compounds are one such coupler.

20.3 CHEMISTRY

Alkyl dimethicone compounds are made by a reaction referred to as the hydrosilylation reaction. In the reaction, an alpha olefin is reacted with a silanic hydrogen-containing polymer.

20.3.1 HYDROSILYLATION REACTION[7,8]

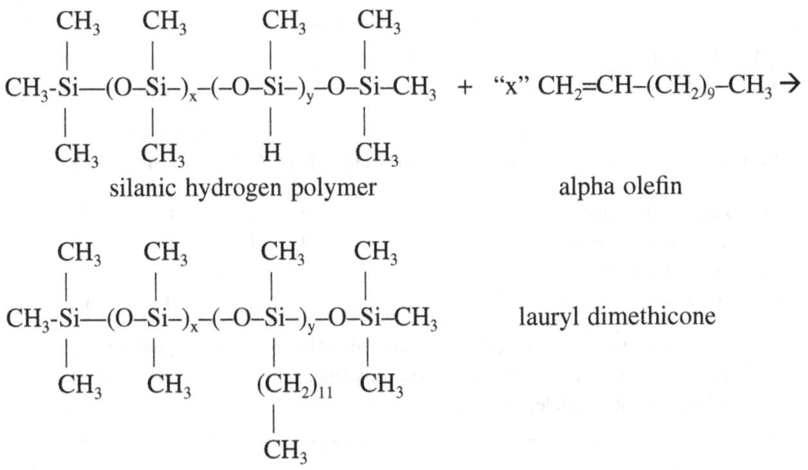

$$
\begin{array}{cccc}
CH_3 & CH_3 & CH_3 & CH_3 \\
| & | & | & | \\
\end{array}
$$

CH_3-Si—(O-Si-)$_x$–(–O-Si-)$_y$–O-Si–CH$_3$ + "x" CH_2=CH–(CH$_2$)$_9$–CH$_3$ →

$$
\begin{array}{cccc}
| & | & | & | \\
CH_3 & CH_3 & H & CH_3 \\
\end{array}
$$

silanic hydrogen polymer   alpha olefin

$$
\begin{array}{cccc}
CH_3 & CH_3 & CH_3 & CH_3 \\
| & | & | & | \\
\end{array}
$$

CH_3-Si—(O-Si-)$_x$–(–O-Si-)$_y$–O-Si–CH$_3$ lauryl dimethicone

$$
\begin{array}{cccc}
| & | & | & | \\
CH_3 & CH_3 & (CH_2)_{11} & CH_3 \\
& & | & \\
& & CH_3 &
\end{array}
$$

While the reaction looks quite straightforward, it is rather complicated and requires the proper selection of catalyst, reaction conditions, and mole ratios. The alkyl groups of interest to the personal care market have between 6 and 45 carbon atoms.

20.4 PHYSICAL PROPERTIES

The alkyl dimethicone product so prepared has very interesting solubility. The compounds are insoluble in water and isopropanol. They are soluble in mineral oil, even with low levels of alkyl groups. Table 20.1 shows some solubility information.

These products, unlike silicone fluids, can be solids, depending upon the length of the alkyl group (z) or the amount of silicone groups (y).

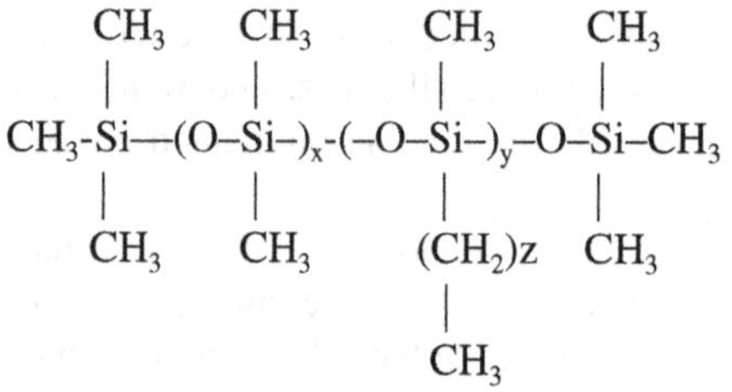

$$
\begin{array}{ccccc}
CH_3 & CH_3 & CH_3 & CH_3 \\
| & | & | & | \\
CH_3\text{-Si}-(O\text{-Si-})_x\text{-}(-O\text{-Si-})_y\text{-O-Si-}CH_3 \\
| & | & | & | \\
CH_3 & CH_3 & (CH_2)z & CH_3 \\
& & | \\
& & CH_3
\end{array}
$$

In general, the larger the value of z, and the smaller the ratio of x/y, the more likely the product will be a paste or solid. Generally, when the value of x/y is less than or equal to 1, and the value of z is equal to or greater than 18, the product will be a paste or solid. The greater the value of x/y, the more liquid the product will tend to be. The melt points of these products can be roughly determined using the following equation:

Melt point =
$-40.246 - 2.423 \times A + 4.076 \times B + 0.031 \times A \times A + 0.034 \times A \times B - 0.018 \times B \times B$

TABLE 20.1
Solubility

Product	Water	Mineral Oil	PG	D-5	Sil Fluid 350 Visc	IPA
D-026 cerotyl dimethicone	I	S	I	D	D	I
J-226 cerotyl dimethicone	I	S	I	D	D	I
H-418 stearyl dimethicone	I	S	I	D	I	I
L-118 stearyl dimethicone	I	S	I	I	I	I

Note: 10% weight of alkyl dimethicone indicated. PG = propylene glycol; D-5 = cyclomethicone; Sil Fluid 350 Visc = 350 viscosity silicone fluid; IPA = isopropanol; I = insoluble; d = dispersible; s = soluble.

TABLE 20.2
Alkyl Silicone Properties

Product	x/y	Length of Alkyl Group	Appearance	Melt Point (Celsius)
Product 1	2	C26	Hard wax	47
Product 2	6	C26	Hard wax	45
Product 3	10	C26	Hard wax	43
Product 4	20	C26	Soft wax	37
Product 5	30	C26	Soft wax	35

where A = ratio of x/y and B = length of alkyl chain.

Table 20.2 shows a series of alkyl dimethicones where the value of x/y varies, but the value of z (the alkyl group) remains the same. As can be seen, the melt point decreases as the ratio x/y increases.

Table 20.3 shows a series of alkyl dimethicones where the value of x/y remains the same, but the value of z (the alkyl group) varies. As can be seen, as the length of the alkyl group increases, the melt point increases as well.

These properties give the formulator of pigmented products the ability to modify the ratio of oil to silicone present in the molecule, the melt point of the molecule, and the softness of the molecule and still maintain the ability to place the molecule in an oil phase. The viscosity and melt point of the oil will have a dramatic impact upon the feel of the product. The play time, drag, and payoff all can be altered by picking a different alkyl dimethicone.

Understanding these trends allows for the selection of a wax for the specific application chosen. All silicone waxes offer improved oil solubility over silicone fluids. Waxes added to oil phases offer an ability to alter the viscosity and skin feel of a formulation. Mineral oil can be gelled by addition of the proper wax. Petrolatum can be thinned out and made less grainy by adding liquid waxes. The play time at

TABLE 20.3
Alkyl Silicone Properties

Product	x/y	Length of Alkyl Group	Appearance	Viscosity (cps)	Melt Point (Celsius)
Product 6	10	C16	Liquid	380	NA
Product 7	10	C18	Liquid	415	NA
Product 8	10	C22	Gel at RT	NA	20
Product 9	10	C26	Soft wax	NA	46
Product 10	10	C32	Hard wax	NA	60

a given melt point can be altered by (1) selecting the specific alkyl chain (melt point) and (2) adding differing amounts of silicone to the molecule (hardness).

Silicone waxes also have an effect upon the ability of an oil to spread on the skin, making them of interest in serum formulations. These products, based upon oils, need to spread easily and efficiently on the skin. This very ability — causing oils to spread — makes these materials invaluable aides to the formulation of pigmented products. These materials facilitate the thorough and efficient wetting of the coating of pigments, resulting in a uniform grinding and a stable emulsion. The ability of these versatile materials to function in the formulation of pigmented products is only now being realized and has not been utilized to the technology's potential.

20.5 PATENTS

The patent literature related to alkyl dimethicone polymers used in personal care is somewhat limited in terms of both number of patents and age of the patents. The oldest patent was issued in 1986 and the most recent in 2004.

1. U.S. Patent 4,574,082, "One-Phase Silicone-Based Cosmetic Products Containing Wax," issued March 4, 1986, to Tietjen et al. — "Cosmetic products which do not suffer phase separation comprise a mixture of a cosmetically acceptable wax with dimethylpolysiloxane and either an organosilane or an organically substituted polysiloxane."

2. U.S. Patent 5,194,260, "Cosmetic Composition for the Hair Contains a Film Forming Polymer and a Silicone Incorporated in a Wax Microdispersion and a Cosmetic Treatment Using the Same," issued March 16, 1993, to Grollier et al. — "A cosmetic composition for the hair contains at least one film forming polymer and at least one silicone incorporated into a support consisting essentially of a wax microdispersion in an aqueous liquid vehicle."

3. U.S. Patent 5,288,482, "Silicone Containing Lip Care Cosmetic Composition," issued February 22, 1994, to Krzysik — "A lip care cosmetic composition containing as ingredients an emollient including castor oil, a wax, a suspending agent, a coloring agent, and as an additional ingredient, an organosilicone compound. The improvement resides in increasing the durability of lip care products by including an alkylmethylpolysiloxane."

4. U.S. Patent 5,478,555, "Cosmetic Composition for the Make-up of the Skin, Containing at Least One Silicone Wax and Process for Its Preparation," issued December 26, 1995, to Bara et al. — "Composition in which the silicone wax(es) is (are) dispersed in an aqueous phase containing two water-soluble acrylic polymers; the first type of polymer(s) consists of at least one copolymer of a C_3-C_6 monoethylenic

acid or of its anhydride, and the second type of polymer(s) consists of at least one acrylic acid polymer or one of its salts. The presence of these two water-soluble acrylic polymers allows the dispersion of silicone wax(es) to be stabilized."

5. U.S. Patent 5,556,613, "Anhydrous Cosmetic or Dermatological Composition Containing the Combination of a Silicone Oil and a Wax Made from an Ethylene Homopolymer or Copolymer," issued September 17, 1996, to Arnaud et al. — "A silicone oil-based anhydrous cosmetic or dermatological anhydrous composition having a homogeneous fatty phase wherein said fatty phase contains a silicone having alkyl groups with between 1 to 30 carbon atoms."

6. U.S. Patent 5,733,533, "Reconstituted Silicone Wax Esters," issued March 31, 1998, to O'Lenick, Jr., et al. — Silicone "wax esters, prepared by the reaction of a silicone polymer and a natural high molecular wax ester selected from the group consisting of beeswax, candelillia, and carnauba wax. These materials are useful in preparation of cosmetic products where their ability to couple organic silicone and other components into a uniform mass is unsurpassed. One major area for the use of these materials is in lipsticks. In addition they are useful in antiperspirants and other formulations which contain both oils and silicones."

7. U.S. Patent 5,750,095, "Anhydrous Cosmetic or Dermatological Composition Containing the Combination of a Silicone Oil and a Wax Made from an Ethylene Homopolymer or Copolymer," issued May 12, 1998, to Arnaud et al. — "A silicone oil-based anhydrous cosmetic or dermatological anhydrous composition having (i) a homogeneous fatty phase wherein said fatty phase contains a silicone oil having alkyl groups with between 1 to 30 carbon atoms, aryl or aralkyl, n represents a whole number between 0 and 100, and m represents a whole number between 0 and 100, provided that the sum of n + m is between 1 and 100; and (ii) a wax in an amount ranging from 3 to 50 percent by weight based on the total weight of said fatty phase."

8. U.S. Patent 6,235,292, "Transfer-Free Make-up or Care Composition Containing an Organopolysiloxane and a Fatty Phase," issued May 22, 2001, to Bara et al. — "A transfer-free composition containing an organopolysiloxane and a fatty phase containing at least one oil which is volatile at room temperature, particularly a make-up or care composition for the lips or a make-up foundation composition both for the human face and the body. This composition is gentle to apply, spreads easily, is non-sticky and does not dry the skin or the lips."

9. U.S. Patent 6,444,212, "Moisturizing and Long-Wearing Make-up Composition," issued September 3, 2002, to Cavazzuti et al. — "A

cosmetic composition which can be used for caring for and/or for making up the human face, in particular, the skin, eyelids, or lips, comprising at least one wax, at least one ester, and at least one long chain alcohol."

10. U.S. Patent 6,72734034, "Fluoro Alkyl Dimethicone Copolyol Esters," issued April 27, 2004, to O'Lenick, Jr. — "Novel dimethicone copolyol ester compounds bearing a fluoro group attached through a hydrophobic ester linkage to silicon. This invention also relates a series of such products having differing amounts of water-soluble groups, silicone soluble groups and fatty soluble groups. By careful selection of the compounds so constructed, very efficient mild conditioning agents may be achieved."

20.6 COMMERCIAL PRODUCTS

One of the best ways to get an idea of the use of a raw material is through a search of the Net (http://www.ewg.org/reports/skindeep/chemhealtheffect). The following shows the use of cetyl dimethicone in commercial products. As will become evident, there are a lot of products from many prominent manufacturers.

20.6.1 PRODUCT CATEGORIES WITH CETYL DIMETHICONE[1]

Cetyl dimethicone is found in 61 products in our database. The specific type of product is shown in Tables 20.4–20.8.

TABLE 20.4

Product Category	Products Count
Sunscreen/tanning oil	20
Foundation	9
Mascara	6
Facial moisturizer/treatment	5
Blush	5
Concealer	2
Powder	2
Antiaging treatment	2
Moisturizer	2
Conditioner	1
Styling product	1
Nail treatments	1
Acne treatment/medication	1

TABLE 20.5
Group 1: Makeup Products Containing Alkyl Dimethicone

Product

Max Factor Facefinity Foundation SPF 15, Almond
Max Factor Facefinity Foundation SPF 15, Buff Beige
Max Factor Facefinity Foundation SPF 15, Cool Bronze
Max Factor Facefinity Foundation SPF 15, Cream Beige
Max Factor Facefinity Foundation SPF 15, Light Ivory
Max Factor Facefinity Foundation SPF 15, Medium Beige
Max Factor Facefinity Foundation SPF 15, Natural Honey
Max Factor Facefinity Foundation SPF 15, Rose Beige
Philosophy the present clear makeup

TABLE 20.6
Group 2: Mascara Products Containing Alkyl Dimethicone

Product

Maybelline Great Lash — Waterproof Mascara, Brown Black
Maybelline Great Lash — Waterproof Mascara, Dark Brown
Maybelline Great Lash — Waterproof Mascara, Soft Black
Maybelline Great Lash — Waterproof Mascara, Very Black
Maybelline Great Lash Curved Brush Mascara, Dark Brown
Maybelline Great Lash Curved Brush Mascara, Velvet Black

TABLE 20.7
Group 3: Concealer Products
Containing Alkyl Dimethicone

Product

Almay Kinetin Skin-Smoothing Concealer, Light
Almay Kinetin Skin-Smoothing Concealer, Medium

TABLE 20.8
Group 4: Powder Products Containing
Alkyl Dimethicone

Product

L'Oreal Feel Naturale Powder, Medium
L'Oreal Feel Naturale Powder, Light

20.6.2 FORMULATIONS[9]

Formulation 1: SPF 15 Cream Foundation Formulation

Ingredients	% Weight
Phase A	
Abil EM 90 (Goldschmidt) (cetyl dimethicone coplyol)	3.2
Isolan GI-34 (Goldschmidt) (polyglyceryl-4 isostearate)	1.0
Tegosoft-OP (Goldschmidt) (ethylhexyl palmitate)	2.0
Abil Wax 9801 (Goldschmidt) (cetyl dimethicone)	2.0
Abil B8839 (Goldschmidt) (cyclopentasiloxane (and) cyclohexasiloxane)	6.0
Permethyl-99A (Presperse) (isododecane)	6.0
Tegosoft OS (Goldschmidt) (ethylhexyl stearate)	2.0
Abil AV-20 (Goldschmidt) (phenyl trimethicone)	1.0
Phase B	
Red Iron Oxide 7080 (Warner Jenkinson) (iron oxide)	0.5
Yellow Iron Oxide 7055 (Warner Jenkinson) (iron oxide)	0.5
Black Iron Oxide 7133 (Warner Jenkinson) (iron oxide)	0.2
Spheron-2000 (Presperse) (silica)	1.0
Sericite PHN (Presperse) (mica)	2.0
Tronox CR-837 (Kerr-Mcgee) (titanium dioxide)	2.0
Phase C	
Deionized water	58.0
Disodium EDTA	0.1
Glycerin	2.0
Magnesium sulfate (Malinckrodt)	0.5
Germaben II (ISP) (methyl paraben (and) propyl paraben (and) propylene glycol)	1.0
Phase D	
Granlux GA145 (Presperse) (titanium dioxide (and) polyglyceryl-4 isostearate (and) cetyl dimethicone copolyol (and) hexyllaruate)	9.0

Procedure: Mix ingredients of phase A into the main beaker and start mixing. Mix phase B ingredients and pass through a pulverizer/blender to ensure uniformity. Pass through a 20-mesh screen and add to phase A. Mix. Heat the mixed phase A/B to 60°C and add phase D; mix thoroughly until uniform. Stop heat and continue mixing. Add deionized water to suitable beaker and add the ingredients of phase C one at a time. Start mixing; continue mixing until clear. Add phase C to phase A slowly. Mix for 10 min. Homogenize the batch for 10 min. Pour into suitable containers. Measure viscosity and recheck viscosity after 24 h.

More info: Presperse, Inc., 635 Pierce St., Somerset, NJ 08873. Tel: 732-356-5200. Fax: 732-356-8350. Website: www.presperse.com.

Formulation 2: Presun Sugar Scrub

Ingredients	% Weight
Phase A	
Apifil (Gattefossé) (PEG-8 beeswax)	8.50
Emulcire 61 WL 2659 (Gattefossé) (cetyl alcohol (and) ceteth-20 (and) steareth-20)	2.00
Compritol 888-ATO (Gattefossé) (glyceryl dibehenate (and) tribehenin (and) glyceryl behenate)	2.50
Hydrogenated castor oil	1.00
DC 2502 (Dow Corning) (cetyl dimethicone)	2.50
DC 345 fluid (Dow Corning) (cyclomethicone)	4.00
Labrafac Hydrophile WL 1219 (Gattefossé) (caprylic/capric triglyceride PEG-4 esters)	4.50
DPPG (Gattefossé) (propylene glycol dipelargonate)	5.00
Softcutol O (Gattefossé) (ethoxydiclycol oleate)	4.00
Vitamin E acetate (DSM) (tocopheryl acetate)	0.50
MOD (Gattefossé) (octyldodecyl myristate)	3.00
Phenonip (Nipa) (phenoxyethanol (and) methyl paraben (and) butyl paraben (and) ethyl paraben (and) propyl paraben)	0.40
Phase B	
Glycerin	14.50
Butylene glycol	13.00
Sodium chloride	6.50
Phase C	
Sepigel 305 (Seppic) (polyacrylamide (and) isoparaffin (and) laureth-7)	2.50
Phase D	
Papaya secrets (Gattefossé) (maltodextrin (and) carica papaya (papaya) fruit extract)	2.00
Phase E	
Perfume Pamplothe CR/1213 (MLW)	0.40
C-Protect (Gattefossé) (*Rosemarinus officinalis* (rosemary) leaf oil (and) *Origanum heracleoticum* flower oil (and) *Eugenia caryophyllus* bud oil (and) *Thymus vulgaris* (thyme) oil (and) *Origanum majorana* flower oil (and) *Curcuma zedoaria* root oil (and) *Helianthus annuus* (sunflower) seed oil (and) *Rosemarinus officinalis* (rosemary) leaf extract	0.20
Phase F	
Coarse cane sugar	23.00

Procedure: Heat phase A to 85°C and phase B to 75°C. Under stirring, add phase A to phase B. Continue rapid mixing (1700 Rd/min) for 5 min. Cool while stirring, and at about 50°C, add Sepigel. At about 35°C, add phases D, E, and F. Complete cooling.

More info: Gattefossé Corp., 650 From Rd., Paramus, NJ 07652. Tel: 201-265-4800. Fax: 201-265-4853. Website: www.gattefosse.com.

Formulation 3: Ethnic Hair Glosser/Extra Conditioner

Ingredient	% Weight
Phase A	
Abil EM-90 (Goldschmidt) (cetyl dimethicone copolyol)	2.0
Petrolatum	6.0
Mineral oil	10.0
Abil Wax 9801 (Goldschmidt) (cetyl dimethicone)	2.0
Tegosoft OP (Goldschmidt) (octyl palmitate)	3.5
Tegosoft P (Goldschmidt) (isopropyl palmitate)	3.0
Lanolin oil (Fanning Corporation)	3.0
Abil AV 20 (Goldschmidt) (phenyl trimethicone)	2.0
Abil Quat 3474 (Goldschmidt) (quaternium-80)	0.5
Phase B	
Fragrance	As desired
Phase C	
Water	64.3
Sodium chloride	0.7
Glycerin	3.0
Preservative	As required

Procedure: Blend the components of phase A together, heating to 50°C. Mix until fully dispersed. Cool to 40 to 45°C with agitation. Add fragrance. In a separate vessel, mix the components of phase C together. Add phase C to phase A–B slowly with a lightening mixer until all water is incorporated into the mixture. Homogenize.

More info: Goldschmidt Chemical Corp., 914 East Randolph Rd., Hopewell, VA 23860. Tel: 800-446-1809. Fax: 804-541-8689.

Formulation 4: Long-Wearing Creamy Lipstick

Ingredients	% Weight
Phase A	
Castor oil	50.05
Tegosoft liquid (Goldschmidt) (cetearyl ethylhexanoate)	3.00
Abil Wax 9801 (Goldschmidt) (cetyl dimethicone)	1.00
Mineral oil	9.00
Candelilla wax	4.35
Carnauba wax	3.00
Ozokerite	3.00
Abil Wax 9810 (Goldschmidt) (alkyl methicone)	3.15
Abil Wax 2440 (Goldschmidt) (behenoxy dimethicone)	2.00
Lanolin alcohol	3.00
BHA	0.05
Phase B	
Pigments	3.00
Abil Wax 9801 (Goldschmidt) (cetyl dimethicone)	0.40
Castor oil	4.00
Phase C	
Titanium dioxide (and) mica	11.00
Phase D	
Fragrance	As desired
Phase F	
Preservative	As required
Fragrance	As desired

Procedure: Melt phase A ingredients together at 80°C. Mix. Grind the pigments of phase B into the oils and waxes of phase B using a triple roll mill. Add to phase A. Mix at 80°C. Add phase C. Cool to 55°C. Add fragrance. Mold.

More info: Goldschmidt Chemical Corp., P.O. Box 1299, Hopewell, VA 23860. Tel: 804-446-1809. Fax: 804-541-8689.

Formulation 5: Sun Protection Lotion with High SPF

Ingredients	% Weight
Phase A	
Abil EM 90 (Degussa/Goldschmidt) (cetyl PEG/PPG-10/1 dimethicone)	2.5
Abil Wax 9801 (Degussa/Goldschmidt) (cetyl dimethicone)	1.0
Tegosoft DEC (Degussa/Goldschmidt) (diethylhexyl carbonate)	6.5
Tegosoft TN (Degussa/Goldschmidt) (C$_{12-15}$ alkyl benzoate)	4.0
Macadamia ternifolia nut oil	2.0
Gilugel OS (Giulini) (octyl stearate (and) aluminum/magnesium hydroxide stearate)	5.0
Tocopheryl acetate	0.5
Tinosorb S (Ciba) (bis-ethylhexyloxyphenol methoxyphenol triazine)	3.0
Parsol SLX (Roche) (benzylidene malonate polysiloxane)	2.0
Ethylhexyl methoxycinnamate	6.5
Phase B	
Allantoin	0.1
GluCare S (Degussa/Goldschmidt) (sodium carboxymethyl betaglucan)	0.2
Glycerin	2.0
Sodium chloride	0.5
Sodium hydroxide (10% in water)	q.s.
Tego Sun TAQ 40 (Degussa/Goldschmidt) (titanium dioxide (and) glycerin (and) isolaureth-4 phosphate (and) vinyl buteth-25 (and) sodium maleate copolymer)	12.2
Water	52.0
Preservative, parfum	q.s.

Procedure: Heat phase A to approximately 80°C. Add phase B (80°C or room temperature) slowly while stirring and homogenize for a short time. Cool with gentle stirring below 30°C and homogenize again.

Comments: SPF 38 (following the Colipa method; 5 persons).

More info: Degussa/Goldschmidt AG, Goldschmidtstrasse 100, D-4512, P.O. Box D-45116, Essen, Germany. Tel: 49-201-173-2854. Fax: 49-201-173-1828. Website: www.degussa-personal-care.com.

Formulation 6: Long-Wearing Eye Shadow

Ingredient	% Weight
Cardre Talc SI (Cardre Corp.) (talc (and) methicone)	42.0–44.0
Silk mica (Rona)	30.0
cc33-2527 (Sun) (red iron oxide)	4.0
cc33-8073 (Sun) (yellow iron oxide)	6.7
cc33-134 (Sun) (black iron oxide)	1.5
Biron ESQ (Rona) (bismuth oxychloride)	5.0
Zinc stearate	3.0
Methyl paraben	0.2
Propyl paraben	0.1
Poly-Pore E200 or L200 (Chemdal)	1.0–3.0
Tegosoft CO (Goldschmidt) (cetearyl octanoate (and) cetyl dimethicone)	4.0
Emerest 2452 (Henkel) (polyglyceryl-3 diisostearate)	0.5

Procedure: Adjust percentage of Poly-Pore with talc usage. Combine the dry ingredients. Pulverize twice through a 0.027-inch screen. Combine Tegosoft CO and Emerest 2457. Spray onto batch. Pulverize once through a 0.027–inch screen.

Properties: Use of Poly-Pore polymer imparts smooth, soft feel to product and increases the product wear time, since polymer is highly effective at adsorbing skin oil.

More info: Chemdal Corp., 1530 E. Dundee Rd., Ste. 350, Palatine, IL 60067-8314. Tel: 847-705-5600. Fax: 847-705-5643.

REFERENCES

1. Floyd, D.T., Organo-modified silicone copolyers for cosmetic use, in *Cosmetic and Pharmaceutical Applications of Polymers*, Geblein, C. et al., Eds., New York: Plenum Press (1991).
2. Floyd, D.T. and Jenni, K.R., Silicone polymers, organo-modified (application in personal care), in *Polymeric Materials Encyclopedia*, Salamone, J.C., Ed., New York: CPC Press (1996).
3. DiSapio, A. and Fridd, P., Silicone glycols for cosmetic and toiletries applications, in *Preprints 15th IFSCC Congress*, 1, 89, London (1988).
4. Schafer, D., The use of silicone surfactants in cosmetic applications, in *Preprints 15th IFSCC Congress*, 1, 103, London (1988).
5. Starch, M. and Krosic, C., Silicones, a new class of cosmetic ingredients, *Cosmetic Technology*, 20, November 1982.
6. O'Lenick, A.J., *Silicone Products for Personal Care,* Carol Stream, IL: Allured Publishing, 2003, p.32.
7. U.S. Patent 4,417,068 to Kollmeier et al., issued November 22, 1983.
8. U.S. Patent 4,609,752 to Giesing et al., issued September 2, 1986.
9. HAPPI formulation website.

21 Esters in Pigmented Products

John A. Imperante
Phoenix Chemical, Inc.

CONTENTS

21.1 INTRODUCTION AND BACKGROUND

Fatty esters have long been used as vehicles for the preparation of pigment dispersions and as oil phases in cosmetic products. The term *esters* covers a variety of products that have different functionality in pigmented systems. In this chapter we shall review the types of esters used in pigment grinding and in pigmented systems generally, as well as review some formulations using these versatile materials.

The proper selection of a material in which to disperse pigments is a complicated undertaking that includes many steps of trial and error. The types of materials available include hydrocarbons, silicone compounds, esters, fatty alcohols, and polyesters.

The selection of materials is complicated by the observation that the vast majority of pigments have some type of coating on them. These coatings are either adsorbed or reacted. The former is transient and can result in long-term instability of the pigment dispersion. The latter is more permanent. In addition to the type of coating, the physical properties of the coating are of prime importance. Pigments can be coated with silicone, hydrocarbons, fatty acids, or fluoro oils. Since many of these coating materials are insoluble in each other, the oil phase used for grinding and dispersion needs to match the pigment in terms of compatibility. Polarity and solubility are key attributes of the oil phase.

The following concept was introduced by Anthony O'Lenick[1] to expand the concept of oil and water solubility. Hydrophobic describes a compound that literally hates water. The type of materials that fit into this category are hydrocarbon loving (oleophilic), silicone loving (siliphilic), and fluoro loving (fluorophilic). Since these three types of hydrophobic materials are mutually insoluble, they make a hydrophobic pigment function quite differently in oil. A truly siliphilic pigment (i.e., one treated with silicone) will not disperse well in hydrocarbon. Under this expanded concept, a coating on a pigment must be compatible with the oil phase chosen for grinding.

Many pigments produce a more stable grind in more polar oil phases. Esters are a member of that class of products that offer this polarity. As a class, fatty esters are used widely in the personal care market. This chapter will address esters used in the pigmented products area.

21.2 CHEMISTRY

In the most basic form, an ester conforms to the following structure:

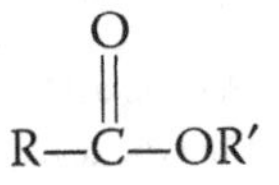

$$R-\overset{\overset{\displaystyle O}{\|}}{C}-OR'$$

The compounds that are important for this chapter, that is, oily esters, are those in which both the R and R' have more than six carbon atoms each. The esters having fewer carbon atoms for the most part do not have the requisite oiliness.

The ester, unlike the hydrocarbon, contains a polar group. That polar group is made up of a carbonyl group and an oxygen group, commonly referred to as an ester linkage. The nature of this polar group alters the properties vis-à-vis hydrocarbons.

As will become evident, there are a number of ester types, each of which results in a variety of solubilities, polarities, and viscosities. Each will have a function in the preparation of stable pigment dispersions.

21.2.1 SIMPLE ESTERS

Simple esters are made by the reaction of a fatty acid and a fatty alcohol. The reaction is as follows:

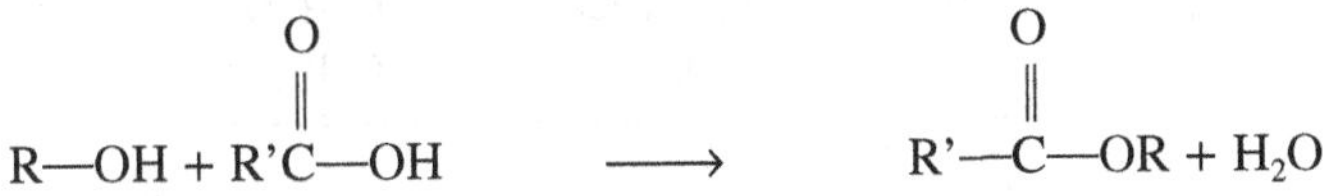

$$R-OH + R'\overset{\overset{\displaystyle O}{\|}}{C}-OH \longrightarrow R'-\overset{\overset{\displaystyle O}{\|}}{C}-OR + H_2O$$

The reaction is conducted at high temperature (typically 180 to 240°C), and the water generated is removed under vacuum. Since the reaction is done at high temperature, the introduction of air during processing will result in significant darkening. Therefore, reactions are often carried out under a nitrogen blanket.

21.2.1.1 Fatty Acid Nomenclature

A shorthand nomenclature for the fatty components used has been adopted.[2] The convention is C-18:1, which means 18 carbon atoms with 1 double bond between carbon atoms. This would commonly be called an oleic acid. This double bond occurs predominantly between the 9th and 10th carbon atoms from the carboxyl acid group. Fatty esters in the cosmetic business use common, rather than International Union of Pure and Applied Chemistry (IUPAC), names (Table 21.1).

The ester is named by taking the name of the fatty acid and changing the ending to *ate* and preceding it with the name of the alcohol's alkyl group.

TABLE 21.1
Common Fatty Acid Names

Designation	Name	Formula
C6	Caproic acid	$C_6H_{12}O_2$
C8	Caprylic acid	$C_8H_{16}O_2$
C10	Capric acid	$C_{10}H_{20}O_2$
C12	Lauric acid	$C_{12}H_{24}O_2$
C12:1	Lauroleic acid	$C_{12}H_{22}O_2$
C14	Myristic acid	$C_{14}H_{28}O_2$
C14:1	Myristoleic acid	$C_{14}H_{26}O_2$
C16	Palmitic acid	$C_{16}H_{32}O_2$
C16:1	Palmitoleic acid	$C_{16}H_{30}O_2$
C18	Stearic acid	$C_{18}H_{36}O$
C18:1	Oleic acid	$C_{18}H_{34}O_2$
C18:2	Linoleic acid	$C_{18}H_{32}O_2$
C18:3	Linolenic acid	$C_{18}H_{30}O_2$
C20	Arachidic acid	$C_{20}H_{40}O_2$
C20:1	Gadoleic acid	$C_{20}H_{38}O_2$
C22	Behenic acid	$C_{22}H_{44}O_2$
C22:1	Erucic acid	$C_{22}H_{42}O_2$
C22:2	Clupanodinic acid	$C_{22}H_{40}O_2$
C24	Lignoceric acid	$C_{24}H_{48}O_2$
C26	Cerotic acid	$C_{26}H_{52}O_2$
C28	Montanic acid	$C_{28}H_{56}O_2$
C30	Myricic acid	$C_{30}H_{60}O_2$
C32	Lacceroic acid	$C_{32}H_{64}O_2$
C34	Geddic acid	$C_{34}H_{68}O_2$

$$CH_3-(CH_2)_{10}-\overset{\overset{\displaystyle O}{\|}}{C}-OH + CH_3-(CH_2)_{17}-OH \longrightarrow CH_3(CH_2)_{10}\overset{\overset{\displaystyle O}{\|}}{C}-O-(CH_2)_{17}CH_3 + H_2O$$

(lauric acid) + (stearyl alcohol) $\longrightarrow$ stearyl laurate and water

21.2.1.2 Alkyl Group

One major factor that has an effect upon the functionality of an ester is the number of carbon atoms in the chain. Other factors include the number and location of double bonds and the presence of additional functional groups. Generally, as one evaluates the tactile properties of an oil on the skin, the lower the molecular weight, the less oily the feel of the compound. The higher the molecular weight, the more greasy the feel. In surfactant preparation, detergent products and high-foaming products generally peak between 12 and 14 carbon atoms. Conditioners and softeners have 16 to 18 carbon atoms. Today there is a growing trend toward using materials with 22 or more carbon atoms for conditioning.

Double bonds, in general, lower the titer point of the triglyceride, resulting in a triglyceride that stays liquid at lower temperatures. Conjugated double bonds (i.e., those with only one carbon between two double bonds ($-C\!\!=\!\!C-C\!\!=\!\!C-$)) are very effective in depressing the titer point, but they can present problems with rancidity. Rancidity is a process by which the double bond is oxidized and ultimately broken. This releases many different molecules, many of which have objectionable odors. Rancidity can be mitigated at times with the addition of antioxidants, prior to the start of the rancidity process.

Finally, many oils, fats, butters, and waxes, upon additional processing, lose their identity as the oil and become known by the fatty name of the predominant species present after the treatment. These processes include preparation of methyl esters, fractionation of the methyl ester, and preparation of a fatty alcohol. For example, if olive oil is completely hydrogenated under high pressure, both reduction of the double bond and hydrogenolysis occur, giving stearyl alcohol, the predominant material in the mixture. In order to preserve the double bond, special catalysts are used.

21.2.1.3 Iodine Value

The iodine value is a measure of the unsaturation present in a particular chemical. The higher the iodine value, the more double bonds present in the molecule. The preferred method is known as the Wijs procedure.[3] This method measures the absorption of iodine monochloride by the sample and is very useful for nonconjugated double bonds. A rule of thumb for iodine values of less than 10 is that the percentage of monounsaturation roughly equals the iodine value. Therefore, a wax with an iodine value of 5 can be predicted to have about 5% unsaturated species present. It is important to note that other components in the composition that can react with iodine monochloride can falsely increase the indicated amount of unsaturation. Generally, as the iodine value increases, the liquidity of the oil increases and the titer point decreases. Some oils have a high iodine value but are surprisingly resistant to rancidity. Meadowfoam seed oil is one such product. The stability is due to the fact that the double bonds are not conjugated and to the presence of natural antioxidants in the oil. Some oil processors add antioxidants to their oils; BHT and BHA are such antioxidants. BHA is declining in its use due to its inclusion in California's Proposition 65 list. Antioxidants can only prevent oxidation; they cannot take a product that has started to oxidize and reverse the reaction. Surprisingly, too much antioxidant can accelerate oxidation.

The structure of this type of ester, that is, one containing a double bond, has a dramatic effect upon skin feel, spreadability and melting point. Esters made with linear saturated alcohols and acids are generally solids if they contain over 32 total carbon atoms. These esters are waxy and are used as emollients. The term *dry time* is used here to indicate the amount of time it takes for 0.5 ml of the ester to feel dry on the skin (back of the hand) when rubbed in with the index finger. The lower the number, the more dry the ester. The opposite of dry has been described as cushion. Esters with cushion are said to have a long playtime.

21.2.2 COMPLEX ESTERS

The most commonly encountered alcohols used to make complex esters are glycerin, ethylene glycol, neopentyl glycol, and pentaerythritol. These alcohols have low equivalent weight and, as such, lead to a molecule that is predominantly fatty acid by weight. An example is pentaerythrityl tetrastearate, which is over 90% by weight stearic acid. The degree of substitution of a polyfunctional alcohol, such as pentaerythritol, is also an issue. There is a potential for any mole ratio of acid to alcohol, from one-to-one to one-to-four equivalents. The hydrophobicity of such esters, their melting points, and functional attributes would differ significantly.

Complex esters can also be made by using polyacids. The most commonly used are citric, dimer, succinic, azelic, and adipic acids.

Complex fatty esters are the result of the reaction of one polyfunctional reactant with a monofunctional reactant. According to this definition, pentaerythritol reactions with monofunctional acids are complex esters. There are many other complex esters that find applications in household and personal care areas as well as in a host of industrial applications.

Complex esters need to be distinguished from polyesters. Although complex esters can have several esters within the molecule, the product is not the result of reaction a polyol and a polyacid. The latter produces polyesters, a series of polymers that have recurring ester groups made up of many repeating units. One such polyester is a product called Zenigloss,[3] a polyester made by the reaction of castor oil (trihydroxy) and succinic acid (diacid). The chemistry of this type of material is covered in another chapter.

Examples of complex esters include:

Pentaerythritol esters (mono-, di-, tri-, and tetraesters)
Glyceryl esters (mono-, di-, and triesters)
Citrate esters (mono-, di-, and triesters)

21.2.2.1 Chemistry

The reaction to make complex esters most commonly uses compounds that contain more than one hydroxyl group. These products are called polyols.

21.2.2.2 Polyols

There are a variety of polyhydroxy compounds or polyols used to make complex esters. The most common are shown below:

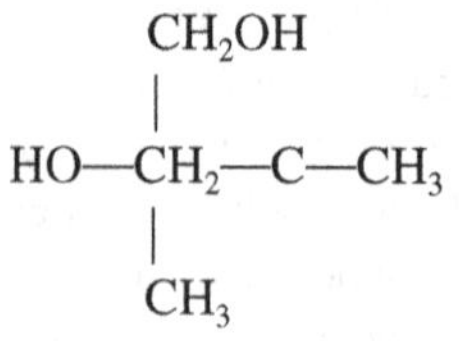

$$CH_2OH$$
$$|$$
$$HO-CH_2-C-CH_3 \qquad \text{Neopentyl glycol (NPG),} \qquad \text{2 hydroxyl groups}$$
$$|$$
$$CH_3$$

CH$_2$OH
|
HO—CH$_2$—C—CH$_2$CH$_3$ trimethylol propane (TMP),   3 hydroxyl groups
|
CH$_2$OH

CH$_2$—OH   glycerin,   3 hydroxyl groups
|
CH—OH
|
CH$_2$—OH

CH$_2$OH
|
HO—CH$_2$—C—CH$_2$—OH   pentaerythritol (PE),   4 hydroxyl groups
|
CH$_2$OH

CH$_2$OH   CH$_2$OH
| |
HO—CH$_2$—C—CH$_2$—OCH$_2$—C—CH$_2$OH di-pentaerythritol (DPE), 6 hydroxyl groups
| |
CH$_2$OH   CH$_2$OH

Polyols are reacted with differing amounts of fatty acid to make the desired product.

CH$_2$OH
|
HO—CH$_2$—C—CH$_2$—OH + 4 CH$_3$—(CH$_2$)$_{16}$—C(O)—OH $\longrightarrow$ 4 H$_2$O
|
CH$_2$OH

CH$_2$OC(O)—(CH$_2$)$_{16}$—CH$_3$
|
CH—(CH$_2$)$_{15-3}$ C(O)O—CH$_2$—C—CH$_2$—O C(O)—(CH$_2$)$_{16}$—CH$_3$ pentaerythrityl tetrastearate
|
CH$_2$O C(O)—(CH$_2$)$_{16}$—CH$_3$

Please note that the nomenclature remains the same; the name of the acid is listed as the last word with *ate* added, and the alcohol is the prefix.

21.2.2.3 Triglycerides

Triglycerides are a very important class of compounds that occur both in nature and as the product of the organic chemist. Triglycerides are the triesters of glycerin with three equivalents of organic acid. Fatty acids are defined as those acids having alkyl or alkylene groups of C-5 and higher. The reaction is as follows:

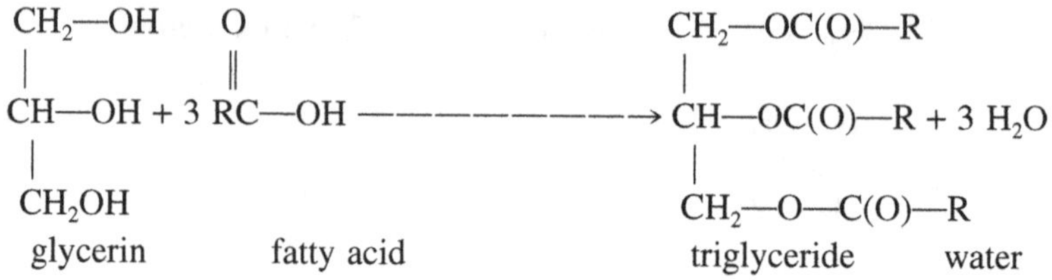

$$
\begin{array}{cc}
\text{CH}_2\text{—OH} & \text{O} \\
| & \| \\
\text{CH—OH} + 3\ \text{RC—OH} & \longrightarrow \\
| & \\
\text{CH}_2\text{OH} & \\
\text{glycerin} & \text{fatty acid}
\end{array}
\qquad
\begin{array}{c}
\text{CH}_2\text{—OC(O)—R} \\
| \\
\text{CH—OC(O)—R} + 3\ \text{H}_2\text{O} \\
| \\
\text{CH}_2\text{—O—C(O)—R} \\
\text{triglyceride} \qquad \text{water}
\end{array}
$$

Triglycerides are commonly encountered as a natural product. Plants use enzymatic systems to make the triglyceride, effectively at ambient temperatures.

21.2.2.4 INCI Nomenclature

INCI names now require the genus and species of the plants or insects that produce a given wax, oil, butter, or fat and all products that are derived from the various oils, fats, butters, and waxes. This is due, in part, to the European Union's use of the Latin names for ingredient listings.

21.2.2.5 Carbon Number

Triglycerides can be classified not only by the source of the product (animal or plant) or the chemistry of the product (triglyceride or ester), but also by the carbon number and unsaturation levels within the groups. Carbon number is a measure of the average number of carbon atoms in the triglyceride. It is the value obtained by multiplying the percentage of a component in a product by the number of carbon atoms in the component, then adding up all the components.

For example, if an oil had the composition as shown in Table 21.2, then the carbon number calculation would be as shown in Table 21.3:

TABLE 21.2
Carbon Number Calculation: Oil Composition

Component	% Weight
C16	20
C18	20
C18:1	20
C20	40
Total	100

TABLE 21.3

Carbon Number Calculation: Oil from Table 21.2

Component (a)	% Weight (b)	Carbon Atoms in Component	Calculation (a × b)
C16	20	16	3.2
C18	20	18	3.6
C18:1	20	18	3.6
C20	40	20	8.0
Total	100		18.4

Note: Carbon number = 18.4.

There are several types of oils that have very similar carbon numbers, which we have then classified by unsaturation, the other salient factor. One can expect derivatives from oils having a very similar carbon number and unsaturation levels to have very similar — often identical — functional properties. The choice of which of the many oils to select in this instance depends upon the economics of the oil or the desire of the formulator to name the oil for label and marketing purposes. As will become clear, there are many different fats, oils, waxes, and butters that, when derivatized, result in compounds of strikingly similar carbon distributions, while having their source oil, wax, fat, or butter be quite different. Thus, naming the material by the predominant species is not very enlightening to the formulator as to the source of the raw material.

It is also quite interesting that nature has provided many triglycerides that have very similar carbon numbers. In fact, of 38 triglycerides presented here, 31 have carbon numbers between 17 and 18. This also explains why the other important variable, unsaturation, is critical in choosing an oil for a specific application.

21.2.2.6 Types of Triglycerides

21.2.3 POLYESTERS

The reaction of polyfunctional alcohols with polyfunctional acids results in polyester. These materials, unlike complex esters, are true polymers, rather than ester

TABLE 21.4

Group 1: Animal-Derived Triglycerides

Triglyceride	Carbon No.	Iodine Value
Milk fat	15.5	39

TABLE 21.5
Group 2: Plant-Derived Triglycerides

Triglyceride	Carbon No.	Iodine Value
Coconut oil	12.8	8
Palm kernel oil	13.3	19
Babassu oil	13.4	15
Sunflower oil	16.0	130
Japan wax	16.3	6
Palm oil	17.1	50
Apricot kernel oil	17.1	102
Tallow	17.3	45
Coca butter	17.5	37
Andiroba oil	17.5	45
Mango butter	17.5	46
Avacado oil	17.6	84
Cottonseed oil	17.6	108
Rice bran oil	17.6	105
Shea butter	17.6	60
Wheat germ oil	17.7	130
Illipe butter	17.7	49
Corn oil	17.8	123
Olive oil	17.8	84
Poppy seed oil	17.8	138
Grape seed oil	17.8	135
Sesame oil	17.8	110
Sweet almond oil	17.9	102
Hazelnut oil	17.9	86
Soybean oil	17.9	130
Safflower oil	17.9	145
Hybrid safflower oil	17.9	140
Walnut oil	17.9	150
Canola oil	17.9	92
Peanut oil	18.0	98
Tall oil	18.0	130
Kokhum butter	18.0	131
Cupuacu butter	18.2	40

TABLE 21.6
Group 3: Drying Triglycerides, Plant Derived

Triglyceride	Carbon No.	Iodine Value
Linseed oil	17.9	190
Tung oil	17.9	170

molecules that contain more than one ester group. In order for molecules to be polymeric, they must contain repeating groups. In order to differentiate complex esters from polyesters, the following examples are offered:

COMPLEX ESTER

$$CH_2OC(O){-}(CH_2)_{16}{-}CH_3$$
$$|$$
$$CH_3{-}(CH_2)_{16}\,C(O)O{-}CH_2{-}C{-}CH_2{-}O\,C(O){-}(CH_2)_{16}{-}CH_3 \quad \text{pentaerythrityl tetrastearate}$$
$$|$$
$$CH_2O\,C(O){-}(CH_2)_{16}{-}CH_3$$

This product is made by the reaction of pentaerythritol (a tetrafunctional polyol) and 4 equivalents of stearic acid. Please note that there are many (four) esters on a single molecule that does not contain repeating groups. This is a complex ester.

POLYESTER

$$\overset{O}{\overset{\|}{CH_3{-}(CH_2)_{16}C}}{-}({-}O{-}CH_2CH_2{-}O{-}\overset{O}{\overset{\|}{C}}{-}CH_2CH_2{-}\overset{O}{\overset{\|}{C}})_x{-}OH$$

This product is made by the reaction of the following:

Reactant 1

$$\overset{O}{\overset{\|}{CH_3{-}(CH_2)_{16}C}}{-}OH \quad \text{stearic acid (a mono acid chain stopper),} \quad 1 \text{ equivalent}$$

Reactant 2

$$HO{-}CH_2CH_2{-}OH \quad \text{ethylene glycol (a difunctional polyol),} \quad x \text{ equivalents}$$

Reactant 3

$$\overset{O}{\overset{\|}{HO{-}C}}{-}CH_2CH_2{-}\overset{O}{\overset{\|}{C}}{-}OH \quad \text{succinic acid (a difunctional acid),} \quad x \text{ equivalents}$$

The presence of the x subscript indicates repeating units and is indicative of a polyester.

21.3 ESTER PROPERTIES AND USE IN PIGMENTED PRODUCTS

21.3.1 Simple Esters

21.3.1.1 S-1: Oleyl Erucate

The use of natural, vegetable-derived ingredients is extremely popular in modern personal care formulations. Jojoba oil is an example of such an ingredient. Availability of jojoba, like many naturally derived materials, can vary and is subject to variations in meteorological and seasonal conditions. Oleyl erucate is a synthetic, vegetable-based jojoba oil substitute. This ester's physical and functional properties are virtually identical to jojoba oil. Oleyl erucate can be used as a total replacement for jojoba or as an economical diluent or supplement to jojoba oil and still retain functionality and marketing claims.

Oleyl erucate is a superb, light emollient having good dry-down and spreading characteristics. It leaves a nonoily, silky, smooth feel on the skin or hair. Its light emolliency makes oleyl erucate a good choice for use in hair care products to promote shine and luster.

Recommended use levels are 1 to 10%.

INCI name: Oleyl erucate
CAS number: 17673-56-2
EINECS number: 241-654-9
Japanese ingredient code: 532030

Structure

$$R—O—C(O)—R'$$

R is C18:1 (oleyl)

R' is C22:1 (erucate)

Specifications

Appearance at 25°C	Clear liquid
Odor	Waxy
Color (Gardner)	3 max.
Hydroxyl value	10 max.
Acid value, mg KOH/g	2.0 max.
Moisture %	0.5 max.

Solubility

Castor oil	m	Propylene glycol	d
Ethanol	i	Isopropyl myristate	m
Volatile silicone	m	Water	i
Mineral oil	m		

Note: m = miscible (soluble at all proportions);
d = dispersible;
i = insoluble.

21.3.1.2 S-2: Isocetyl Behenate

Isocetyl behenate is a 100% active, low-viscosity, stable, vegetable-derived, liquid ester. It is both odorless and tasteless and exhibits excellent emolliency and skin spreadability characteristics.

Isocetyl behenate exhibits broad solubility in oils and silicone, and is useful as a melting point modifier in lipstick and makeup systems. It also imparts emolliency and sheen to lipsticks, and is suitable for anhydrous skin products or emulsion systems. Use levels of 2 to 5% are indicated in skin products, and 5 to 10% in lipstick and lip products.

INCI name: Isocetyl behenate
CAS number: 94247-28-6
EINECS number: 304-205-9

Structure

$$R\text{—}O\text{—}C(O)\text{—}R'$$

R is C16 (Guerbet)   R' is C22 (Behenic)

Specifications

Appearance at 25°C	Clear, slightly yellow liquid
Odor	Bland
Color (Gardner)	4 max.
Acid value	3 max.
Saponification value	70—95

Solubility

Castor oil	m
Ethanol	i
Volatile silicone	m
Mineral oil	m
Propylene glycol	i
Isopropyl myristate	m
Water	i

Note: m = miscible (soluble at all proportions);
　　　d = dispersible;
　　　i = insoluble.

Safety

Primary eye irritation	Nonirritating
Primary skin irritation	Nonirritating
Acute oral toxicity	Nontoxic
Comedogenicity	Noncomedogenic

21.3.1.3 S-3: Octyldodecyl Erucate

Octyldodecyl erucate is an oil-soluble, 100% active, liquid ester. It is completely vegetable derived. For a long-carbon-chain-length ester (42 carbon atoms), it is surprisingly very low in viscosity and has excellent shelf-life and clarity at low temperatures. It is readily absorbed into skin, leaving a soft, smooth, nongreasy, dry feel. Octyldodecyl erucate also rapidly absorbs into leather surfaces.

INCI name: Octyldodecyl erucate
CAS number: 132208-25-4
Japanese code number: 520172

Structure

$$R—O—C(O)—R'$$

R is C20 (Guerbet)

R' is C22:1 (erucate)

Specifications

Chemical name	Eicosyl erucate
Color (Gardner)	3 max.
Acid value (mg KOH/g)	1.0 max.
Residual alcohol (%)	1.5 max.
Water (%)	0.05 max.

Solubility

Castor oil	m
Ethanol	i
Volatile silicone	m
Mineral oil	m
Propylene glycol	i
Isopropyl myristate	m
Water	i

Note: m = miscible (soluble at all proportions);
d = dispersible;
i = insoluble.

Applications

Octyldodecyl erucate is suitable for use in:

- Lipstick
- Makeup products
- Nail cuticle treatments

Safety

Toxicity studies have shown octyldodecyl erucate to be extremely safe; results are summarized below:

Primary eye irritation	Nonirritating
Primary skin irritation	Nonprimary irritant
Acute oral toxicity	Orally nontoxic
Comedogenicity	Noncomedogenic

21.3.1.4   S-4: Isostearyl Behenate

Isostearyl behenate is a 100% active ester and exists as a soft, opaque, off-white paste at ambient temperatures. It melts at skin temperature and imparts an extremely emollient and soft feel to skin. Isostearyl behenate is generally soluble in oil and insoluble in water. It is an effective moisture barrier and imparts "slip" to powders.

INCI name: Isostearyl behenate
CAS number: 125804-16-2

Structure

R-O-C(O)-R'

R is C18 (isostearic)
R' is C22 (behenic)

Specifications

Chemical name	Isostearyl behenate
Appearance at 25°C	Soft paste
Color	White to off-white
Acid value	3.0 max.
Saponification value	80—100
Melting point	31—37°C

Solubility

Castor oil	s
Ethanol	i
Volatile silicone	s
Mineral oil	s
Propylene glycol	i
Isopropyl myristate	m
Water	i

Note: m = miscible (soluble at all proportions);
　　　d = dispersible;
　　　i = insoluble.

Applications

Isostearyl behenate is silicone compatible and is useful in lotions and creams, lipsticks, mascara, liquid eye makeup, eye shadow, and powder makeup.

Safety

Isostearyl behenate in an extremely safe ester. Toxicity studies are summarized as follows:

Primary eye irritation	Nonirritating
Primary skin irritation	Nonirritating
Acute oral toxicity	Nontoxic
Comedogenicity	Noncomedogenic

21.3.2 COMPLEX ESTERS

21.3.2.1 C-1: Trioctyldodecyl Citrate

Trioctyldodecyl citrate is a clear, oil-soluble, slightly yellow, slightly viscous triester. It is, in fact, surprisingly low in odor for a citrate triester. It is substantive to skin and extremely emollient. The hydroxyl functionality in trioctyldodecyl citrate makes it a uniquely effective wetting agent for pigments. In addition to its compatibility with castor oil, trioctyldodecyl citrate is a very effective pigment-wetting and -grinding vehicle for anhydrous pigment systems containing mineral oil, petrolatum, or microcrystalline wax, due to trioctyldodecyl citrate's compatibility with hydrocarbons.

Trioctyldodecyl citrate also has the unique property of being miscible with cyclomethicone, the resulting solution being extremely silky and soft in feel.

INCI name: trioctyldodecyl citrate
CAS number: 126121-35-5
Japanese code number: 532050

Structure

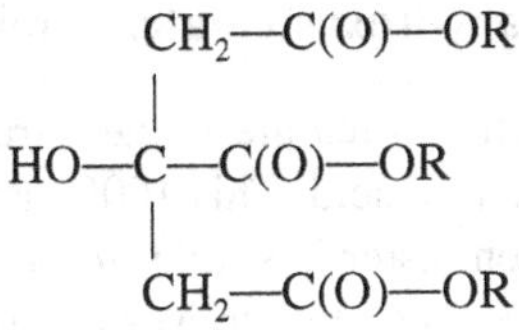

$$CH_2—C(O)—OR$$
$$|$$
$$HO—C—C(O)—OR$$
$$|$$
$$CH_2—C(O)—OR$$

R is octyldodecyl (Guerbet)

Specifications

Chemical name	Trioctyldodecyl citrate
Appearance at 25°C	Clear to hazy oily liquid
Color (Gardner)	3 max.
Acid value	5 max.
Saponification value	135 — 165

Solubility

Castor oil	m
Ethanol	i
Volatile silicone	m
Mineral oil	m
Propylene glycol	i
Isopropyl myristate	m
Water	i

Note: m = miscible (soluble at all proportions);
d = dispersible;
i = insoluble.

Applications

Trioctyldodecyl citrate is useful in skin preparations where cushion is desired and is silicone compatible for such end products as creams and lotions, makeup products, lipstick and lip products, hair products (conditioners, oils, and gels), and pressed powders.

Safety

Trioctyldodecyl citrate is an extremely safe ester. Toxicity studies are summarized as follows:

Primary eye irritation	Nonirritating
Primary skin irritation	Nonirritating
Acute oral toxicity	Nontoxic

21.3.2.2　C-3: Dipentaerythrityl Tetrahydroxystearate/Tetraisostearate

Dipentaerythrityl tetrahydroxystearate/tetraisostearate is the tetraester of dipentaerythrityl and hydroxystearic acid/isostearic acid. This 100% active, hydrophobic, occlusive, skin-conditioning, emollient ester is similar to lanolin in feel and consistency. Dipentaerythrityl tetrahydroxystearate/tetraisostearate is a paste with excellent water-holding capacity, due to the presence of hydroxyl groups in the molecule.

These characteristics make dipentaerythrityl tetrahydroxystearate/tetraisostearate an ideal ester for use in:

- Lipstick
- High-Performance creams and lotions
- Mascara

Recommended use levels are 1 to 10%.

INCI name: Dipentaerythrityl tetrahydroxystearate/tetraisostearate
CAS number: 220716-33-6
EINECS: Polymer exempt
Japanese ingredient code: 508055

Specifications

Appearance at 25°C	Yellow paste
Odor	Odorless
Acid value	1.5 max.
Saponification value	155—180
Hydroxyl value	155—185

Solubility

Castor oil	d
Ethanol	d
Volatile silicone	i
Mineral oil	d
Propylene glycol	i
Isopropyl myristate	d
Water	i

Note: m = miscible (soluble at all proportions);
d = dispersible;
i = insoluble.

21.3.2.3 C-4: Trimethylolpropane Triisostearate

Trimethylolpropane triisostearate is a 100% active, liquid triester of trimethylolpropane and isostearic acid. It is unique in its sensory and visual properties. Trimethylolpropane triisostearate has excellent cushion and playtime; it is non-tacky, light, glossy on skin, and improves application of solid delivery systems such as lipsticks and makeup products.

Trimethylolpropane triisostearate also exhibits broad solubility properties, dissolving in silicone as well as esters. It forms solid systems with esters such as glyceryl behenate. Glyceryl behenate is a solid ester melting at about 70°C. Glyceryl behenate, when melted, can be blended with trimethylolpropane triisostearate to form lubricious, homogeneous, stable systems with any degree of softness required by the formulator. Similar systems are possible with other solid esters, such as behenyl behenate, low concentrations of which will form very lubricious gels melting at skin temperature.

Trimethylolpropane triisostearate has been found to gel in mixtures with 12-hydroxy stearic acid by merely stirring the two components with heat until they mutually dissolve and allowing the mixture to come to ambient temperatures. While firm opaque gels are formed in ratios of 70% trimethylolpropane triisostearate and 30% 12-hydroxy stearic acid, for example, virtually clear firm gels are formed in ratios of 99% trimethylolpropane triisostearate and 1% 12-hydroxy stearic acid. Applications for these gels are particularly seen in lipstick and lip products.

These excellent properties make trimethylolpropane triisostearate an ester of choice for use in a broad range of cosmetic products, such as in lipsticks and lip products, makeups, skin creams and lotions, and massage oils.

Recommended use levels are 2 to 8%.

INCI name: Trimethylolpropane triisostearate
CAS number: 68541-50-4
EINECS number: 271-347-5
Japanese ingredient code: 503098

Structure

$$CH_3CH_2-C-(CH_2OR)_3$$

R is isostearic

Specifications

Appearance at 25°C	Clear, viscous liquid
Color (Gardner)	2 max.
Moisture content (%)	0.5 max.
Acid value	2.0 max.
Saponification value	175—195
Iodine value (Hanus)	4.0 max.

Solubility

Castor oil	m
Ethanol	i
Volatile silicone	m
Mineral oil	m
Dimethicone	d
Propylene glycol	i
Isopropyl myristate	m
Water	i

Note: m = miscible (soluble at all proportions);
d = dispersible;
i = insoluble.

Safety

Primary Eye Irritation	Nonirritating
Primary Skin Irritation	Nonirritating

21.3.2.4   C-5: Tri C$_{12-13}$ Alkyl Citrate

Tri C$_{12-13}$ alkyl citrate is a 100% active, virtually odorless, water white triester of citric acid and C$_{12-13}$ alcohols. It is castor oil compatible and an effective pigment-wetting and -dispersing agent. It can be used in place of castor oil in pigmented systems for low odor or fragrance-free products.

Tri C$_{12-13}$ alkyl citrate can be gelled with 12-hydroxystearic acid. It will form translucent gels in the 1.5 to 6% 12-hydroxystearate range. As the concentration of 12-hydroxystearic acid increases above 6%, the gels become opaque rather than translucent. The most important property of these gels is their extremely luxurious feel, while at the same time evidencing little to no payout.

These properties make Tri C_{12-13} alkyl citrate an ester of choice for transfer-proof lipstick, lip balms, and other lip and transfer-resistant makeup products.

Tri C_{12-13} alkyl citrate can also be formulated into clear, fragrance-free skin products. Having CAS, EINECS, and Japanese registration numbers, tri C_{12-13} alkyl citrate is suitable for global cosmetic products.

Recommended use levels are 3 to 20%.

INCI name: Tri alkyl C_{12-13} citrate
CAS number: 93573-19-4
EINECS number: 297-554-0
Japanese registration number: 532251

Structure

R is C_{12-13} alcohol

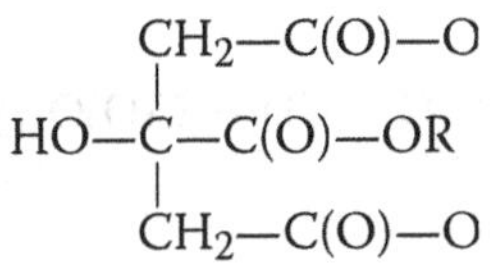

$$CH_2-C(O)-O$$
$$HO-\underset{|}{\overset{|}{C}}-C(O)-OR$$
$$CH_2-C(O)-O$$

Specifications

Appearance at 25°C	Clear oily liquid
Color (Gardner)	1 max.
Moisture, %	0.5 max.
Acid value	5.0 max.
Saponification value	205–235

Solubility

Castor oil	m
Ethyl alcohol	i
Volatile silicone	m
Mineral oil	m
Propylene glycol	i
IPM	m
Water	i

Note: m = miscible (soluble at all proportions);
     d = dispersible;
     i = insoluble.

21.3.2.5 C-6: Pentaerythrityl Tetaisostearate

Pentaerythrityl tetaisostearate is a rapidly absorbed emollient. It possesses cushion and a slight amount of drag. In addition to these attributes, it has an extremely bland taste, making it particularly useful to lipstick and lip treatment formulas. For applications where shine is undesirable, pentaerythrityl tetaisostearate performs well because of its matte appearance on the skin.

It is supplied as a 100% active, clear, straw-colored liquid that is compatible with a variety of personal care raw materials. This medium-viscosity emollient is a valuable addition to the palettes of both color cosmetic and skin care formulators.

INCI name: Pentaerythrityl petraisostearate
CAS number: 62125-232-8
EINECS number: 263-423-1
Japanese ingredient code: 520782

Structure

$$C-(CH_2-C(O)OR)_4$$

R is isostearate (C_{18} iso)

Solubility

Castor oil	m
Ethanol	i
Volatile silicone	m
Mineral oil	m
Propylene glycol	i
Isopropyl myristate	m
Water	

Note: m = miscible (soluble at all proportions);
     d = dispersible;
     i = insoluble.

Specifications

Appearance at 25°C	Clear liquid
Color (Gardner)	2 max.
Moisture, %	0.1 max.
Acid value	2 max.

Safety [Repeat Insult Patch Test (skin irritation)]

An RIPT study with 50 human subjects has revealed pentaerythrityl tetaisostearate to be both nonirritating and nonsensitizing.

21.3.2.6 C-7: Triisostearyl Citrate

Triisostearyl citrate is recommended as a pigment-wetting and -dispersing agent. It helps impart spreadability and gloss in lipstick and makeup products. It is a virtually odorless and tasteless product, making it an ideal candidate for color cosmetics.

INCI name: Trisiostearyl citrate
CAS number: 113431-54-2

Structure

R is isostearyl (C_{18} iso)

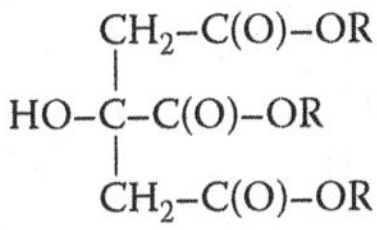

$$CH_2-C(O)-OR$$
$$HO-C-C(O)-OR$$
$$CH_2-C(O)-OR$$

Specifications

Appearance at 25°C	Viscous liquid
Color (APHA)	150 max.
Acid value	2.0 max.
Iodine value	3.0 max.
Saponification value	150–165

Solubility

Castor oil	m
Ethanol	i
Volatile silicone	m
Mineral oil	m
Propylene glycol	i
Isopropyl myristate	m
Water	i

Note: m = miscible (soluble at all proportions);
d = dispersible;
i = insoluble.

21.3.2.7 C-8: Diisostearyl Malate

Diisostearyl malate is a 100% active liquid diester of an alpha-hydroxy acid. This ester exhibits excellent skin feel characterized by cushion and emolliency, leaving the skin soft and supple. Diisostearyl malate is oil and silicone soluble and can be formulated with these materials in a variety of cosmetic products. Diisostearyl malate is suitable for lipstick and lip products as well as makeup and skin formulations. Recommended use levels are 2 to 10%.

INCI name: Diisostearyl malate
CAS number: 67763-18-2
EINECS number: 267-041-6
Japanese ingredient code: 502172

Specifications

Appearance at 25°C	Clear yellow liquid
Color (APHA)	100 max.
Odor	Typical
Acid value	5.0 max.
Saponification value	165–180

21.3.2.8   C-9: Tridecyl Trimellitate

Tridecyl trimellitate is the tritridecyl ester of trimellitic acid. It is a 100% active, hydrophobic, emollient ester, with good skin substantivity. Solubility characteristics for tridecyl trimellitate indicate its use in lipstick, lip products, makeup, and in skin formulations of various types.

Tridecyl trimellitate is recommended for use in the 2 to 10% range.

Specifications

Appearance at 25°C	Slightly yellow, liquid[a]
Odor	Essentially odorless
Color (Gardner)	1.0 max.
Acid value	1.0 max.
Saponification value	235–255

[a]Temperature dependent. Product is liquid at ambient temperatures but will develop gelatinous flock or become soft solid on cooling. Product returns to liquid state upon warming. Physical state is reversible without deleterious consequences.

Solubility

Castor oil	m
Ethanol	m
Volatile silicone	m
Mineral oil	m
Water	i

Note: m = miscible (soluble at all proportions);
    d = dispersible;
    i = insoluble.

21.3.2.9 C-10: Trimethylolptopane Triethylhexanonate

Trimethylolpropane triethylhexanoate is a 100% active, liquid, synthetically derived ester. It is categorized as a medium to light emollient oil with exceptional playtime. It is also hydrophobic, nontacky, and substantive to skin. Trimethylolpropane triethylhexanoate is also useful in lipstick and makeup products at 10 to 30% use levels.

INCI name: Trimethylolpropane triethylhexanoate
CAS number: 26086-33-9
Japanese code number: 503099

Specifications

Appearance at 25°C	Clear, viscous liquid
Color (Gardner)	1 max.
Moisture content (%)	0.5 max.
Acid value	1.0 max.
Saponification value	300–330

Solubility

Castor oil	m
Ethanol	m
Cyclomethicone	m
Mineral oil	m
Propylene glycol	i
Isopropyl myristate	m
Water	i

Note: m = miscible (soluble at all proportions);
    d = dispersible;
    i = insoluble.

21.3.3 POLYESTERS

21.3.3.1 P-1: Polyhydroxystearic Acid

Polyhydroxystearic acid is a 100% active, all-vegetable-derived polyester. It is a viscous, substantive, yellow liquid at ambient temperatures and, as with any polymer, will tend to fractionate on cooling. Product clarity and homogeneity are restored on heating and stirring with no adverse effect on the product.

Polyhydroxystearic acid has many polar sites and, although oil soluble, will complex water via hydrogen bonding on the skin surface. It will therefore function as a skin conditioner and humectant. Its substantivity and solubility profile strongly suggests its use in color cosmetics. Polyhydroxystearic acid also functions as a superior pigment-wetting, -grinding, and -coating agent.

Polyhydroxystearic acid retains single terminal hydroxy and carboxy groups, allowing for derivatization into many complex esters, which will be the subject of patented technology.

Polyhydroxystearic acid is a true polymeric ester; we can postulate that specific polar sites on the polymer chain will form a film in solution via hydrogen bonding with adjacent molecules to form multilayered micelles in a polymeric liquid crystal pattern. It is this associative gel matrix formation that accounts for the superior liquid crystal emulsification properties of polyhydroxystearic acid.

> INCI name: Polyhydroxystearic acid
> CAS number: 27924-99-8
> EINECS number: Polymer exempt
> Japanese code number: 532305

Applications

Polyhydroxystearic acid is used in concentrations as much as 50% in lipsticks, and its use is highly recommended in lipsticks, mascara, foundations, and skin conditioners.

21.3.3.2 P-2: Dimer Dilinoleyl Dimer Dilinoleate

Dimer dilinoleyl dimer dilinoleate is a 100% active, hydrophobic, completely vegetable derived polyester formed by the reaction of dimer dilinoleyl alcohol and dimer dilinoleic acid. It possesses interesting properties and can be characterized as:

- Tasteless
- Substantive
- Odorless
- Glossy

Structure

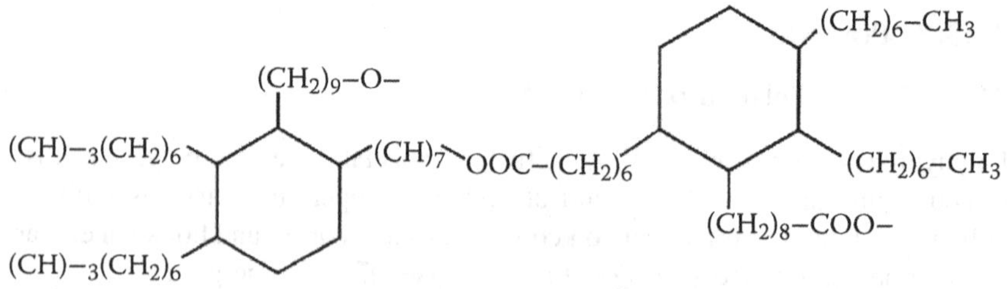

wherein n is 1 to 9

INCI name: Dimer dilinoleyl dimer dilinoleate
CAS number: 378789-58-3
EINECS number: Polymer exempt

21.4 FORMULATIONS

In order to demonstrate the effectiveness of the above esters in pigmented products, the following formulations are offered. The formulations were developed by Sun Chemical and make use of Phoenix Chemical's esters. Both companies have graciously allowed them to be used in this book. The formulations are given as illustrative; neither company makes any warranties about the formulation or its ability to be used free of any patents.

Formulation 1: Pressed Face Powder (Tan)

Ingredient	% Weight
Part A	
Talc	43.95
Zinc stearate	7.00
Polyethylene B-6	7.00
Magnesium carbonate	4.00
Timica silk white	25.00
Titanium dioxide	2.00
Red iron oxide	0.50
Black iron oxide	0.15
Yellow iron oxide	0.40
Part B	
Mineral oil	7.00
Octyldodecyl stearoyl stearate	3.00
Total	100.00

Process:
1. Mix Part A as a dry blend and disperse through a hammer mill.
2. Blend Part B.
3. Spray Part B on Part A in dry mix. Mix at medium speed for 30 min.
4. Press well-mixed batches into pan.

Formulation 2: Pressed Powder Blush (Terracotta)

Ingredient	% Weight
Part A	
Talc	20.00
Zinc stearate	7.00
Polyethylene B-12	9.00
Calcium silicate	2.00

Formulation 2: Pressed Powder Blush (Terracotta) (continued)

Ingredient	% Weight
Bismuth oxychloride	10.00
D&C 7 Ca Lake	2.00
Titanium dioxide	1.00
FD&C Yellow 5 Al Lake	2.00
Manganese violet	1.00
Methyl paraben	0.20
Propyl paraben	0.10
BHT	0.05
Sodium dehydroacetate	0.15
Part B	
Mica SVA	20.00
Nylon 12	6.00
Serecite GMS	7.00
Part C	
Trioctanoin	6.00
Octyldodecyl stearoyl stearate	2.00
Dimethicone and trimethylsiloxysilicate	3.50

Process:
1. Mix Part A as a dry blend and disperse through a hammer mill.
2. Blend Part A and Part B in a mixer. Mix at medium speed for 30 min. Scrape mixer sides and mix at medium speed for an additional 30 min.
3. Spray liquids on Part C into dry mix. Mix at medium speed for 30 min.
4. Press well-mixed batches into pans.

Formulation 3: Cosmetic Extruded Eyeliner

Ingredient	% Weight
Part A	
Japan wax	8.00
Caprylic capric stearic triglycerides	11.00
Carnauba wax	5.00
Hydrogenated coco glycerides	35.00
Hydrogenated castor oil	5.00
Caprylic capric triglycerides	6.00
Part B	
Nylon 12	2.50
Kaolin	3.00
Mica UF	4.00
Black iron oxide	9.00
Red iron oxide	2.00

Formulation 3: Cosmetic Extruded Eyeliner (continued)

Ingredient	% Weight
Yellow iron oxide	2.50
Russel iron oxide	3.00
Chromium oxide green	4.00

Process:
1. Weigh in and melt into a mixer the ingredients in Part A.
2. Heat to 85°C while mixing with slow sweep.
3. Once melted to clear liquid, add dry materials in Part B, mixing continuously and slowly so   as not to incorporate air into mass.
4. Once batch is homogeneous, remove liquid/molten product from mixer and disperse through   3-roll mill until pigments are fully dispersed.
5. Allow to cool to 25°C. Product is ready to extrude into pencils.

Formulation 4: Liquid Makeup

Ingredient	% Weight
Part A	
Titanium dioxide	9.00
Yellow iron oxide	0.75
Red iron oxide	0.50
Black iron oxide	0.05
Talc	5.00
Part B	
Distilled water	61.95
Triethanolamine	1.00
Polysorbate 60	0.60
Part C	
Magnesium aluminum silicate	1.00
Glycerin	2.00
Propylene glycol	2.00
PVP/hexadecane polymer	3.00
Part D	
Methyl paraben	0.20
Propyl paraben	0.10
Disodium EDTA	0.05
Germall 15	0.30
Part E	
Beeswax	4.00
Lanolin alcohol	2.00
Pentaerythritol tetraisostearate	2.00
Sorbitan isostearate	2.00
Cetyl alcohol	0.50

Formulation 4: Liquid Makeup (continued)

Ingredient	% Weight
Stearic acid	<u>2.00</u>
	100.0

Process:

1. Premill pigments together with talc in Part A through a hammer mill.
2. Using a homogenizer, combine milled dry color premix (Part A) to ingredients of Part B. Heat to 80°C to homogenize.
3. Add Part C in order shown, maintaining temperature at 80°C.
4. Add Part D, sequentially, while mixing.
5. Combine ingredients of oil phase (Part E) in a separate mixer. Mix and melt while using sweep action mixing. Heat to 80°C.
6. When both phases are homogeneous and both at 80°C, add oil phase (Part E) to water phase (Parts A to D), under homogenizing agitation.
7. Cool to below 45°C and fill.

Formulation 5: Gloss in a Tube

Material	% Weight
Acetylated lanolin	5.00
Triisostearyl citrate	20.00
Polyglycerol-3-diisostearate	5.00
Octyldodecanol	5.00
Lanolin	10.00
Petrolatum	11.00
Polybutene 100	20.00
Beeswax	6.50
Isopropyl lanolate	15.00
D&C Red 7 Ca Lake	2.00
D&C Red 27 Al Lake	<u>0.50</u>
	100.0

Process:

1. Premix and disperse pigments, triisostearyl citrate, and isopropyl lanolate, passing mixture through a 3-mill roll.
2. Combine all ingredients, heat to 80°C, and mix all melted ingredients until homogeneous.
3. Cool to 60°C and fill.

Formulation 6: Concealer in a Tube

Material	% Weight
Isostearyl neopentanonate	51.00
Ozokerite	5.00
Beeswax	2.00
Carnuba	3.00
Silica	10.00

Formulation 6: Concealer in a Tube (continued)

Material	% Weight
Titanium dioxide	20.00
Yellow iron oxide	1.50
Red iron oxide	0.75
Black iron oxide	0.10
Mica UF	6.60
BHT	<u>0.05</u>
	100.00

Process:
1. Premix isostearyl neopentanoate and pigments. Disperse pigments by passing through a 3-roll mill.
2. Mix and melt waxes at 80°C.
3. Add color blend and mix until homogeneous.
4. Add silica and mica, mix slowly with sweeping action.
5. Cool to 55 to 60°C to fill.

Formulation 7: Lash-Thickening Mascara

Ingredient	% Weight
Part A	
Petroleum distillate	70.00
Polyethylene AC 617A	12.00
Dihydroabietyl behenate	5.00
Candelilla wax	2.40
Part B	
Aluminum stearate	0.50
Butyl paraben	0.10
Part C	
Black iron oxide	<u>10.00</u>
	100.00

Process:
1. Heat Part A to 85°C, with medium agitation.
2. Sprinkle in Part B while mixing.
3. Add Part C and disperse at high speed for 45 min at 85°C.
4. Cool to 40°C and fill.

Formulation 8: Moisturizing Lipstick (Cranberry)

Ingredient	% Weight
Part A	
Octyldodecyl ricinoleate	10.20
Castor oil	18.00
Tridecyl trimellitate	3.00
Octyldodecanol	4.00
Lanolin wax	6.00
Lanolin oil	6.00
Hydroxylated milk glycerides	5.00
Hydrogenated coco triglycerides	3.00
Acetylated lanolin	5.00
Pentaerythritol tetraisonanonate	4.00
Ozokerite wax	5.00
Candelilla wax	5.00
Carnuba wax	1.00
Synthetic wax	3.00
Part B	
BHA	0.05
Propyl paraben	0.15
Part C	
FD&C Yellow 6 Al Lake	2.50
Castor oil dispersion (1:2)	
FD&C Red 7 Ca Lake	7.50
Castor oil dispersion (1:2)	
FD&C Red 21 Al Lake	1.00
Castor oil dispersion (1:2)	
Black iron oxide	0.60
Castor oil dispersion (1:2)	
Red iron oxide	2.00
Castor oil dispersion (1:2)	
Part D	
Serecite GMS	3.00
Pearl Flamenco Super Gold	3.00
Pearl Duochrome RY	2.00
	100.00

Process:

1. Individually premix each pigment (Part C) and disperse through a 3-mill roll.
2. Mix and melt Part A, heating to 85°C.
3. Mix in preservatives (Part B) until fully dispersed.
4. Add premilled pigments and castor oil dispersions (Part C); mix until homogeneous.
5. Add Part D; gently blend pearls and mica into batch.
6. Allow batch to cool to 55 to 60°C.
7. Pour into molds.

Formulation 9: High-Gloss Lipstick

Ingredient	% Weight
Part A	
Castor oil	14.00
Isononyl isonanonate	16.00
Pentaerythrityl tetracaprylate/tetracaprate	8.00
Octyldodecanol	5.00
Lanolin oil	10.90
Caprylic/capric/stearic triglyceride	6.50
Candelilla wax	8.50
Carnuba wax	3.00
Polybutene H-100	7.00
Ozokerite	2.00
Lanolin wax	1.00
Part B	
Methyl paraben	0.20
Propyl paraben	0.10
BHT	0.05
Part C	
Russel iron oxide	7.00
Castor oil dispersion (1:2)	
FD&C Red 7 Ca Lake	3.00
Castor oil dispersion (1:2)	
FD&C Yellow 5 Al Lake	2.00
Castor oil dispersion (1:2)	
FD&C Yellow 6 Al Lake	1.00
Castor oil dispersion (1:2)	
D&C Red 28 Al lake	0.75
Castor oil dispersion (1:2)	
Part D	
Silk mica (Timica silk white)	<u>4.00</u>
	100.00

Process:

1. Individually premix each pigment (Part C) and disperse through a 3-mill roll.
2. Mix and melt Part A, heating to 85°C.
3. Mix in preservatives (Part B) until fully dispersed.
4. Add premilled pigments and castor oil dispersions (Part C); mix until homogeneous.
5. Add Part D; gently blend pearls and mica into batch.
6. Allow batch to cool to 55 to 60°C.
7. Pour into molds.

21.5 PATENTS

One of the best indications of the state of the art is patent literature. There are several reasons for this. First, patent law requires that an inventor disclose the best mode of an invention. This means that an inventor cannot hold back information from the patent office related to how a technology works. Second, patents are becoming more and more important to the personal care industry. Twenty years ago, they were curiosities. Today, there does not seem to be a Tuesday morning (the date new patents are published) when new inventions related to personal care are not disclosed. Companies that do not patent are at a serious disadvantage. The patents below were chosen to highlight the use of esters in cosmetic products.

21.5.1 MASCARA

1. U.S. Patent 5,486,356 to Defossez et al., issued January 23, 1996, discloses an invention entitled "Cosmetic Make-Up Composition Containing a Transparent Titanium Oxide and Silicon Oxide Pigment". It states, "A cosmetic make-up composition containing, in a suitable cosmetic carrier, a transparent pigment consisting of at least 60 wt% laminar titanium oxide and at most 10 wt% silicon oxide, wherein the average pigment size is 1–300 mm and the thickness is 0.001–0.3 mm. Excellent cosmetic properties regarding pearlizing, coverage, spreadability and smoothness are obtained." Not surprisingly, it makes use of esters. The patent states, "Among the binding agents, there may be … esters such as isopropyl myristate, isopropyl palmitate, butyl stearate, hexyl laurate, isononyl isononanate, 2-ethylhexyl palmitate, 2-hexyldecyl laurate, 2-octyldecyl palmitate, 2-octyldodecyl myristate, 2-diethylhexyl succinate, diisostearyle malate, 2-octyldodecyl lactate, glycerin triisostearate, diglycerin triisostearate and the like."

2. U.S. Patent 5,614,200 to Bartholomey et al., issued March 25, 1997, discloses an invention entitled "Mascara Compositions." It provides mascara compositions having improved application characteristics. Said improvement is attributed to incorporation of a setting rate agent that delays the setting of the composition long enough to provide sufficient time to distribute the mascara in semiliquid form onto the lashes, as well as contribute to lash-thickening properties while avoiding negative aesthetics. It states: "Examples of fatty acid esters useful in the present invention include the glyceryl esters of higher fatty acids such as stearic and palmitic such as glyceryl monostearate, glyceryl distearate, glyceryl tristearate, palmitate esters of glycerol, C.sub.18-36 triglycerides, glyceryl tribehenate and mixtures thereof."

3. U.S. Patent 6,214,329 to Brieva et al., issued April 10, 2001, discloses an invention entitled "Mascara Compositions and Method for Curling Lashes." It demonstrates a pigmented emulsion composition for application to eyelashes or eyebrows comprising an aqueous phase and a

nonaqueous phase, wherein the nonaqueous phase consists of at least one organic, solid, nonpolymeric gelling agent, which is capable of gelling the pigmented emulsion composition to a viscosity of 4000 to 2,000,000 centipoise at 25°C, and a method for lengthening, coloring, and curling eyelashes using said composition.

Claim 1 outlines the required components:

1. A pigmented emulsion composition for application to eyelashes or eyebrows comprising 0.1–99.5% aqueous phase and 0.1–99% non-aqueous phase, wherein the non-aqueous phase comprises at least one organic, solid, non-polymeric gelling agent selected from the group consisting of:

a. N-acyl amino acids, or esters, or amides thereof;

b. 12-hydroxystearic acid and esters and amides thereof,

c. fatty acid esters of di- or tri-functional alcohol dimers;

d. alkylamides of di- and tricarboxylic acids; and

e. mixtures thereof

which is capable of gelling the pigmented emulsion composition to a viscosity of 4,000 to 2,000,000 centipoise at 25°C.

21.5.2 LIPSTICK

Esters are very commonly used and critically important materials in both long-wear and traditional lipsticks. Several patents teach the importance of these materials.

1. U.S. Patent 5,225,186 to Castrogiovanni et al., issued July 6, 1993, discloses an invention entitled "High Cosmetic Powder Lipstick Composition." This is one of several key patents that disclose a stick-shaped lipstick composition that comprises a higher loading of cosmetic powders than those available in prior art compositions. The composition includes between about 10% and about 65% of at least one cosmetic powder. At least one low-viscosity liquid carboxylic acid ester, present in a concentration of between about 10% and about 65%, is also included. A third component of the composition is at least one high-viscosity surface oil included in an amount of between about 1% and about 18%. The composition additionally comprises between about 2% and about 15% of at least one plasticizing agent. All of the above-mentioned percentages are by weight, based on the total weight of the composition. The high concentration of cosmetic powder provides a unique finish, texture, and feel lipstick heretofore unavailable in convenient stick shape.

The teaching on the importance of the ester is very enlightening. The patent states:

Another essential component of the stick shaped lipstick composition is at least one liquid, low viscosity carboxylic acid ester. The ester component, present in the composition in a concentration of between about 10% and about 65% by weight, based on the total weight of the lipstick composition, is preferably characterized by a viscosity, at 25°C, in the range of between about 5 centipoise (cp) and about 100 cp. More preferably, the liquid low viscosity carboxylic acid ester is present in a concentration of between about 25% and about 45% by weight.

The carboxylic acid ester component serves to wet out the cosmetic powder component and significantly contribute to the light, dry, silky and powdery texture of the final lipstick product. In addition, the liquid ester component performs in such a way to promote better adhesion and wear of the lipstick composition to the lips of the user. The ester component further contributes to the moisturizing effect of the lipstick composition on the lips to which it is applied.

Among the liquid, low viscosity carboxylic acid esters that can be used in the lipstick composition are isotridecyl isononanoate, isostearyl neopentanoate, cetyl octanoate, glyceryl trioctanoate, isodecyl oleate and isodecyl neopentanoate, ingredients mentioned in the CTFA Ingredient Dictionary, 3rd Edition incorporated herein by mentioned reference. In addition, mixtures of these esters, as well as PEG-4 diheptanoate, tridecyl neopentanoate, isohexyl neopentanoate and tridecyl octanoate.

2. U.S. Patent 5,093,111 to Baker et al., issued March 3, 1992, discloses an invention entitled "Lipstick Composition Comprising Cetearyl Isononanoate, a Sesquistearate and Isopropyl Hydroxystearate." It provides very specific esters useful in lipstick applications, specifically a lipstick composition comprising by weight from 8 to 20% of waxes, 30 to 80% of oils, 3 to 30% of colorants, 8 to 20% of cetearyl isononanoate, 1 to 10% of a sesquistearate, and 2 to 20% of isopropyl hydroxystearate. The lipstick has the aesthetic performance characteristics of a regular lipstick, but more effectively soothes and protects the lips.

3. U.S. Patent 5,225,186 to Castrogiovanni et al., issued July 6, 1993, discloses an invention entitled "High Cosmetic Powder Lipstick Composition." It states:

A stick shaped lipstick composition which comprises a higher loading of cosmetic powders than those available in prior art compositions is disclosed. The composition includes between about 10% and about 65% of at least one cosmetic powder. At least one low viscosity liquid carboxylic acid ester, present in a concentration of between about 10% and about 65%, is also included. A third component of the composition is at least one high viscosity surface oil included in an amount of between about 1% and about 18%. The composition additionally comprises between about 2% and about 15% of at least one plasticizing agent. All of the above mentioned percentages are by weight, based on the total weight of the composition. The high concentration of cosmetic powder provides a unique finish, texture and feel lipstick heretofore unavailable in convenient stick shape.

Specifically, the ester is present at "between about 25% and about 45% of a liquid carboxylic acid ester selected from the group consisting of isotridecyl isononanoate, isostearyl neopentanoate, cetyl octanoate, glyceryl trioctanoate, isodecyl oleate, isodecyl neopentanoate, PEG-4 diheptanoate, tridecyl neopentanoate, isohexyl neopentanoate, tridecyl octanoate and mixtures thereof."

4. U.S. Patent 5,593,662 to Deckner et al., issued January 14, 1997, discloses an invention entitled "Moisturizing Lipstick Compositions." It teaches a long-lasting, physically stable, moisturizing lipstick composition essentially free of water. Said lipsticks contain lipophilic materials with high levels of moisturizers distributed throughout. They resist separation of the moisturizing material from the body of the lipstick. This invention uses esters, among other ingredients. The inventor specifies:

The fatty acid esters useful in the present invention are fatty acids whose active hydrogen has been replaced by the alkyl group of monohydric and polyhydric alcohols (the fatty acid esters of the polyhydric alcohol glycerol being triglycerides). In the present invention the fatty acid esters are selected from the group consisting of cetyl ricinoleate, cetyl acetate, glycerol oleate, glycerol monostearate, isopropyl lanolate, isopropyl linoleate, isopropyl myristate, isopropyl palmitate, isopropyl oleate, isopropyl stearate, ethyl glutimate, ethyl laurate, ethyl linolenate, ethyl methacrylate, ethyl myristate, ethyl palmitate, and mixtures thereof. The preferred fatty acid ester is selected from the group consisting of isopropyl myristate, isopropyl palmitate, isopropyl oleate, isostearate, and mixtures thereof.

5. U.S. Patent 5,690,918 to Jacks et al., issued November 25, 1997, discloses an invention entitled "Solvent-Based Non-drying Lipstick." It teaches a long-wearing, durable, nonsmearing-type wax-based pigmented lipstick product including volatile solvents, a nonvolatile silicone polymer, an oil-soluble liquid phase, and a dry powder phase, and is made to have improved moisturizing properties by incorporating a mixture of moisturizers that includes essential fatty acids provided by diisoarachidyl dilinoleate, fatty acid ester of alpha-tocopherol, cholesteryl/behenyl/octyldodecyl/lauroyl glutamate complex, and lauryl pyrrolidone carboxylic acid ester.

6. U.S. Patent 6,036,947 to Barone et al., issued March 14, 2000, discloses an invention entitled "Transfer Resistant High Lustre Lipstick Compositions." Barone, considered by many to be the father of the transfer-resistant lipstick, and his group disclose "an anhydrous cosmetic stick composition with improved transfer resistance and luster finish comprising, by weight of the total composition: a) 10–70% of a volatile solvent having a viscosity of 0.5 to 20 centipoise at 25°C, b) 0.5–40% of a guerbet ester, and c) 0.1–20% of a siloxysilicate polymer." They also disclose: "It has been unexpectedly discovered that cosmetic compositions containing the combination of a volatile solvent, a Guerbet

ester, and siloxy silicate polymer provide a high lustre lipstick composition which exhibits transfer resistance which is equivalent if not better than the traditional matte formulas."

Examples of Guerbet esters are as set forth in U.S. Patent 5,488,121, which is hereby incorporated by reference. Suitable fluoro-Guerbet esters are set forth in U.S. Patent 5,312,968, which is hereby incorporated by reference. Most preferred is a Guerbet ester having the tentative CTFA name fluoro-octyldodecyl Meadowfoamate. This reference clearly delineates the interrelationship between silicone resin and ester.

7. U.S. Patent 6,090,396 to Deckner et al., issued July 18, 2000, discloses an invention entitled "Moisturizing Lipstick Compositions." It discloses long-lasting, physically stable, moisturizing lipstick compositions essentially free of water. Said lipsticks contain lipophilic materials with high levels of moisturizers distributed throughout. They resist separation of the moisturizing material from the body of the lipstick. The patent teaches:

The fatty acid esters useful in the present invention are fatty acids whose active hydrogen has been replaced by the alkyl group of monohydric and polyhydric alcohols (the fatty acid esters of the polyhydric alcohol glycerol being triglycerides). In the present invention the fatty acid esters are selected from the group consisting of cetyl ricinoleate, cetyl acetate, glycerol oleate, glycerol monostearate, isopropyl lanolate, isopropyl linoleate, isopropyl myristate, isopropyl palmitate, isopropyl oleate, isopropyl stearate, ethyl glutimate, ethyl laurate, ethyl linolenate, ethyl methacrylate, ethyl myristate, ethyl palmitate, and mixtures thereof. The preferred fatty acid ester is selected from the group consisting of isopropyl myristate, isopropyl palmitate, isopropyl oleate, isostearate, and mixtures thereof.

8. U.S. Patent 6,143,283 to Calello et al., issued November 7, 2000, discloses an invention entitled "Glossy Transfer Resistant Lipstick Compositions." It discloses "a cosmetic composition having improved transfer resistance comprising: a) from about 0.1–60% of a copolymer which is an adhesive at room temperature, b) from about 0.1–60% by weight of a volatile solvent having a viscosity of 0.5 to 20 centipoise at 25°C, c) 0.1–60% by weight of a nonvolatile oil, d) 0.1–80% dry particulate matter.

The nonvolatile oil may comprise esters of the formula RCO–OR', wherein R and R' are each independently a C_{1-25}, preferably a C_{4-20} straight- or branched-chain alkyl, alkenyl, or alkoxycarbonylalkyl or alkylcarbonyloxyalkyl. Examples of such esters include isotridecyl isononanoate, PEG-4 diheptanoate, isostearyl neopentanoate, tridecyl neopentanoate, cetyl octanoate, cetyl palmitate, cetyl ricinoleate, cetyl stearate, cetyl myristate, coco-dicaprylate/caprate, decyl isostearate, isodecyl oleate, isodecyl neopentanoate, isohexyl neopentanoate, octyl palmitate, dioctyl malate, tridecyl octanoate, myristyl myristate, octododecanol, and fatty alcohols such as oleyl alcohol, isocetyl alcohol, and the like, as well as the esters disclosed on pages 24 to 26 of the CTFA *Cosmetic Ingredient Handbook*, 1st Edition, 1988, which is hereby incorporated by reference.

9. U.S. Patent 6,585,985 to Sakuta, issued July 1, 2000, discloses an invention entitled "Lipstick Composition Containing Hydrophilic Crosslinked Silicon." It discloses a composition for molding a lipstick capable of exhibiting an excellent cosmetic finishing effect with remarkable sustainability and a comfortable feeling of use. The most characteristic ingredient of the composition is a cross-linked hydrophilic organopolysiloxane insoluble in organic solvents obtained by the hydrosilation reaction between an organohydrogenpolysiloxane and an alkenyl-terminated polyoxyalkylene compound, which is combined with a liquid oily compound, solid or semisolid oily or waxy compound, and pigments in specified weight proportions.

Also disclosed is:

The component (b) in the inventive lipstick composition is an oily liquid at room temperature which can be selected from the group consisting of liquid hydrocarbon compounds such as liquid paraffin, squalane and pristane, fatty acid esters having 6 to 50 carbon atoms in a molecule such as cetyl isooctanoate, octyldodecyl myristate, isopropyl palmitate, isocetyl stearate and octyldodecyl oleate, triglyceride oils such as glycerin trioctanoate and glycerin triisostearate, higher fatty acids having 6 to 50 carbon atoms in a molecule such as isostearic acid, oleic acid, hexanoic acid and heptanoic acid, aliphatic higher alcohols having 6 to 50 carbon atoms in a molecule, such as isostearyl alcohol and oleyl alcohol, cyclic or straightly linear organopolysiloxanes such as octamethyl cyclotetrasiloxane, decamethyl cyclopentasiloxane, dimethylpolysiloxane oils and methylphenylpolysiloxane oils. These oily compounds can be used either singly or as a combination of two kinds or more, if compatible, as the component (b). These oily compounds should have a viscosity in the range from 1.0 to 1000 mm²/second at 25°C.

21.5.3 COSMETIC POWDER

1. U.S. Patent 5,814,311 to Le Bras-Roulier et al., issued September 29, 1998, discloses an invention entitled "Cosmetic Composition in the Form of a Compact Powder and Process for Preparing It." The invention relates to a cosmetic composition in the form of a compact powder comprising a fatty phase and a pulverulent phase. The said pulverulent phase comprises a first incompatible filler and at least a second filler, which may be compatible or incompatible; these two fillers are of different types. The composition preferably has an internal porosity of greater than 2 m²/g. The composition is obtained by preparing an oil-in-water type emulsion of the fatty phase in an aqueous phase, dispersing the pulverulent phase in the emulsion, casting the dispersion obtained in a mold, and freeze drying the dispersion.

The invention discloses the use of "fatty esters, such as isopropyl myristate, isopropyl palmitate, butyl stearate, hexyl laurate, isononyl isononoate, 2-ethylhexyl palmitate, 2-hexyldecyl laurate, 2-octyldecyl palmitate, 2-octyldodecyl myristate or lactate, 2-diethylhexyl succinate, diisostearyl malate, glycerin or diglycerin triisostearate."

2. U.S. Patent 6,132,743 to Kuroda et al., issued October 17, 2000, discloses an invention entitled "Zinc Oxide Powder with Suppressed Activity and Cosmetic Preparation." It teaches: "A zinc oxide powder having a suppressed photocatalytic activity and prepared by coating a zinc oxide powder with at least one silicone compound in a non-gaseous state and firing the coated zinc oxide powder in an oxidizing atmosphere at a temperature of 600 to 950°C. A cosmetic preparation containing this zinc oxide powder is excellent in feel, sebum resistance, and protection against ultraviolet light."
The inventors also teach:

As the oily agent, mention may be made of higher alcohol such as cetyl alcohol, isostearyl alcohol, lauryl alcohol, hexadecyl alcohol, and octyldodecanol, fatty acids such as isostearic acid, undecylenic acid and oleic acid, polyhydric alcohols such as glycerol, sorbitol, ethylene glycol, propylene glycol and polyethylene glycol, esters such as myristyl myristylate, hexyl laurylate, decyl oleate, isopropyl mirystylate, hexyldecyl dimethyloctanoate, monostearic acid glycerol, dimethyl phthalate, monostearic acid ethylene glycol and octyl oxystearate, hydrocarbons such as liquid paraffin, Vaseline and squalane, waxes such as lanolin, reduced lanolin and carnauba wax, oils and fats such as mink oil, cacao butter, coconut oil, palm kernel oil, tsubaki oil, sesame oil, castor oil and olive oil, etc.

3. U.S. Patent 6,517,820 to Robert et al., issued October 17, 2000, discloses an invention entitled "Cosmetic Composition in the Form of a Powder Comprising a Specific Ester." It teaches:

A cosmetic composition in the form of a powder containing a particulate phase and a fatty phase, characterized in that the fatty phase contains at least one fatty acid ester or at least one fatty alcohol ester, the carbonaceous chain of the fatty acid or alcohol being branched and saturated, and containing 24 to 28 carbon atoms. It also relates to the cosmetic applications of such a composition.

Claim 1 is very enlightening:

1.A cosmetic composition in the form of a powder comprising:

a particulate phase and

a fatty phase,

wherein the fatty phase comprises at least one fatty acid ester or at least one fatty alcohol ester, the at least one fatty acid ester or the at least one fatty alcohol ester being saturated and branched, and comprising at least two carbonaceous chains comprising 24 to 28 carbon atoms, wherein the at least one fatty acid ester or at least fatty alcohol ester is a polyester.

The inventors have found, unexpectedly, that the use as a powder binder of at least one specific oily ester, composed of saturated and branched (C_{24} to C_{28}) fatty acids or fatty alcohols, makes it possible to obtain a powder that not only exhibits excellent cosmetic properties, but also exhibits an improved hold.

The present invention is therefore directed to a cosmetic composition in the form of a powder comprising a particulate phase and a fatty phase, characterized in that the fatty phase comprises at least one fatty acid ester or fatty alcohol ester, the carbonaceous chain of the fatty acid or alcohol being saturated and branched and comprising 24 to 28 carbon atoms.

21.5.4 PIGMENT EXTENDERS

1. U.S. Patent 5,486,233 to Mitchell et al., issued January 23, 1996, discloses an invention entitled "Pigment Extenders." It teaches:

A pigment composition includes a pigment extender which optionally contains a pigment, and further includes a non-hydrogenated phospholipid material, such as non-hydrogenated lecithin, and a surface modifying agent. Suitable modifying agents are selected from fatty acids, fatty acid esters or fatty acid triglycerides, silicones and mixtures thereof.

The surface modifying agent may include oleic, palmitic, stearic, linoleic or linolenic acid, or mixtures thereof. The fatty acid esters may include, or be selected from the group consisting of, isocetyl stearate, diisopropyl dimerate, neopentanoate, isocetylstearyl stearate, isopropyl isostearate, diisostearyl dilinoleate octadecyl palmitate, and mixtures thereof. For example, isocetyl stearyl stearate and diisopropyl dimerate have been found to be suitable.

REFERENCES

1. O'Lenick, A.J., *Journal of Surfactants and Detergents*, 3(3), 388(2000).
2. O'Lenick, A.J., *Surfactants Properties and Applications*, Carol Stream, IL: Allured Publishing, 1999, p. 96.
3. Zenitech LLC Analytical Procedure ZAM-5, Appendix 1.

22 Hydrolysis-Resistant Esters

John A. Imperante
Phoenix Chemical, Inc.

CONTENTS

Oil phase materials are of interest to the cosmetic chemist in a variety of applications, including in pigmented products. These materials function as potential oils in which pigments may be ground, or oil phases used in emulsions. The type of products that are useful include poly alpha olefin (PAO), esters, Guerbet alcohols, and mineral oils (all of which are discussed in a separate chapter). The selection of the proper material for use depends upon many factors, one of which is the polarity of the oil. PAO and mineral oils are very nonpolar. The introduction of an oxygen, if either a hydroxyl group or an ester group, increases the polarity of the oil. The selection of a more polar oil for the creation of a pigment dispersion can be highly desirable in many instances, because the pigment can be considered a polar material. All chemistry students remember being admonished that likes dissolve likes. The negative attribute of using esters is that the materials can be hydrolytically unstable, breaking down at a pH of below 5 or over 10. This chapter deals with a new class of esters that are hydrolytically stable. This allows the formulator the ability to chose the polarity of the oil phase to optimize dispersion particle size and stability.

22.1 CHEMISTRY

Esters are a well-known class of compounds both to the organic chemist and to the cosmetic chemist. There are a number of subclasses of esters that differ in both functionality and structure.[1] These include (1) simple fatty–fatty esters, (2) complex esters, (3) polyesters, (4) Guerbet esters, and (5) water-soluble esters. Each subclass provides specific functionality in cosmetic formulations.

The chemistry of the ester class of compounds is as follows:[1]

$$R^1\text{---}C(O)OH + R^2OH \rightarrow R^1\text{---}C(O)\text{---}OR^2 + H_2O$$

fatty acid + fatty alcohol   ester and water

As the reaction proceeds, water is generated and is removed by distillation. The esterification reaction is generally conducted at high temperatures (150 to 250°C) in the presence of a variety of catalysts.[2] The product of interest to the cosmetic formulator has a very low acid value (free acid), low hydroxyl value (free alcohol), and high saponification value (high ester content). This requires that the reaction be driven to completion.

In order to drive the reaction, most esters are made with an excess of the alcohol. This excess can run from 5 to 15% by weight. Consequently, the acid value of the product will be low and the hydroxyl value somewhat higher. In addition, there are often refining steps used to lower the acid value of the ester. These can include washing the product with mild alkali to remove unreacted acid.

The names used for fatty acids are shown in Table 22.1.

Even using the recommended excess and refining processes, there are circumstances when getting the purity of the ester high enough, sometimes due to steric hindrance, can be a challenge, often resulting in protracted reaction times. This is a major issue when either the acid or alcohol used as a raw material has unsaturation. The presence of unsaturation, most importantly conjugated unsaturation, will result in dark color and malodor. This is due to oxidation of the double bond and formation of aldehydic and ketonic intermediates.

There are two critical values used to evaluate the applicability of a triglyceride to make acids and ultimately esters. One is carbon number, and the other is iodine value.

Carbon number is an important classification for acids and, consequently, for esters. Carbon number is the value obtained by multiplying the percentage of a component in a product by the number of carbon atoms in the component, then adding up all the components.

Iodine value is an analytical procedure used to measure unsaturation. Table 22.2 lists the iodine value of various oils. Fatty acids derived from these oils will likewise have high iodine values.

Esters are more polar than hydrocarbon compounds, which explains their properties. This added polarity relates to the oxygen atoms present in the molecule.

$$R^1\text{---}O\text{---}C(O)\text{---}OR^2$$

TABLE 22.1
Fatty Acid Names

Designation	Name	Formula
C6	Caproic acid	$C_6H_{12}O_2$
C8	Caprylic acid	$C_8H_{16}O_2$
C10	Capric acid	$C_{10}H_{20}O_2$
C12	Lauric acid	$C_{12}H_{24}O_2$
C12:1	Lauroleic acid	$C_{12}H_{22}O_2$
C14	Myristic acid	$C_{14}H_{28}O_2$
C14:1	Myristoleic acid	$C_{14}H_{26}O_2$
C16	Palmitic acid	$C_{16}H_{32}O_2$
C16:1	Palmitoleic acid	$C_{16}H_{30}O_2$
C18	Stearic acid	$C_{18}H_{36}O$
C18:1	Oleic acid	$C_{18}H_{34}O_2$
C18:2	Linoleic acid	$C_{18}H_{32}O_2$
C18:3	Linolenic acid	$C_{18}H_{30}O_2$
C20	Arachidic acid	$C_{20}H_{40}O_2$
C20:1	Gadoleic acid	$C_{20}H_{38}O_2$
C22	Behenic acid	$C_{22}H_{44}O_2$
C22:1	Erucic acid	$C_{22}H_{42}O_2$
C22:2	Clupanodinic acid	$C_{22}H_{40}O_2$
C24	Lignoceric acid	$C_{24}H_{48}O_2$
C26	Cerotic acid	$C_{26}H_{52}O_2$
C28	Montanic acid	$C_{28}H_{56}O_2$
C30	Myricic acid	$C_{30}H_{60}O_2$
C32	Lacceroic acid	$C_{32}H_{64}O_2$
C34	Geddic acid	$C_{34}H_{68}O_2$

22.2 HYDROLYSIS

The presence of the ester linkage in the molecule not only results in some desirable properties vis-à-vis formulation properties, but also results in some problems related to hydrolytic instability. Esters are susceptible to a retrograde reaction in which water reacts with the molecule to break down the molecule into its component parts.

22.2.1 GENERAL HYDROLYSIS

$$R^1—C(O)—OR^2 + H_2O \longrightarrow R^1—C(O)OH + R^2OH$$

ester + water $\qquad$ fatty acid + fatty alcohol

The rate of hydrolysis is dependent upon the water solubility of the ester and the pH of the formulation. The rate of hydrolysis of the ester increases at either high (above 10) or low (below 5) pH values.

TABLE 22.2
Plant-Derived Triglyceride Composition

	Triglyceride	Carbon No.	Iodine Value
1	Coconut oil	12.8	8
2	Palm kernel oil	13.3	19
3	Babassu oil	13.4	15
4	Sunflower oil	16.0	130
5	Japan wax	16.3	6
6	Palm oil	17.1	50
7	Apricot kernel oil	17.1	102
8	Tallow	17.3	45
9	Coca butter	17.5	37
10	Andiroba oil	17.5	45
11	Mango butter	17.5	46
12	Avacado oil	17.6	84
13	Cottonseed oil	17.6	108
14	Rice bran oil	17.6	105
15	Shea butter	17.6	60
16	Wheat germ oil	17.7	130
17	Illipe butter	17.7	49
18	Corn oil	17.8	123
19	Olive oil	17.8	84
20	Poppy seed oil	17.8	138
21	Grape seed oil	17.8	135
22	Sesame oil	17.8	110
23	Sweet amond oil	17.9	102
24	Hazelnut oil	17.9	86
25	Soybean oil	17.9	130
26	Safflower oil	17.9	145
27	Walnut oil	17.9	150
28	Canola oil	17.9	92
29	Peanut oil	18.0	98
30	Kokhum butter	18.0	131
31	Cupuacu butter	18.2	40

22.2.2 BASE-CATALYZED HYDROLYSIS

$$R^1\text{—}C(O)\text{—}OR^2 + H_2O \xrightarrow{\text{KOH}} R^1\text{—}C(O)O\text{—}K^+ + R^2OH$$

ester + water   fatty soap + fatty alcohol

22.2.3 ACID-CATALYZED HYDROLYSIS

The reaction products are the same as for the general hydrolysis scheme, but the rate of hydrolysis is more rapid with acid present.

$$R^1\text{—}C(O)\text{—}OR^2 + H_2O \xrightarrow{\text{H}^+} R^1\text{—}C(O)H + R^2OH$$

22.2.4 ANALYTICAL HYDROLYSIS

In fact, susceptibility of esters to hydrolyze is the basis of the saponification value analysis. The saponification value is a measure of the equivalent molecular weight of an ester, and in order to be accurate, the ester needs to hydrolyze completely in the presence of the strong base used in the process.

Unfortunately, there are a number of formulations used in personal care applications where the pH of the formulation is below 5 or above 10, and hydrolysis of the ester makes their use impractical. It is therefore a desirable thing to make esters that provide emolliency, have the polarity lacking in hydrocarbon, and yet are applicable to both low and high pH values.

22.2.5 NONHYDROLYZABLE ESTERS

The synthesis and commercialization of esters that are stable at the extremes of pH would allow the formulator to produce elegant products that are currently not available. Such products have been synthesized, developed, patented, and made available commercially. They make use of the following diol reaction sequence:

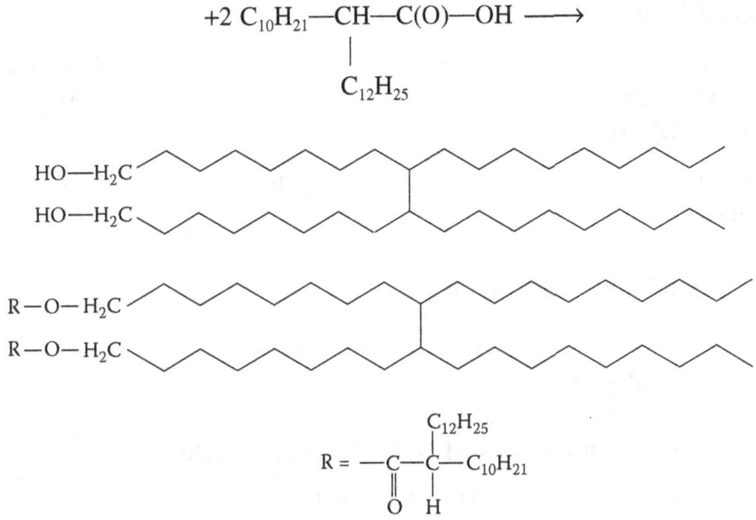

$$+2 \ C_{10}H_{21}\text{—}CH\text{—}C(O)\text{—}OH \longrightarrow$$
$$\underset{C_{12}H_{25}}{|}$$

HO—H_2C

HO—H_2C

R—O—H_2C

R—O—H_2C

$$R = \underset{\overset{\|}{O} \ \overset{|}{H}}{\text{—C—C—}} C_{10}H_{21}$$
$$\overset{C_{12}H_{25}}{|}$$

There are two patents covering the compounds.[2,3] The products are commercially available and are described in Table 22.3 and 22.4. The patents provide novel ester compositions, based upon dimer alcohol. This type of ester exhibits outstanding stability at high and low pH values, heretofore unattainable. One patent uses Guerbet acids, a specific class of fatty acids, and the other makes use of regular fatty acids. The products made from the Guerbet acids have superior liquidity, even at high molecular weight.

Products covered by these patents exhibit extraordinary resistance to hydrolysis on both the acidic and alkaline pH values. This is most easily seen when one attempts to run a saponification value. The saponification value is an analytical technique that allows one to determine the molecular weight of an ester, by breaking down the ester with base (KOH). In standard esters, the amount of KOH consumed in the analysis is measured and is stoichiometric with the molecular weight of the ester. Surprisingly, the esters of the present invention do not have the expected saponification value. In fact, they have essentially no saponification value, since the ester must hydrolyze to provide the saponification value.

The analysis is conducted with excess KOH, and the difference between the starting amount of KOH and the residual KOH is titrated with standardized acid. The amount of KOH consumed is stoichiometric, and the saponification value is reported as milligrams of KOH per gram of sample tested.

Hydrolytic Stability of Dimer Diol Di-Esters

Product	Theoretical Value	Observed Result	% Hydrolyzed
PELEMOL® 362924	124	6.2	5.0%
PELEMOL 362932	90	0.3	0.3%
PELEMOL 362936	77	2.6	3.3%

Standard Ester

Product	Theoretical Value	Observed Result	% Hydrolyzed
Behenyl behenate (PELEMOL BB)	86.6	86.4	99.8
Oleyl oleate (Pelemol OO)	102.2	101.9	99.8

22.2.6 COMMERCIAL PRODUCTS

TABLE 22.3
PELEMOL 362924
INCI: Dioctadecanyl Didecyltetradecanoate

Trade name:	PELEMOL 362924
Chemical name:	Dioctadecanyl didecyltetradecanoate
CAS #:	500208-76-4

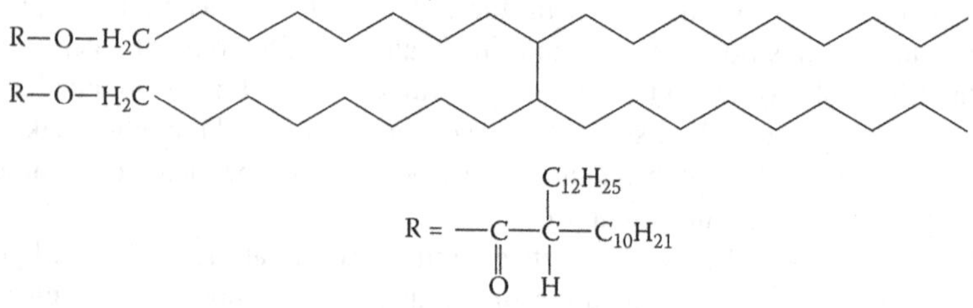

$$R = -\overset{\displaystyle}{\underset{\displaystyle O}{C}} - \overset{\displaystyle C_{12}H_{25}}{\underset{\displaystyle H}{C}} - C_{10}H_{21}$$

TABLE 22.4
PELEMOL 362932
INCI: Dioctadecanyl Dioctadecyltetradecanoate

Trade Name:	PELEMOL 362932
Chemical Name:	Dioctadecanyl Dioctadecyltetradecanoate
CAS #:	500208-75-3

22.2.7 Formulation Properties

These esters possess outstanding stability at high pH. Tested at pH 13.5, they appear to have the greatest stability out of a series of esters with similar chemistry. The esters also exhibit stability at pH 3, giving them broad application potential.

22.3 ANALYTICAL METHODOLOGY

22.3.1 Saponification Value Method

This method is applicable to all fats and oils, as well as products derived from them, such as esters and fatty acids. The saponification value is the amount of alkali necessary to saponify a definite quantity of the sample. It is expressed as the number of milligrams of potassium hydroxide (KOH) required to saponify 1 g of the sample. A sample is refluxed in 0.5 N methanolic KOH for 1.5 h and titrated using 0.5 N HCl. Materials needed are:

1. Potassium hydroxide (KOH), methanolic 0.5 N
2. Hydrochloric acid (HCl), 0.5 N
3. Phenolphthalein indicator solution, 0.1% in ethanol

The procedure is as follows:

1. Melt the sample, if not a liquid, and mix thoroughly to ensure homogeneity. Weigh the appropriate amount of sample into an Erlenmeyer flask. Record the weight.
2. Pipette 50 ml of 0.5 N KOH into the flask, add some boiling stones, and reflux for 1.5 h. Make sure that there is cold water going through

the condensers to aid in the condensing of the sample back into the Erlenmeyer flasks.

3. Prepare and run a blank simultaneously with the samples by pipetting 50 ml of 0.5 N KOH into an empty flask, adding some boiling stones, and refluxing alongside the samples.

4. After 1.5 h of refluxing, rinse the inside of the condensers with about 25 ml of deionized water and catch the rinsings in the Erlenmeyer flasks. Remove the flasks from the condensers and allow the sample solutions to cool to room temperature.

5. To each flask, add three to five drops of phenolphthalein indicator and a stir bar. Titrate, while mixing, with 0.5 N HCl until the pink color disappears. Record the respective titration volumes used to reach each endpoint.

6. Using Equation 22.1, calculate the SAP value of the samples analyzed. Report the results to one decimal place.

7. The ester value of a product can be determined using Equation 22.2, if the acid value is also known.

$$\text{SAP value} = \frac{(\text{mL Blank} - \text{mL Sample}) \, (\text{N of HCl}) \, (56.1)}{(\text{wt. of sample})} \qquad (22.1)$$

$$\text{Ester value} = \text{saponification value} - \text{acid value} \qquad (22.2)$$

Precision: The relative standard deviation for saponification value determinations was determined to be ±0.5% when one sample was analyzed 36 times by different chemists on different days within the same laboratory. This relative standard deviation was determined on a sample with an average saponification value of 336.0.*

*Reference: A.O.C.S. Official Method Cd 3c-91.

REFERENCES

1. O'Lenick, A.J., *Surfactants Chemistry and Properties*, Allured Publishing, 1999.
2. U.S. Patent 6,706,259, March 16, 2004; assigned to Phoenix Research Corporation.
3. U.S. Patent 6,537,531, March 23, 2003; assigned to Phoenix Research Corporation.

23 Branched Esters as Oil Phases in Pigmented Products

Anthony J. O'Lenick, Jr.
Siltech LLC

CONTENTS

23.1 INTRODUCTION

Low-viscosity oil phases have always been of interest in formulating pigmented products. Included in this group are poly-alpha olefin (PAO), mineral oils, esters, and other oils. The large variety of oily materials find application in pigmented products, including as vehicles for the grinding of pigments and as oil phases in emulsions. Highly hydrophobic materials that are liquid to low temperature, possess little or no odor, and have a cosmetically acceptable taste are highly prized raw materials. This chapter will deal with two classes of materials used in these applications. The first are Guerbet alcohols and the second branched esters made by the introduction of a limited number of moles of propylene oxide. Other chapters deal with other types of raw materials. All need to be considered when selecting raw materials for incorporation into personal care products.

23.2 GUERBET ALCOHOLS AND DERIVATIVES

Despite the fact that people are constantly rediscovering them, Guerbet alcohols have been known for over 100 years now. Marcel Guerbet pioneered the basic chemistry in the 1890s. These products are regiospecific beta-branched hydrophobes that can be prepared to high purity, have little or no smell and taste, and are growing in cosmetic usage. The ability to capitalize upon this reaction sequence and develop derivatives has resulted in many materials that find use in applications where liquidity and lubrication are important. The chemistry results in a unique class of materials that remain underutilized to this day.

23.2.1 CHEMISTRY

Guerbet alcohols, the oldest and best understood material in the class of compounds, have been known since the 1890s when Marcel Guerbet[1] first synthesized them. The reaction sequence, which bears his name, is related to the Aldol reaction and occurs at high temperatures under catalytic conditions. The overall reaction can be represented by the following equation:

$$CH_3(CH_2)_9OH \xrightarrow[\text{Catalyst}]{} CH_3(CH_2)_9\overset{\displaystyle (CH_2)_7CH_3}{\underset{\displaystyle |}{C}}HCH_2OH$$

The product is an alcohol with twice the molecular weight of the reactant alcohol minus a mole of water. The reaction proceeds by a number of sequential steps. These steps are as follows:

A. Oxidation of alcohol to aldehyde
B. Aldol condensation after proton extraction
C. Dehydration of the Aldol product
D. Hydrogenation of the allylic aldehyde

The following information is known about the sequence of reactions:[2]

1. The reaction takes place without catalyst, but it is strongly catalyzed by addition of hydrogen transfer catalysts.
2. At low temperatures (130 to 140°C), the rate-limiting step is the oxidation process (i.e., formation of the aldehyde).
3. At somewhat higher temperatures (160 to 180°C), the rate-limiting step is the Aldol condensation.
4. At even higher temperatures, other degradative reactions occur and can become dominant.

Many catalysts have been described in the literature as effective for the preparation of Guerbet alcohols. These include nickel, lead salts (U.S. Patent 3,119,880), oxides of copper, lead, zinc, chromium, molybdenum, tungsten, and manganese (U.S. Patent 3,558,716). Later, U.S. patents include palladium (U.S. Patent 3,979,466) and silver (U.S. Patent 3,864,407) compounds. There are advantages and disadvantages for each type.

The Cannizzaro reaction[3] is a major side reaction and is described as the disproportionation of two molecules of an aldehyde brought about by the action of sodium or potassium hydroxide to yield the corresponding alcohol and acid.[4]

23.2.2 RAW MATERIALS FOR THE PREPARATION OF GUERBET ALCOHOLS

Most often the alcohols used to produce Guerbet alcohols are of natural origin, they are straight-chain, even-carbon, primary alcohols. Guerbet alcohols are beta-branched primary alcohols. Oxo alcohols can also be used, but the reaction rate and conversions are reduced.

Guerbet alcohols also undergo a series of postreaction steps that remove (a) unreacted alcohol (vacuum stripping), (2) unsaturation (hydrogenation), (3) Cannizzaro soap (filtration), and (4) color/odor bodies. These operations add to the cost of the product and in many applications can be minimized or eliminated.[4]

23.2.3 GUERBET ALCOHOL PROPERTIES

Guerbet alcohols are high molecular weight; hence,[5]

1. They have low irritation properties.
2. They are branched, and therefore liquid to extremely low temperatures.
3. They have low volatility.
4. They are primary alcohols, and hence are reactive and can be used to make many derivatives.
5. They are useful as superfatting agents.
6. They are good lubricants.

Guerbet alcohols are essentially saturated; hence,

1. They exhibit very good oxidative stability at elevated temperatures.
2. They have excellent color initially and at elevated temperatures.
3. They exhibit improved stability over unsaturated products in many applications.

23.2.4 GUERBET ACIDS

A relatively new Guerbet derivative is the Guerbet acid. It is prepared by the oxidation of Guerbet alcohols to produce primary carboxylic acids. One method by which this can be achieved is the dehydrogenation of the alcohol with alkali metal salts, called oxidative alkali fusion, which gives excellent yields of carboxylic acids.[6–8]

$$
\begin{array}{ccc}
(CH_2)_9CH_3 & & (CH_2)_9CH_3 \\
| & & | \\
CH_3(CH_2)_7CHCH_2{-}OH & \xrightarrow{\ NaOH\ } & CH_3(CH_2)_7CHC(O){-}OH + 2\ H_2 \\
\text{octyldodecanol} & & \text{octyldodecanoic acid}
\end{array}
$$

The regiospecificity, purity, and liquidity of the starting Guerbet acid make these materials good candidates for the evaluation of the effects of branching.

When comparing the melting point of Guerbet acids and Guerbet alcohols having the same number of carbon atoms, the Guerbet alcohol has a lower titer point (Table 23.1).

The melting points of the acids are higher than those of the alcohol with the same number of carbon atoms present (Table 23.2). This is because the carboxylic acid is able to form two hydrogen bonds with another acid, while the corresponding alcohol is able to form only one. This is well known.[9] Figure 23.1.

23.2.5 GUERBET ESTERS[10]

One of the desired effects of Guerbet branching introduced into ester molecules is to make esters that are liquid to very low temperatures. With the availability

TABLE 23.1
Melting Points of Various Alcohols

Carbon Number	Linear	Guerbet
C12	24°C	−30°C
C16	50°C	−18°C
C18	58°C	−8°C
C20	62°C	0°C
C24	69°C	19°C

TABLE 23.2
Melting Points of Various Acids

Carbon Number	Linear	Guerbet
12	44°C	–15°C
16	63°C	17°C
20	75°C	35°C
24	84°C	48°C

of Guerbet acids and alcohols, branching can be introduced into (1) the alcohol, (2) the acid, or (3) both. The titer point of esters was evaluated. The ester being tested is heated to clarity and allowed to slowly cool until the first development of haze of solid occurs. This temperature is recorded as the titer point. The titer point can differ from the solidification point in that some esters do not become solid, but become a slushy semisolid (Tables 23.3 and 23.4).

Clearly, the lowest titer point products are obtained by having the Guerbet branching pattern in both the acid and alcohol portions of the molecule. The next lowest titer point is obtained when the Guerbet branch is placed in the acid. The highest titer point is obtained when the branch is placed in the alcohol. It should be noted that there is a substantial difference between the product based upon linear acid and linear alcohol and the product based upon linear acid and Guerbet alcohol. Specifically, the former is a rock-hard solid and the latter a liquid with a snowy precipitate.[11]

23.2.6 SOLUBILITY

The various Guerbet derivatives are shown in Tables 23.5 and 23.6. Solubility of the introduction of the Guerbet branch into the ester molecule did not result in an alteration of the solubility. .

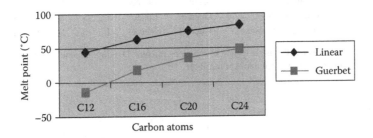

FIGURE 23.1 Melting Point of Acids (°C).

TABLE 23.3
Esters Having 32 Carbon Atoms

Designation	Acid Structure	Alcohol Structure	Appearance	Titer Point
Cetyl palmitate	Linear	Linear	White solid	34°C
Hexyldecyl palmitate	Linear	Guerbet	Slushy liquid	50°C
Cetyl hexyldecanonate	Guerbet	Linear	Yellow liquid	9°C
Hexyldecyl hexyldecanonate	Guerbet	Guerbet	Yellow liquid	<0°C

TABLE 23.4
Esters Having 40 Carbon Atoms

Designation	Acid Structure	Alcohol Structure	Appearance	Titer Point
Eicosanoyl eicosanate	Linear	Linear	White solid	38°C
Octyldodecyl eicosanate	Linear	Guerbet	White solid	48°C
Eicosanoyl octyldodeconate	Guerbet	Linear	Yellow liquid	34°C
Octyldodecyl octyldodeconate	Guerbet	Guerbet	Yellow liquid	<0°C

TABLE 23.5
Esters Having 32 Carbon Atoms

Designation	Alcohol	Acid	A	B	C	D	E
Cetyl palmitate	Linear	Linear	I	S	S	I	S
Hexyldecyl palmitate	Linear	Guerbet	I	S	S	I	S
Cetyl hexyldecanonate	Guerbet	Linear	I	S	S	I	S
Hexyldecyl hexyldecanonte	Guerbet	Guerbet	I	S	S	I	S

Note: A = water; B = isopropanol; C = cyclomethicone; D = dimethicone (350 Visc); E = mineral oil; s = soluble; i = insoluble.

TABLE 23.6
Esters Having 40 Carbon Atoms

Designation	Alcohol	Acid	A	B	C	D	E
Eicosanoyl eicosanate	Linear	Linear	I	S	S	I	S
Octyldodecyl eicosanate	Linear	Guerbet	I	S	S	I	S
Eicosanoyl octyldodeconate	Guerbet	Linear	I	S	S	I	S
Octyldodecyl octyldodeconate	Guerbet	Guerbet	I	S	S	I	S

Note: A = water; B = isopropanol; C = cyclomethicone; D = dimethicone (350 Visc); E = mineral oil; s = soluble; i = insoluble.

23.2.7 GUERBET PATENTS

The tremendous versatility of Guerbet chemistry can be seen in the great diversity of patents covering new compositions of matter, applications, and processes for making and using Guerbet derivatives.

23.2.7.1 Compounds (Composition of Matter)

1. **6,093,856, Polyoxyalkylene Surfactants**, issued July 2000; inventors: Cripe, T., Conner, D., Vinson, P., Burckett, L., James, C., Willman, J.; assigned to Procter and Gamble Co.
2. **5,786,389, Guerbet Castor Esters**, issued July 1999; inventors; O'Lenick, Jr., A., Parkinson, J.K.
3. **5,744,626, Complex Guerbet Acid Esters**, issued April 1999; inventor: O'Lenick, Jr., A.
4. **5,717,119, Polyoxyalkylene Glycol Guerbet Esters**, issued February 1999; inventor: O'Lenick, Jr., A.
5. **5,646,321, Guerbet Meadowfoam Esters**, issued July 1997; inventor: O'Lenick, Jr., A.
6. **5,488,121, Di-Guerbet Esters**, issued January 1996; inventor: O'Lenick, Jr., A.
7. **5,312,968, Fluorine Containing Guerbet Citrate Esters**, issued May 1994; inventors: O'Lenick, Jr., A., Buffa, C.W.
8. **4,830,769, Propoxylated Guerbet Alcohols and Esters Thereof**, issued May 1989; inventors: O'Lenick, Jr., A., Bilbo, R.E.
9. **4,800,077, Guerbet Quaternary Compounds**, issued January 1989; inventors: O'Lenick, Jr., A., Smith, W.C.
10. **4,767,815, Guerbet Alcohol Esters**, issued August 1988; inventor: O'Lenick, Jr., A.; assigned to GAF Corporation.
11. **4,425,458, Polyguerbet Alcohol Esters**, issued January 1984; inventors: Lindner, R., O'Lenick, Jr., A.; assigned to Henkel Corporation.

23.2.7.2 Applications (Formulations)

1. **6,036,947, Transfer Resistant High Lustre Lipstick Composi-tions**, issued March 2000; inventors: Barone, S., Krog, A., Jose, N., Ordino, R.
2. **5,837,223, Transfer Resistant High Lustre Cosmetic Stick Compo-sitions**, issued November 1998; inventors: Barone, S., Krog, A., Jose, N., Ordino, R.
3. **5,736,571, Guerbet Meadowfoam Esters in Personal Care**, issued April 1998; inventor: O'Lenick, Jr., A.
4. **5,686,087, Cosmetic and/or Pharmaceutical Formulations with an Improved Feeling on the Skin Based on Mixed Guerbet Alcohols**, issued November 1997; inventors: Ansmann, A., Kawa, R., Mohr, K., Koester, J.
5. **5,639,791, Di-Guerbet Esters in Personal Care Applications**, issued June 1997l inventor: O'Lenick, Jr., A.
6. **5,494,938, Oil-in-Water Emulsions**, issued February 1996; inventors: Kawa, R., Ansmann, A., Weurth, M., Tessman, H., Foerster, T.; assigned to Henkel Kgaa.

23.2.7.3 Process

1. **5,777,183, Process for the Production of Guerbet Alcohols**, issued July 1997; inventors: Mueller, G., Gutsche, B., Schmid, K., Bougardt, F., Jeromin, L., Peukert, E., Frankenbach, H.
2. **5,218,134, Process for Esters**, issued June 1993; inventors: Pruett, R., Mozeleski, E.
3. **5,068,469, Process for Preparation of Condensed Alcohols by Alkoxide Catalysts**, issued November 1991; inventors: Young, D., Jung, J., McLaughlin, M.
4. **4,518,810, Process for Preparation of Guerbet Alcohols**, issued May 1985; inventors: Matsauda, M., Horio, M.
5. **4,011,273, Method for the Production of Guerbet Alcohols Utilizing Insoluble Lead Catalysts**, issued March 1977; inventors: Abend, G., Leenders, P.

23.3 PROPOXYLATED ESTERS

Another approach to obtaining liquid products is to introduce branching into the product. Specifically, short branching (including methyl ranching) can be introduced into a molecule as a consequence of the process used to make an alcohol. The oxo process, for example, introduces the methyl group into the molecule.

Oxo alcohols are prepared by the reaction of alpha olefin with hydrogen and carbon monoxide using a catalyst, commonly cobalt compounds. The reaction occurs in two parts: (1) the preparation of the aldehyde and (2) the reduction of the aldehyde to the alcohol. What is very important is the fact that two different aldehyde compounds, one linear, the other with a methyl branch, form in the first part of the reaction. Both then rearrange into alcohols.

23.3.1 REACTION

$$R\text{—}CH\text{=}CH_2 + CO + H_2 \longrightarrow R\text{—}CH_2CH_2\text{—}\overset{\overset{\displaystyle O}{\|}}{C}H \text{ and } R\text{—}\underset{\underset{\displaystyle CH_3}{|}}{C}H\text{—}\overset{\overset{\displaystyle O}{\|}}{C}H$$

$$R\text{—}CH_2CH_2\text{—}CH_2OH \text{ and } R\text{—}\underset{\underset{\displaystyle CH_3}{|}}{C}H\text{—}CH_2OH \longleftarrow$$

A particularly potent branch pattern that can be introduced is the Guerbet branch. Guerbet alcohols have been known since the 1890s, when Marcel Guerbet first synthesized these materials. The reaction sequence that bears his name is related to the Aldol reaction and occurs at high temperatures under catalytic conditions.

While a very interesting process and, if properly chosen, a very effective one in making liquid products, the Guerbet products suffer from high costs. This is due not only to the technical sophistication of the Guerbet process, but also to the high cost added to products by the various postprocess sequences used to refine and purify them. These steps include, but are not limited to, distillation (to increase purity), hydrofinishing (to lower unsaturation), washing (to remove soap), and filtration (to remove catalyst).

There is a need for a cost-effective method to obtain a series of products that are liquid and have a range of melting points for cosmetic and other applications. In order to address these needs, we chose to undertake a project that studied the effectiveness of methyl branching introduced into an ester by the propoxylation of an alcohol prior to esterification.

23.3.2 MELTING POINT

In order for a material to be a crystalline solid, the particles need to be arranged in a very regular, symmetrical manner so as to make up the repeating unit of the crystal. Liquid materials, on the other hand, are random in their order and move about freely. Melting is the change from orderly arrangement of a solid into a random liquid form. To the extent the forces that lead to an ordered system are destroyed, the melting point of a material decreases. Stated another way, the amount of energy necessary to disrupt the organized structure of a solid, making it a liquid (i.e., melting it), decreases for those molecules that have structural features that tend to prevent disruption of the crystalline structure. This is the precise reason that branching lowers the melting point. The branched molecule rotates more rapidly as the temperature increases until the crystalline structure is destroyed. A particularly striking example of the effect of symmetry on the melting point is seen by comparing the melting point of benzene with that of toluene. The presence of the methyl group in the toluene lowers the melting point from 5 to $-95°C$. With this in mind, our study was undertaken to see if the introduction of a methyl branch via propoxylation of stearyl alcohol could dramatically reduce the melting point of the resultant compounds.

23.3.2.1 Raw Materials

$$CH_3—(CH_2)_{16}CH_2OH \qquad \text{stearyl alcohol}$$

$$CH_3(CH_2)_9—CH—CH_2—OH \qquad \text{Guerbet alcohol}$$
$$\qquad\qquad\quad |$$
$$\qquad\qquad (CH_2)_7—CH_3$$

$$CH_3—(CH_2)_{15}CHOH \qquad\qquad \text{methyl branched alcohol}$$
$$\qquad\qquad\quad |$$
$$\qquad\qquad CH_3$$

$$CH_2—CH—CH_3 \qquad\qquad \text{propylene oxide}$$
$$\quad \backslash \quad /$$
$$\qquad O$$

23.3.2.2 Propoxylation of Stearyl Alcohol

The propoxylation reaction is carried out by reacting propylene oxide with stearyl alcohol under a base catalyst. The product that results is a methyl branched alcohol having three more carbon atoms, an additional oxygen atom, and a new ether linkage. Just as important, the new molecule has a secondary hydroxyl group $(—CH—(CH_3)OH)$, rather than the primary one $(—CH_2OH)$ that previously was present. As will hopefully become clear, the presence of the methyl group and the number of moles of propylene oxide added (the n value) will determine to a large degree the melting point of the ester produced by reacting the propoxylated alcohol with various fatty acids.

Propoxylation of stearyl alcohol:

$$CH_3—(CH_2)_{16}CH_2OH \quad + \quad n\ CH_2—CH—CH_3 \longrightarrow$$
$$\qquad\qquad\qquad\qquad\qquad \backslash \quad /$$
$$\qquad\qquad\qquad\qquad\qquad O$$

$$CH_3—(CH_2)_{16}CH_2O—(CH_2—CH—O)n\ H$$
$$\qquad\qquad\qquad\qquad\qquad |$$
$$\qquad\qquad\qquad\qquad\quad CH_3$$

23.3.2.3 Experimental

Stearyl alcohol was propoxylated to make the following compounds:

$$CH_3—(CH_2)_{16}CH_2O—(CH_2—CH—O)_n\ H$$
$$\underset{CH_3}{|}$$

The various products are shown Table 23.7.

TABLE 23.7
Designation n Value

O	0.0
A	0.7
B	1.5
C	2.2

The properties of these esters are shown in 23.8.

TABLE 23.8
Analysis of Propoxylated Alcohol

	O	A	B	C
Color (Gardner)	1	1	1	1
Appearance 50°C	Clear	Clear	Clear	Clear
pH 1% aqueous	7.0	7.0	6.9	6.8
Acid value	0.0	0.06	0.05	0.03
Hydroxyl value	208.7	181.2	161.2	139.3
Moisture (%)	0.1	0.1	0.1	0.1
Titer point (°C)	49	38	31	27

23.3.2.4 Stearate Esters

The resulting propoxylated alcohols were then reacted with stearic acid using a tin catalyst. The properties are shown in Table 23.9.

$$CH_3—(CH_2)_{16}CH_2O—(CH_2—CH—O)n\ H + CH_3—(CH_2)_{16}—C—OH$$
$$\underset{CH_3}{|} \qquad\qquad \underset{O}{\|}$$

stearyl propoxylate stearic acid

$$CH_3—(CH_2)_{16}CH_2O—(CH_2—CH—O)n—C—(CH_2)_{16}CH_3 + H_2O$$
$$\underset{CH_3}{|} \quad \underset{O}{\|}$$

stearyl-ppg-stearate water

TABLE 23.9
Analysis of Propoxylated Stearyl Stearate

	S-O	S-A	S-B	S-C
Color (Gardner)	5	4	3	3
Appearance 50°C	Clear	Clear	Clear	Clear
Acid value	2.0	3.1	2.9	3.8
Hydroxyl value	7.6	6.8	8.0	7.0
Saponification value	104.5	97.2	89.7	84.0
Titer point (°C)	51	41	38	29

23.3.2.5　Isostearate Esters

The resulting propoxylates were then reacted with stearic acid using a tin catalyst.

$$CH_3—(CH_2)_{16}CH_2O—(CH_2—CH—O)n\ H + R—C—OH$$
$$\phantom{CH_3—(CH_2)_{16}CH_2O—(CH_2—CH—O)n\ H}|\|$$
$$\phantom{CH_3—(CH_2)_{16}CH_2O—(CH}CH_3O$$

stearyl propoxylate　　isostearic acid

$$CH_3—(CH_2)_{16}CH_2O—(CH_2—CH—O)n—C—R + H_2O$$
$$\phantom{CH_3—(CH_2)_{16}CH_2O—(CH_2—CH—O)n}|\|$$
$$\phantom{CH_3—(CH_2)_{16}CH_2O—(CH}CH_3O$$

stearyl-ppg-isostearate　　　　　water

The properties are shown in Table 23.10.

TABLE 23.10
Analysis of Propoxylated Stearyl Isostearate

	i-S-O	i-S-A	i-S-B	i-S-C
Color (Gardner)	4	4	3	3
Appearance 50°C	Clear	Clear	Clear	Clear
Acid value	3.0	4.1	3.7	2.8
Hydroxyl value	7.9	8.2	7.7	6.8
Saponification value	104.8	98.3	89.9	85.0
Titer point (°C)	26	20	15	12

23.3.2.6   2-Ethyl Hexanoic Esters

The resulting propoxylated products were then reacted with stearic acid using a tin catalyst.

$$CH_3—(CH_2)_{16}CH_2O—(CH_2—CH—O)_n\,H + R—C—OH$$

$$\underset{\text{stearyl propoxylate}}{\overset{\displaystyle |}{CH_3}} \qquad \underset{\text{2-ethyl hexanoic acid}}{\overset{\displaystyle ||}{O}}$$

$$CH_3—(CH_2)_{16}CH_2O—(CH_2—CH—O)n—C—R + H_2O$$

$$\underset{\text{stearyl-ppg-2-ethylhexanoate}}{\overset{\displaystyle |}{CH_3}} \qquad \underset{\text{water}}{\overset{\displaystyle ||}{O}}$$

TABLE 23.11
Analysis of Propoxylated Stearyl 2-Ethyl Hexonate

2EH-O	2EH-A	2EH-B	2EH-C	
Color (Gardner)	4	4	3	3
Appearance 50°C	Clear	Clear	Clear	Clear
Acid value	2.6	3.2	4.1	3.8
Hydroxyl value	7.6	7.2	6.4	7.7
Saponification value	141.3	129.0	116.0	106.7
Titer point (°C)	41	31	29	27

23.3.2.7   Conclusions

1. The propoxylation of stearyl alcohol prior to esterification results in the lowering of the melting point for all the compounds studied. This confirmed the effect of branching upon the melting point. Melting points of the alcohol were dropped by over 20°C by adding 2.2 mol of propylene oxide to the stearyl alcohol. Likewise, significant melting point reductions were encountered when esters were evaluated.

2. The current study added up to 2.2 mol of propylene oxide to the hydrophobe. The melting points of the propoxylate and all derived

esters were still dropping at the 2.2 mol level (relative to the lower levels). This was a surprise, since it was felt that at the 2.2 mol level the effectiveness of the oxide on liquidity would begin to drop essentially to zero. It is interesting to note that at 2.2 mol the percentage of propylene oxide added is 32.4% by weight.

3. It was also a surprise that the esterification of the stearyl propoxylate resulted in only a very modest increase in melting point, relative to the starting alcohol propoxylate. A very significant increase in molecular weight occurred, but a marginal change in the melting point was noticed.

4. The 2-ethyl hexyl esters were less efficient in lowering the melting point of the resulting esters than the isostearate. This was a surprise, since the 2-ethyl hexanoic acid is both lower in molecular weight (C8) and more branched than the C-18-branched isostearate. The propoxylated stearyl alcohol isostearate compounds had the lowest melting point of any of the homologous series studied.

5. We believe that the reaction of fatty alcohols with propylene oxide, then subsequent derivization, will allow for the synthesis of a new class of compounds with very desirable properties on the skin.

23.4 CONCLUSION

Guerbet chemistry offers a unique set of materials that can be used to prepare highly effective oil phases for use in pigmented products. Despite the fact that the basic chemistry has been known for 100 years, the ability to use these materials in high-performance products is a relatively new phenomenon.

Likewise, the introduction of propoxylated groups into esters offers an economic approach to obtain liquid high molecular weight products for use in pigmented products.

REFERENCES

1. Guerbet, M., *C.R. Acad. Sci. Paris*, 128, 1002 (1899).
2. Veibel, S. and Nielsen, J., *Tetrahedron*, 23, 1723–1733 (1967).
3. Cannizzaro, S., *Ann. Chem. Liebigs*, 88, 129, (1853).
4. Geissman, T.A., *Organic Reactions*, Vol. II, Wiley, New York (1944), p. 94.
5. O'Lenick, Jr., A.J. and Bilbo, R.E., *Guerbet Alcohols, Versatile Hydrophobes*, SCCS, April 1987.
6. Henkel, K., *Fatty Alcohols, Raw Materials, Process and Applications*, Henkel KGaA (1982), p. 163.
7. Stein, W., *Method Chim.*, 5, 563–573 (1975).
8. German Patent 538,388, October 1931.
9. Morrison, R. and Boyd, R., *Organic Chemistry*, 3rd ed. (1973), p. 582.
10. O'Lenick, A.J., *Surfactants Chemistry and Properties*, Allured Publishing, Carol Stream, IL (1999), pp. 28–30.
11. Sunwoo, C. and Wade, W.H., *J. Dispersion Sci. Technol.*, 13, 491 (1992).

Index

N

Printed in the United States
by Baker & Taylor Publisher Services